A.A.O.S.

Symposium on

Arthroscopy and arthrography
of the knee

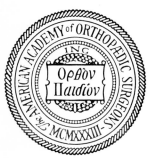

American Academy
of
Orthopaedic Surgeons

Symposium on
Arthroscopy and arthrography of the knee

with 499 illustrations, including 188 in full color

The C. V. Mosby Company

Saint Louis   1978

The C. V. Mosby Company
11830 Westline Industrial Drive, St. Louis, Missouri 63141

Library of Congress Cataloging in Publication Data

Symposium on Arthroscopy and Arthrography of the Knee.

    At head of title: American Academy of Orthopaedic Surgeons.
    Bibliography: p.
    Includes index.
    1. Arthroscopy—Congresses. 2. Knee—Radiography—
Congresses. 3. Knee—Diseases—Diagnosis—Congresses.
I. American Academy of Orthopaedic Surgeons.
RC932.S88 1978   616.7'2   78-17015
ISBN 0-8016-0056-1

GW/U/B   9 8 7 6 5 4 3 2 1

Contributors

Alan L. Bass, F.R.C.P. (Ed.), F.R.C.P. (C)

Director, Service of Rehabilitation, Department of Medicine, Henderson General Hospital; Clinical Professor, Department of Medicine, McMaster University, Hamilton, Ontario

Robert C. Bechtol, M.D.

Consultant, Department of Orthopedic Surgery, Santa Rosa Memorial Hospital, Santa Rosa, California

Benjamin E. Bierbaum

Chairman, Department of Orthopedic Surgery, New England Baptist Hospital; Clinical Professor of Orthopedic Surgery, Boston, Massachusetts

S. Ward Casscells, M.D.

Attending Chief, Orthopedics, Wilmington Medical Center; Consultant at Alfred I. duPont Institute, Wilmington, Delaware

Murray K. Dalinka, M.D.

Professor of Radiology, University of Pennsylvania, Philadelphia, Pennsylvania

Kenneth E. DeHaven, M.D.

Associate Professor of Orthopaedics and Head, Section of Athletic Medicine, University of Rochester School of Medicine, Rochester, New York

Robert E. Eilert, M.D.

Chairman, Department of Orthopaedics, The Children's Hospital; Assistant Clinical Professor, Department of Orthopaedic Surgery, University of Colorado Medical Center, Denver, Colorado

Houshang Farahver, M.D.

Attending Orthopaedist, St. Mary of Nazareth Hospital, Chicago, Illinois

Harry J. Griffiths, M.D.

Associate Professor, Radiology and Orthopedics, University of Rochester Medical Center, Rochester, New York

Michael Harty, M.A., M.Ch., F.R.C.S.

Professor of Anatomy and Orthopaedic Surgery, University of Pennsylvania, Philadelphia, Pennsylvania

Robert W. Jackson, M.D., M.S., F.R.C.S. (C)

Chief, Division of Orthopaedic Surgery, Toronto Western Hospital; Associate Professor, Department of Surgery, University of Toronto, Toronto, Ontario

Lanny L. Johnson, M.D.

Clinical Professor of Surgery, College of Human Medicine, Michigan State University, East Lansing, Michigan

John J. Joyce III, M.D.

Associate Clinical Professor of Orthopaedic Surgery, University of Pennsylvania School of Medicine, Philadelphia, Pennsylvania

Jeremy J. Kaye, M.D.

Associate Professor of Radiology; Associate Professor of Orthopedics and Rehabilitation, Vanderbilt University, Nashville, Tennessee

Ralph T. Lidge, M.D.

Clinical Associate Professor of Orthopaedic Surgery, Abraham Lincoln School of Medicine, University of Illinois at the Medical Center, Chicago, Illinois

John B. McGinty, M.D.

Clinical Professor of Orthopaedic Surgery, Tufts University School of Medicine, Boston, Massachusetts

Richard L. O'Connor, M.D.

Orthopaedic Surgeon, West Covina, California

Rochelle Prescott, B.S.Ch.

Principal Research Scientist, Dyonics, Inc., Woburn, Massachusetts

Preface

During the past 3 years the American Academy of Orthopaedic Surgeons has sponsored continuing medical education courses on arthroscopy and arthrography of the knee. The programs have been conducted eight times in cities across the United States. The response has been enthusiastic, and many physicians have participated in the course more than once.

The purpose of this text is to provide, in greater part, the lectures given by members of the faculty, some of whom represent the pioneers of arthroscopy in North America. It is through their efforts that this volume has been made possible.

Arthroscopy is presented as a technique that requires specialized psychomotor and interpretive skills. Diagnostic findings are illustrated.

Arthroscopy is developing as a modality of treatment, with marked growth of endoscopic surgery expected during the next decade. The procedure decreases morbidity, saves many hours of patients' time through an earlier return to work following surgery, and results in an economic reduction in hospitalization costs.

Arthrography is an accepted diagnostic method and antedates arthroscopy in the United States and Canada. Technical aspects of arthrography are easier than arthroscopy; however, more interpretive data are provided by the latter.

We believe the contents of this text are representative of current fundamental knowledge that will be helpful to all of us in the continuous development of arthroscopy, arthrography, and intraarthroscopic surgery.

We express gratitude to the faculty members who have so generously taken time to produce these courses and to submit papers for this text; and to the secretaries who have devoted many hours in helping plan these programs and prepare subsequent manuscripts, our thanks. We express appreciation, last but not least, to the many physicians who have served as instructors in the laboratory of the arthroscope and other teaching aids.

John B. McGinty
Ralph T. Lidge

Contents

A.A.O.S.

Symposium on

Arthroscopy and arthrography
of the knee

1. Historical perspectives

History of arthroscopy

John J. Joyce III
Robert W. Jackson

DEVELOPMENT OF ENDOSCOPY—EARLY PIONEERS

Although the Hebrews are said to have used vaginal specula, and proctoscopes are said to have been found in the ruins of Pompeii, it remained for Bozzini[8,9] of Frankfurt-am-Main to produce his Lichtleiter in 1805 (Fig. 1-1). The apparatus consisted of a bifid tube which was attached to a light chamber that was divided by a thin, longitudinal partition. A candle, which acted as a light source, was on one side, while the examiner peered through a hole on the other. When this primitive but ingenious device was presented before the Viennese Medical Society in 1806 it was considered "a mere toy" (Fig. 1-2).

Other instruments of improved design followed Bozzini's effort. It remained, however, for Desormaux[8,9] in 1853 to produce the gastrogen endoscope (Fig. 1-3).

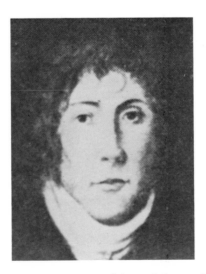

Fig. 1-1. Philip Bozzini (1773-1809), designer of the Lichtleiter. (From Jackson, R. W., and Dandy, D. J.: Arthroscopy of the knee: modern orthopedic monographs, New York, 1976, Grune & Stratton.)

1

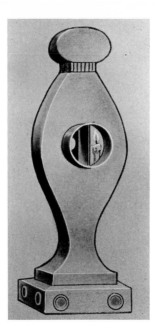

Fig. 1-2. Bozzini's Lichtleiter (1805). (From O'Connor, R. L., editor: Arthroscopy: a scope® publication, Kalamazoo, Mich., 1977, The Upjohn Co.)

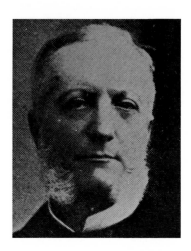

Fig. 1-3. A. J. Desormaux (1815-1882), father of modern cystoscopy, designer of gastrogen endoscope. (From Jackson, R. W., and Dandy, D. J.: Arthroscopy of the knee: modern orthopedic monographs, New York, 1976, Grune & Stratton.)

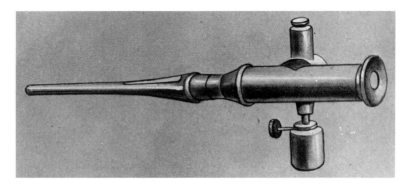

Fig. 1-4. Desormaux's gastrogen endoscope. (From O'Connor, R. L., editor: Arthroscopy: a scope® publication, Kalamazoo, Mich., 1977, The Upjohn Co.)

Many historians consider this device to be the true forerunner of our modern cystoscopes. The apparatus consisted of a gas lamp to which a series of tubes could be attached for insertion into the urethra (Fig. 1-4). A concave, perforated reflector directed the light down the tube and allowed the examiner to peer through the eyepiece into the bladder and urethra. The publication of the results of Desormaux's extensive studies established the value of endoscopy.

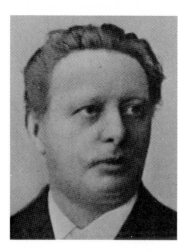

Fig. 1-5. Max Nitze (1848-1906), designer of modern cystoscope. First person to photograph bladder's interior through an endoscope. (From Jackson, R. W., and Dandy, D. J.: Arthroscopy of the knee: modern orthopedic monographs, New York, 1976, Grune & Stratton.)

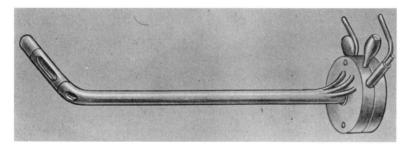

Fig. 1-6. Early model of Nitze cystoscope. (From O'Connor, R. L., editor: Arthroscopy: a scope® publication, Kalamazoo, Mich., 1977, The Upjohn Co.)

Until the advent of electricity, it was necessary to reflect light into the bladder from an outside source. In 1876 Max Nitze[8,9] developed an instrument that closely resembled the modern cystoscope (Fig. 1-5). A platinum loop encased in a water-cooled goose quill, which glowed when electricity was passed through it, provided the first light source *within* the bladder. Edison's development of the incandescent lamp in 1880 was refined sufficiently by 1886 so that it could be substituted for the platinum wire. The addition of a lens system provided a wider and clearer visual field (Fig. 1-6). Rapid improvement of small electric lamps as well as optical systems ensued. By the beginning of the twentieth century the cystoscope had become an important urologic tool. The device was so far advanced that photographs of the bladder were possible.

ARTHROSCOPY

Prof. Kenji Takagi[6,9] of Tokyo University must be considered a father of arthroscopy (Fig. 1-7). In 1918 he viewed a cadaver knee joint through a cystoscope. He was pleased with the extent and clarity of the visual field. Stimulated by his findings this ingenious observer designed a series of instruments better suited for use within joints. His first device, developed in 1920, had a diameter of 7.3 mm, making it impractical for routine use in the knee joint. The field of vision was also quite narrow. Takagi was, however, able to inspect the interior of a tuberculous knee. In 1931 continued efforts enabled this indefatigable pioneer to produce an instrument that was 4 mm in diameter (Fig. 1-8). By this time synovial biopsies had been taken under arthroscopic guidance, and by the mid 1930s Takagi had produced yet another arthroscope, through which the first color photographs were taken. A second light source introduced through a separate incision was required for this remarkable feat.

In 1921 Eugen Bircher[1,2] of Switzerland used a Jacobeus laparoscope to examine a knee that was distended with oxygen or carbon monoxide and reported his findings (Fig. 1-9). Several other reports were made by the same author in subsequent years.

Philip Kreuscher[7] in 1925 published a plea for the use of the arthroscope in the early recognition of meniscal lesions. Although the article provided a picture of the instrument, the author gave no details regarding the device or the technique of its use.

The first paper discussing the use of the arthroscope in joints other than the knee appeared in the 1931 issue of the Journal of Bone and Joint Surgery. Dr. Michael Burman[3,4] not only reported his experiences in the examinations of the hip, knee, and ankle joints but also of the shoulder, elbow, and wrist (Fig. 1-10). This article

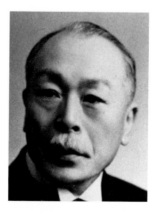

Fig. 1-7. Kenji Takagi, first person to view the knee's interior through an endoscope. (From Jackson, R. W., and Dandy, D. J.: Arthroscopy of the knee: modern orthopedic monographs, New York, 1976, Grune & Stratton.)

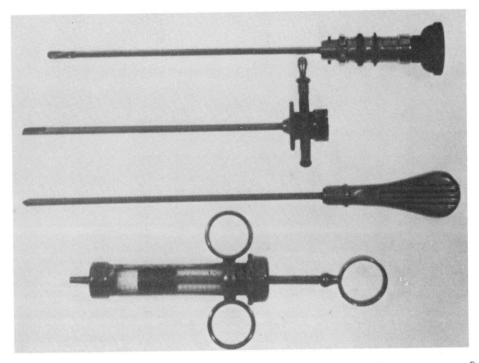

Fig. 1-8. Early Takagi arthroscope. (From O'Connor, R. L., editor: Arthroscopy: a scope® publication, Kalamazoo, Mich., 1977, The Upjohn Co.)

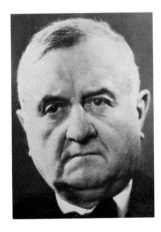

Fig. 1-9. Eugen Bircher (1882-1956), author of several articles on endoscopy of the knee. He used a Jacobeus laparoscope. (From Jackson, R. W., and Dandy, D. J.: Arthroscopy of the knee: modern orthopedic monographs, New York, 1976, Grune & Stratton.)

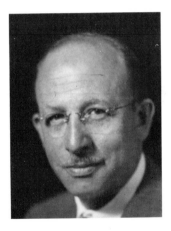

Fig. 1-10. Michael Burman (1901-1975), first person to describe arthroscopic appearance of other joints as well as the knee.

describes the fundamental principles of arthroscopy and remains a classic to this date. Although this ingenious man's arthroscope was a new addition to the field and had many original features, technical problems in the device caused Burman's colleagues to regard it with some skepticism. Unfortunately, his text for a planned monograph on arthroscopy remains unpublished.

In the mid 1900s Drs. Mayer, Finkelstein, and Burman,[4,5] all of the Hospital for Joint Diseases in New York, also collaborated on the publication of a number of significant articles on the subject.

In the German literature, Sommer[10] in 1937 and Vaubel[11] in 1938 reported on their experiences with the procedure.

Although World War II did not produce many articles on this developing technique, interest was revived in 1955 by Hurter who, in the French literature, described arthroscopy as a "new" method of examining joints. Further papers by Imbert also appeared in the French literature in 1956 and 1957.

Stimulated by Takagi's efforts, Dr. Masaki Watanabe (Fig. 1-11) continued to develop new instruments. His persistence and patience finally resulted in the Watanabe no. 21 arthroscope. This remarkable instrument has a diameter of 6.5 mm. The field of vision is 100°. It has a tungsten light source, and excellent photographs can be obtained.

In 1957 the first edition of Watanabe and associates' *Atlas of Arthroscopy* was published.[12] This beautifully documented and illustrated book was revised in 1969. In the meantime Watanabe has written many further reports on the subject.

Since the early 1970s well-documented reports by various authors have firmly established the value of arthroscopy as a diagnostic tool. At the time of this writing further interest has been stimulated by the recent development of operating arthroscopes by several manufacturers.

In 1973 the first seminar on the subject was held at the University of Pennsylvania

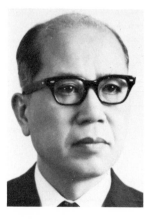

Fig. 1-11. Masaki Watanabe, designer of Watanabe no. 21 arthroscope and Selfoc arthroscope. (From Jackson, R. W., and Dandy, D. J.: Arthroscopy of the knee: modern orthopedic monographs, New York, 1976, Grune & Stratton.)

under the direction of Drs. Michael Harty and John J. Joyce. A second session was held in 1974. At the same time the International Arthroscopy Association was founded. Dr. Masaki Watanabe of Tokyo was elected president, Dr. Robert W. Jackson of Toronto, vice-president, Dr. S. Ward Casscells of Wilmington, Delaware, secretary and Dr. Richard O'Connor of Covina, California, treasurer.

Following these two memorable events a number of postgraduate seminars on the subject were held throughout the United States and Europe.

More recent developments in photography and videotaping techniques have produced reliable documentation of arthroscopic observations.

So rapid have been the developments in the field that it is difficult to predict the ultimate future of arthroscopy. Certainly it has become an invaluable modality to aid in the diagnosis and treatment of joint lesions. Further and still more advanced developments will undoubtedly have arisen by the time this volume is in print.

References

1. Bircher, E.: Die Arthroendoskopie, Zentralbl. Chir. **48**:1460-1461, 1921.
2. Bircher, E.: Beitrag zur Pathologie (Arthritis deformans) und Diagnose der Meniscusverletzungen (Arthroendoskopie), Bruns' Beiträge zur Klinischen Chirurgie **127**:239-250, 1922.
3. Burman, M. S.: Arthroscopy or direct visualization of joints: an experimental cadaver study, J. Bone Joint Surg. **13**(4):669-695, 1931.
4. Burman, M. S., Finkelstein, H., and Mayer, L.: Arthroscopy of the knee joint, J. Bone Joint Surg. **16**:255-268, 1934.
5. Finkelstein, H., and Mayer, L.: The arthroscope. A new method of examining joints, J. Bone Joint Surg. **13**:583-588, 1931.
6. Jackson, R. W., and Dandy, D. J.: Arthroscopy of the knee: modern orthopedic monographs, New York, 1976, Grune & Stratton.
7. Kreuscher, P. H.: Semilunar cartilage disease: a plea for early recognition by means of the arthroscope and early treatment of this condition, Ill. Med. J. **47**:290, 1925.
8. McCrea, L. E.: Clinical cystoscopy, Philadelphia, 1949, F. A. Davis Co., pp. 3-13.
9. National Museum for the History of Science, Leiden, the Netherlands: From Lichtleiter to fiber optics, Catalogue prepared on the occasion of the XVIth Congress of the International Society for Urology.
10. Sommer, R.: Die Endoskopie des Kniegelenkes, Zentralbl. Chir. **64**:1692-1697, 1937.
11. Vaubel, E.: Die Arthroskopie (Endoskopie des Kniegelenkes) Ein Betrag zur Diagnostik der Gelenkenkrankheiten. Der Rheumatismus B. 9, herausgegeben von Prof. Rudolf Jurgens, Dresden und Leipzig, 1938, Theodore Steinkopf.
12. Watanabe, M., Takeda, S., and Ikeuchi, H.: Atlas of arthroscopy, ed. 2, Tokyo, 1969, Igaku Shoin Ltd.

Suggested readings

Eikelaar, H. R.: Arthroscopy of the knee. Thesis for a doctorate in orthopaedic surgery at the University of Groningen, 1975, The Netherlands Royal United Printers Hoitsema, B. V.
Joyce, J. J.: Arthroscopy: asset or liability? Thesis for American Orthopaedic Association, 1974.
Okazaki, H.: On the clinical significance of arthrography and arthroscopy to the diagnosis of internal derangements of the knee, Rinsho-Seikeigera (Clin. Orthop. Surg.) **3**:1046, 1968.

Okmura, T.: An arthroscopic study of the traumatic disorders of the knee joint, J. Japan. Orthop. Assoc. **23**:28, 1945.

Robles, G. J., Katona, G., and Barroso, M. R.: Arthroscopy as an aid to diagnosis and investigation, Excerpta Medica, International Congress Series **143**:6, 1968.

History of knee arthrography

Jeremy J. Kaye

Arthrography of the knee has now become a thoroughly accepted technique in the examination of the patient with a suspected internal derangement of the knee. As primarily an outpatient procedure, it can be simply and safely performed. The technique of arthrography is becoming available in more and more institutions and is being taught in most major training programs. The diagnostic radiologist should be able to perform and interpret this examination with proficiency; the referring surgeon ordinarily does not concern himself with the technical aspects of the examination but should be able to interpret them accurately and judge their technical sufficiency.

A detailed review of the history of knee arthrography is beyond the scope of this symposium. The interested reader is directed to works by Dalinka and associates,[4] Lindblom,[7] and Ricklin and associates.[8]

Arthrography was an early application of roentgenology to the study of joints. The initial knee arthrograms reported by Werndorff and Robinson[9] in 1905 came only about 10 years after the initial report by Roentgen of the discovery of the x-ray. Gas arthrography was popularized during the early 1920s and the 1930s.[2] In the United States the experience of Kleinberg[6] discouraged the use of this technique due to the near-fatal pulmonary gas embolus, which we now know was due to technical factors. In the 1930s iodinated contrast materials were initially tried as contrast materials for arthrography, but this practice was soon discontinued, as the earlier contrast materials were too toxic.

It was not until the late 1930s and the 1940s that water-soluble contrast materials became available and were utilized for arthrography. Lindblom[7] probably did more than any single individual to propagate and promulgate the technique of knee arthrography, in this instance with the single positive–contrast technique. Arthrography was thereafter established as safe and reliable.

In the interval since that time, the majority of advances has been related to arthrography for the knee. The first major advance was the double-contrast technique, initially described with the horizontal beam by Andren and Wehlin.[1] This technique utilized the horizontal radiographic beam. This was introduced and popularized in North America by Freiberger and associates.[5] The next major technical advance was the introduction, in North America, of the fluoroscopic double-contrast method by Butt and McIntyre[3] in 1969. This method was also popularized by Ricklin and associates[8] in Europe.

This latter technique of double-contrast arthrography performed with fluoroscopic control and spot-filming is now the technique accepted by the authors of the arthrography section of this symposium. It is particularly advantageous for the examination of the menisci and articular cartilage.

References

1. Andren, L., and Wehlin, L.: Double-contrast arthrography of the knee with horizontal roentgen ray beam, Acta Orthop. Scand. **29:**307, 1960.
2. Bircher, E.: Pneumoradiographic des Knies und der anderen Gelenke, Schweiz. Med. Wochenschr. **50:**1210, 1931.
3. Butt, W. P., and McIntyre, J. L.: Double-contrast arthrography of the knee, Radiology **92:**487, 1969.
4. Dalinka, M. K., Coren, G. S., and Wershba, M.: Knee arthrography, CRC Crit. Rev. Clin. Radiol. Nucl. Med. **4:**1, 1973.
5. Freiberger, R. H., Killoran, P. J., and Cardona, G.: Arthrography of the knee by double contrast method, Am. J. Roentgenol. Radium Ther. Nucl. Med. **97:**736, 1966.
6. Kleinberg, S.: Pulmonary embolus following oxygen injection of the knee, J.A.M.A. **89:**172, 1927.
7. Lindblom, K.: Arthrography of the knee: roentgenographic and anatomical study, Acta Radiol. [Suppl.] 74, 1948.
8. Ricklin, R., Ruttimann, A., Del Buono, M. S.: Meniscus lesions; practical problems of clinical diagnosis, arthrography, and therapy, New York, 1971, Grune & Stratton.
9. Werndorff, K. R., and Robinson, I.: Uber intraarticulare and interstitielle Sauerstoff-insufflation zu radiologischen, diagnostichen and theraputischen Zwecken, Kongress-verhandlungen Deutschen Gesellschaft Orthopaedie, 1905.

2. Arthroscopists and arthrographers

Arthroscopist

Ralph T. Lidge

Who is an arthroscopist? This is an exciting question and should provoke thoughts, some new and some old, as well as stimulate self-analysis. Can you qualify for this job description?

The arthroscope of today, like the microscope of yesterday, is a breakthrough in the diagnosis and treatment of disease. At this time the arthroscope is still in an infant stage of development. However, it must be recognized as having arrived and should be considered as an important means not only of educating the doctor but also of facilitating care of the patient.

It has befallen the orthopedic surgeon to proceed into a new area, a learning experience totally foreign to most at this time. The physician should realize that the arthroscope, with its rapid refinements, together with ancillary instrumentation, is achieving a tremendous impact in diagnostic accuracy. He becomes aware of the living anatomy of the joint at rest and in action. The knee serves as a useful laboratory for observing and making studies for medical and surgical management. End results can be observed and documented.

Certain skills are demanded. The arthroscopist must be able to employ manual techniques that involve sensory input of visual modalities, including position and depth perception, together with tactile sensation. Both visual and tactile sensation must be continually fed to the brain for interpretation. Facts must undergo concomitant analysis with instantaneous interpretation, resulting in an output of motor function. This requires manual dexterity. There is a continuous flow of information in need of interpretation, retrieval, and command, with manual and visual interplay. One cannot exaggerate the importance of keen observation and accurate interpretation. Fatigue and wishful thinking must be avoided. Results should be honestly defined.

The beginning arthroscopist goes through several phases of learning in the course of mastering arthroscopy.

The early beginner's phase can be termed the "phase of enthusiasm." The majority of individuals in the United States and Canada who have become involved with arthroscopy have attended a course sponsored by the American Academy of Orthopaedic Surgeons. Sooner or later the physician makes a decision to purchase an arthroscope. He usually has beginner's luck, wisely selecting a knee of known pathology, such as one with a torn meniscus. He finds the diagnosis confirmed by arthrotomy and then looks for new knees to conquer.

The late beginner's phase can be termed the "phase of dejection." The majority of budding arthroscopists usually have minimal difficulty with the first few cases, but after 10 to 15 patients the physician may tend to wander or stumble into various situations, such as white-out or red-out, and many times he is unable to find an ongoing solution, to visually interpret, or to perform with manual dexterity. One can coin this period the "arthropause," since at this time the physician must make a decision as to whether to proceed in spite of adversity, hoping that he will improve with time. Error may be repeated without being aware of same.

The intermediate phase usually occurs after 25 to 30 patients. The arthroscopist senses a new feeling, which appears to surge from within. For the first time he develops a sense of confidence and looks back to his early cases with a better understanding of how he can avoid the pitfalls of error in technique and diagnosis.

The advanced phase takes place once the 100 mark has been reached. The arthroscopist develops a feeling not only of renewed confidence but also of euphoria and even wonderment. He has gotten his second wind, and with each additional 100 cases he develops an increasing feeling of equanimity. He realizes, however, that he is constantly learning, and each joint brings with it a new experience, in many instances, the unexpected. Being aware of the latter possibility, he is able to adjust accordingly and usually can arrive at an intelligent answer.

Finally, as the arthroscopist gains experience he realizes that this procedure is an invaluable method of arriving at the truth. He must continue to have a restless feeling to acquire information that may be of help not only to the patient but also to himself.

Arthrographer
Jeremy J. Kaye

An arthrographer is an individual interested in the study of joints by roentgenographic techniques. This usually involves the injection of contrast materials into the joint. These may be either negative-contrast materials (gasses) or positive-contrast materials (iodinated contrast materials). His primary interest is in the diagnosis of intraarticular disease by roentgenographic means. These may be diseases of the meninsci, the articular cartilage, or the ligamentous or synovial structures.

The definition of an arthrographer is by no means restricted to radiologists, although because of their particular technical expertise this is usually the case. In some locations and particular situations, the orthopedic surgeon has chosen, because of his particular interest or expertise, to become involved in this evaluation of the knee. In the usual situation the surgeon need not concern himself with these problems but may refer the patient to the radiologist for an adequate evaluation.

When should the patient be sent for an arthrogram, and when should he have arthroscopy? Should an arthrogram proceed every arthroscopy? Should the patient have an arthrogram only after a negative arthroscopy? What are the relative values of arthroscopy and arthrography in the evaluation of the knee and other joints? Does one examination obviate the need for the other? What are the relative values in terms of diagnostic information, simplicity for the patient, cost to the patient, and disability? These are the questions that we would like to raise at this point, prior to the formal discussion of arthrography. The answers to these questions must be left to the surgeons and radiologists who read this symposium, in terms of their individual practices.

3. Optical design and care of the endoscope

Rochelle Prescott

From an optical standpoint all modern arthroscopes have some features in common: they have an objective, which determines the angle of the field of view; they may or may not have a prismatic element, which inclines the direction of the field of view to the axis of the instrument; and they have a system of relay optics that conveys the image along the tube and an eyepiece through which the final image is viewed.

One can interpret the function of the arthroscope in either of two ways: the image of the interior of the joint is brought outside for viewing or, better, the eye is effectively brought inside the cavity, not only allowing the joint to be seen but to be seen from a unique viewpoint. That is, the arthroscopist now sees the joint as though his eye was at the tip of the arthroscope. There are additional effects in all arthroscopes: the objective looks at a field of view of, say, 40° to 100°, and the eye sees this field of view covering an apparent field of 5° to 10°. As a result of these two effects the novice arthroscopist is faced with the problem of learning to visualize anatomy from a viewpoint with an entirely different perspective. He must go through a period in which he trains his visual centers to adapt to the perspective of the endoscopic system. He should take every opportunity to use the instrument and should carefully scan the entire area to be viewed. It is probably most helpful to scan slowly when going from one area to another in order to connect the images in the visual centers of the brain. The lack of binocular perception must be made up for by the changing perspective as the movement of the tip of the endoscope causes the point of view to change. During this period of learning the arthroscopist must concentrate on the entire task and be constantly aware (1) of the position of the instrument tip (and hence the eye) within the body cavity and (2) of the direction of view.

In order to become proficient in the practice of any form of endoscopy the physician must not only be knowledgeable and practiced in the medical science and skills related to his specialization, but he should also become knowledgeable and practiced in the areas of science and technology relating to endoscopy and to the accessories of endoscopic equipment that he will use.

An endoscope is an optical instrument. Its function is to allow the physician to see   ⋅

13

within the body as clearly as possible with a minimum of trauma. Modern endoscopes range in size from less than 2 mm to somewhat over 10 mm in diameter. They not only have an optical system for bringing the image of the internal areas of the body out to be viewed by the eye of the physician, but they also carry into the body sufficient illumination so that both photography and color television can easily be used for recording with all but the smallest endoscopes.

The first optical endoscope (Nitze, 1879) designed for cystoscopy was only 7 mm in diameter, with the illumination provided by a glowing platinum wire. Progress since that time has taken advantage of the many advances in technical optics to greatly increase the performance of both the imaging system and the illuminating system.

IMAGING OPTICS

There are three basic optical systems used in rigid endoscopes (flexible endoscopes, having found no place in arthroscopy, will not be discussed here). These three systems are shown schematically in Fig. 3-1. The first system (Fig. 3-1, A) consists of an objective to form an image of a wide field of view within the body cavity, a periscopic system of relay lenses to bring this image a convenient distance through the narrow channel of the instrument, and an eyepiece to give the eye a suitably enlarged image for viewing. Endoscopes with this system of optics were the first type made and have been enormously improved by a number of advances in optical technology. New optical glass types, low-reflection coatings for lenses, and advances in optical design and computation have all contributed to the vast improvement of the imaging quality of modern endoscopes of this type.

The second type of endoscopic system, the rod-lens system (Fig. 3-1, B), provides a number of advantages in construction and performance.[4] This design contrasts to that of the conventional system (Fig. 3-1, A) in that the rod-lens system has extremely thick glass lenses (rod lenses) and thin air spaces, just the opposite of the thin glass lenses and long air spaces of the conventional system.

The third type of system, the graded index (GRIN) lens system (Fig. 3-1, C), made possible by the recent development of a glass element in which the refractive index can be varied in a reproducible way,* has the entire objective and relay system in a single glass component consisting of two elements, which are each slender (nominal 1 mm diameter) cylinders of glass and are cemented end to end. The extreme slenderness of this optical system allows an entire system, including the illuminating elements, to be enclosed in a hypodermic tubing as small as 16-gauge (1.7 mm).† In order to allow the eye to comfortably view the image produced by this system a relatively long ocular is used, which enlarges the apparent diameter of the image to some 30 mm. This long ocular also allows the surgeon to comfortably bring his eye close to the eyepiece, while his hand, holding the arthroscope, is some distance from the unsterile area around his face (Fig. 3-2).

---

*Selfoc, Nippon Sheet Glass, Japan.
†Needlescope, Dyonics, Inc., Woburn, Mass.

In comparing these three basic systems we found that the rod-lens system has certain basic advantages, both optical and mechanical, over the classic lens system; these advantages become more important as the diameter of the endoscope is reduced. The GRIN lens system, correspondingly, has certain advantages, also both optical and mechanical, which become more important as the diameter of the system becomes very small (the diameter of this last system is nominally 1 mm, and it is available in a 0.7 mm diameter).

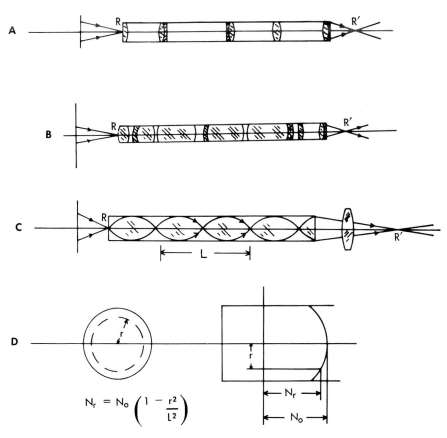

Fig. 3-1. Three basic endoscopic optical systems used in rigid endoscopes. **A,** Classic thin lens system in which lenses are thin in comparison with their diameters and separations. **B,** Rod-lens system designed by Hopkins, in which thicknesses of lenses are large compared to their diameters, and air spaces are small. **C,** Graded index (GRIN) lens systems, in which entire system consists of a slender rod of glass, in which refractory index decreases from axis to periphery, according to a specific mathematical relationship. **D,** Thus rays of light entering lens from a particular point in object space follow helioid paths and come to a focus in an image periodically along rod, **C.** In all systems, point of view of an observer with his eye at R' is transferred to R. (From Prescott, R.: J. Med. Primatol. **5:**133-147, 1976.)

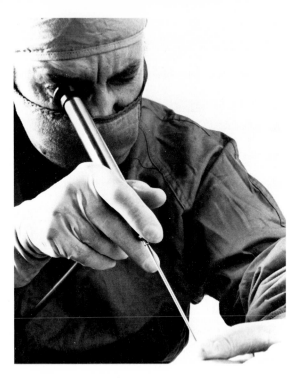

Fig. 3-2. Long ocular of this small arthroscope allows comfortable viewing with eye well removed from sterile area.

ENDOSCOPES
Optical characteristics

There are certain parameters that determine the optical characteristics of an endoscope. For a detailed treatment, the reader is referred to my article, "Optical Principles of Endoscopy."[3] It will be easier to understand the following paragraphs if one has an endoscope to examine while reading.

Angle of field of view. The angle in degrees included between lines drawn from the tip of the endoscope and the extremes of a diameter of the field of view (Fig. 3-3) is the angle of field of view. This is reduced about 30% in water or saline when compared to air. This is due to the refraction that occurs at the entrance window of the endoscope, which is always a plane surface (if this surface were not plane the focus and power of the endoscope would change when immersed into or removed from water). The effect is shown in Fig. 3-3. The refractive index of the glass window has no influence on this. As a first approximation the same diameter of field of view may be seen by increasing the distance by about one third. The actual values for available fields of view range from 35% to 43%.

Direction of view. The direction of view of an endoscope is nominally the angle between the axis of the endoscope and the line connecting the tip of the endoscope

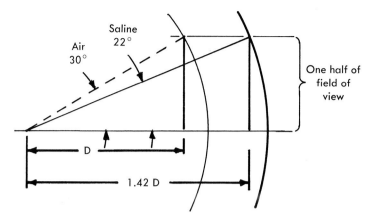

Fig. 3-3. Schema shows how field of view of endoscope is reduced by refraction when used in saline and how increase in distance is required to restore diameter of field viewed.

and the center of its field of view. In arthroscopy this is normally 0°, 30°, or 60°. These lines are shown schematically for a 60° angle-of-field-of-view endoscope (Fig. 3-4). In the forward looking instrument, rotation does not change the area viewed, while for the other two types rotation has a scanning effect (the image does not rotate). The 30° instrument is often termed a "forward oblique" as it always sees directly ahead as well as laterally, and the 60° instrument is called a "lateral" as it sees to the side but does not see directly ahead. The forward and forward-oblique directions of view are most often used in arthroscopy.

Angle of apparent field of view. The angle of the apparent field of view is the angle in degrees included between the two lines drawn from the eye to points at the opposite extremes of a diameter of the apparent field of view (Fig. 3-5).

Exit pupil. If one looks at, not into, the eyepiece of an endoscope which is pointed at a bright field, a circular disk can be seen on the optical axis near the eyepiece. This is the exit pupil, also known as the eyepoint or Ramsden disk. It is an image of the entrance pupil of the instrument, and all of the image-forming light passes through it with the light from each point in the field of view uniformly distributed over it. The distance from this disk to the eyepiece is the "eye relief."

The diameter of the exit pupil determines, to a large degree, both the brightness and the sharpness of the apparent field of view. According to theoretic optics the maximum resolution of which the eye is capable cannot be reached by an instrument whose exit pupil diameter is not at least 2 mm; however, under ordinary viewing conditions one does not discern a lack of sharpness in resolution of detail until the exit pupil diameter is well below this value, perhaps 1.2 to 1 mm. Correspondingly the brightness of the image seen through an instrument should be apparently reduced if the exit pupil diameter is reduced below the diameter of the eye pupil, which may be about 3 mm under the conditions encountered in endoscopy. This does not occur,

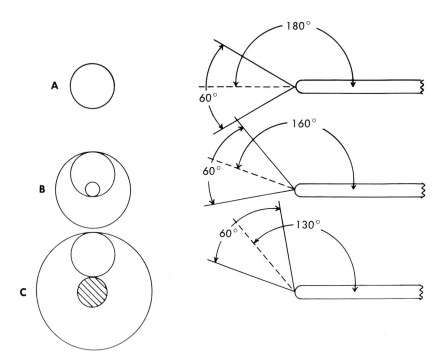

Fig. 3-4. Comparison of fields of view through three endoscopes. In each instance, largest circle to left indicates field of view covered by rotating endoscope. All have a 60° field of view. Rotation of 180° endoscope about its own axis does not change field of view, **A.** Rotation of 160° endoscope, **B,** causes scanning effect that increases area viewed by nearly three times while keeping 20° area *(small circle)* centered on axis constantly in view. Such an endoscope is termed "forward oblique." Rotation of 130° endoscope, **C,** scans an area nearly seven times that of 180° endoscope but never sees what is in 40° area *(hatched circle)* directly ahead of it. It should be noted that in no case does image rotate. (From Prescott, R.: J. Med. Primatol. **5:**133-147, 1976.)

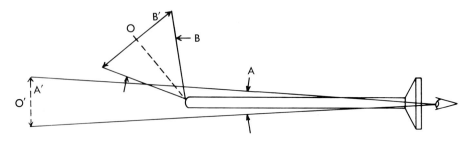

Fig. 3-5. Apparent field of view of endoscope is angle, *A,* from eye, subtended by a diameter of field, *A',* when centered on object, *O'.* Real field of view is angle, *B,* from tip of endoscope subtended by diameter of field, *B',* when centered on object, *O.* Apparent field of view is usually between 5° and 10°, and real field of view is usually between 40° and 100°. (From Prescott, R.: J. Med. Primatol. **5:**133-147, 1976.)

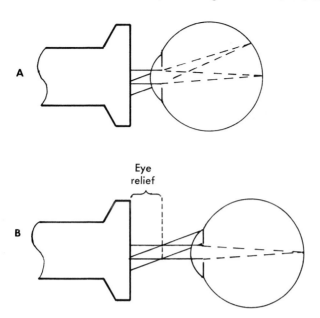

Fig. 3-6. A, Schema of eye at eyepoint of endoscope. Light from all parts of field passes through iris to form image at back of eye. **B** shows what happens when eye is not brought close enough to eyepoint. Only light from central portion of field passes through iris. Periphery of field is occluded, and eye must be moved laterally to scan entire field.

and no noticeable loss of apparent image brightness occurs until the exit pupil is reduced to about 1.2 mm or smaller.

When an endoscope is being used the eye should be brought close enough to the eyepoint so that light from all parts of the image enters the pupil (Fig. 3-6, *A*). If this cannot be done because the eyepoint is too short (Fig. 3-6, *B*), then the observer cannot see the entire field of view without moving the eye laterally and must "knothole" to scan the entire image.

The exit pupil must also serve as the aperture for the camera lens when one is photographing through the endoscope, and here it is even more important that vignetting not occur, due to the entrance pupil of the camera (the diaphragm) being behind the exit pupil plane. This problem is usually solved by opening the camera aperture completely (Fig. 3-7, *A*) or by the use of special lens systems that match the exit pupil of the endoscope (Fig. 3-7, *B*). The latter is the better solution as the special lens mount will also be designed to clamp the eyepiece of the endoscope in the correct position.

Visual accommodation. The image that one sees through an endoscope is at a particular apparent distance. For practical reasons, this distance is adjusted at the time of manufacture and cannot be changed by the user. Until the last decade all instrument manufacturers adjusted such instruments to give an image at infinity. Unfortunately a large portion of the population does not focus best at infinity, whether or not they wear corrective lenses. As it is not practical for the endoscopist

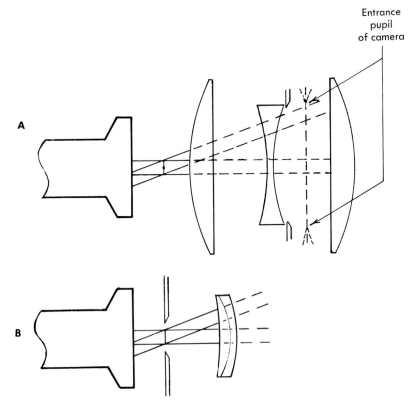

Entrance
pupil
of camera

Fig. 3-7. A, Path of light bundles from center and from edge of field of view when ordinary camera lens is used with endoscope. Unless aperture stop is opened wide, light from peripheral regions of field of view will be stopped, resulting in vignetted photograph, showing only central region. **B,** Lens design in which aperture stop falls in front of glass components, thus allowing it to be mounted adequately close to eyepiece. In either case effective aperture of lens is determined by diameter of exit pupil of endoscope.

to maintain sterility and to don or remove glasses during an endoscopic examination, it would seem that a practical solution to this problem is to adjust the apparent distance of the image to a convenient distance for the other visual tasks associated with the examination and to wear glasses, if necessary, to give this visual correction. A convenient value is 50 cm. A pair of glasses of suitable prescription (not bifocals) will greatly reduce the discomfort of viewing through the arthroscope the great variety of positions required, for example, in a complete arthroscopic examination of the knee joint (Fig. 3-8).

   Resolution. The resolution of an endoscope is often referred to the object space, but it will then be a function of the object distance. It is more convenient to refer the resolution to the apparent image, where a number can be given for the line pairs that can be resolved across the entire field. This is the same value (to a reasonable approximation) for all object distances and might be compared to the case for a

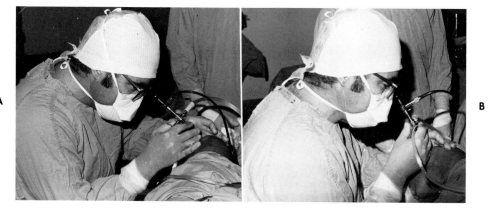

Fig. 3-8. Photographs taken during arthroscopy of knee joint show some positions assumed by arthroscopist during examination. It is clear that use of bifocal spectacles would cause difficulties.

television image. We have all seen a zoom shot, where a figure almost invisible on a broad panoramic screen is brought up to fill the entire screen with great detail and fidelity. In this case the resolution remains constant due to the 525-line format of the video screen. In arthroscopy the lens is fixed, but it is usually easy to zoom in on a detail of interest until it fills the whole field of view. In this case the magnification is proportional to the reciprocal of the distance. There are three factors that limit the closeness with which the endoscopist can approach an object without it going out of focus. One of these is the initial focal adjustment of the endoscope; at what distance is it focused? Another factor is the accommodation of the arthroscopist; as the object gets nearer the tip of the arthroscope the image approaches the arthroscopist, and his accommodation is limited by his visual correction and his age. The last factor, and one that is very important in endoscopy, is the depth of focus; how far can an object be from the point of best focus before its image is noticeably degraded?

The initial focal adjustment of an endoscope is fixed at the time the endoscope is manufactured. It has been customary to focus on an object at a long distance and to set the eyepiece accommodation for an emmetropic eye at its far point, infinity. The individual's accommodation is then used to focus on the image of near objects. Due to the optical properties of the endoscope, this focusing effect or accommodation allows objects at surprisingly small distances to be brought into perfect focus.

There is a trend now by optical instrument manufacturers to adjust the instrument for nearer object and image points for several reasons: the endoscopist must do other visual tasks in the related procedures that require good visual acuity at short range; hence he should be visually corrected to a nearer image; and the objects in the field of view in arthroscopy, for instance, are not more than 5 cm from the tip of the endoscope, so there is no need to have a good image of an object at large distances.

The visual accommodation of an individual, whether he wears corrective glasses or not, varies as a function of age in the same way for every person. The values range from about 10 diopters at age 20 to about 1 diopter at age 65. Fortunately for the endoscopist the optical characteristics of the endoscopic optical system multiply this accommodation by a large factor, ranging from 25 to 100 times. This effect will actually allow a young person with normal vision to accommodate perfectly through an endoscope for objects from infinity to a distance as small as 1 mm. For the average mature surgeon the near point will be several millimeters, but this is still a tremendous range.

The depth of focus is also of importance in endoscopy. As in a camera system the smaller the aperture, the greater the depth of focus, and, as we now know, the aperture of an endoscope is extremely small. On the other hand the depth of focus is relatively small at short distances. In endoscopy these two effects act in opposite directions, so we find that the depth of focus is quite different in different endoscopes. For example, if we adopt a strict criteria, as did Rayleigh, we find that for a $^1/_5$ mm aperture focused on infinity, an object at about 36 mm is not objectionably out of focus. Conversely if the instrument is focused for 36 mm then objects from infinity to 18 mm are in good focus. Thus the endoscopist's depth of focus has added about 28 diopters in each direction to his depth of field. When these effects are properly balanced in the design and adjustment of an endoscope objects from about 1 mm to infinity are in sharp visual focus.

Care

An endoscope is a delicate instrument and must be treated as such at all times. It may be damaged by misuse, but it is likely that most damage occurs in cleaning and sterilization. This task should only be entrusted to well-trained, responsible personnel. A damaged endoscope cannot usually be used at all, and unless a backup instrument is available, procedures must be cancelled until the equipment is repaired or replaced.

The endoscopic equipment is best cleaned immediately after a procedure before blood and body fluids have dried. Each piece should be carefully washed and inspected, and assembled where applicable. The equipment should then be dried sufficiently to look through and sterilized.

Although some endoscopes can be cleaned by a steam autoclave, most cannot and are irreparably damaged by such treatment. Even those endoscopes that are autoclavable require very special preparation for this treatment. The opinion has been expressed that autoclaving any endoscope presents a danger to all endoscopes, as mistakes will occur.

Fortunately, a large body of medical opinion based on hospital and clinical experience indicates that cold soaking of endoscopes* from 10 to 30 minutes for routine sterilization is adequate.[1] Opinions as to the desirability of gas sterilization on occasion, such as receipt of new instruments or following unclean procedures, vary. There are also varied opinions as to the need for steam autoclaving ancillary instru-

---

*Cidex, Arbrook, Arlington, Tex., is most often recommended.

ments, such as cannulas, trocars, obturators, and light guides, which are not sensitive to heat. Some groups recommend that it be done and some that it is not necessary. Experience in laparoscopy is much greater than in arthroscopy with many groups reporting on thousands of cases; however, arthroscopy experience supports the above viewpoints.[2]

Illumination

Many methods have been tried for the illumination of endoscopes, but today only two are still in use. One method uses the tungsten lamp, which is inserted into the body cavity as an integral part of the endoscope or, at least, through the same cannula. The second is the fiber optic light guide, which brings the light from a remotely situated tungsten or arc light down through the endoscope.

The tungsten bulb, which has been in use for several generations, is far superior to all other illumination methods, with the exception of fiber optics. The tungsten bulb has five principal shortcomings:

1. The heat generated in producing the light is approximately 100 times the energy in the light itself, and in general less than 10% of the light produced is directed at the field of view. This large amount of heat must be continuously removed, and this requires a copious flow of saline during arthroscopy to prevent discomfort and even pain or injury to the patient.

2. The tungsten bulb is rather bulky and occupies a diameter approximately equal to the diameter of the instrument. This is particularly unwieldy for insertion between the condyles for examination of remote regions of the knee joint.

3. The bulb has a finite life and hence cannot be an integral part of the arthroscope. It and its carrier are somewhat fragile and liable to breakage or damage.

4. The electric current may cause problems if electric leakage occurs.

5. The saline corrodes the electric connections with resultant problems.

On the other hand, fiber optics is extremely functional as an endoscope illumination method. Only the light energy required to illuminate the field of view is brought down to the area being examined. If desired, even the near infrared may be, and usually is, removed from the light used. This means that large, high-brightness sources can be used with no problems at all in dissipating the energy at the site. The light fibers are an integral part of the endoscope and efficiently fit into the annular or crescent-shaped cross sections around the imaging optics of the endoscope. The light guide is one of the most durable and trouble-free parts of the entire instrument.

A schema of one type of fiber optic light source is shown in Fig. 3-9. The light source is situated in a small metal package with a suitable transformer, a fan to carry away the heat, and so on. The light is focused on the end of the fiber optic light guide, which is usually 1.5 to 2 m in length and which consists of a bundle of special glass fibers. Each fiber, less than the diameter of a human hair, is of a clear optical glass with a thin coating of a glass of a lower refractive index. The fibers at each end of the bundle are packed closely together, set in epoxy cement, and the bundle end ground flat and polished. Most endoscopes have their own fiber optic light guide, which

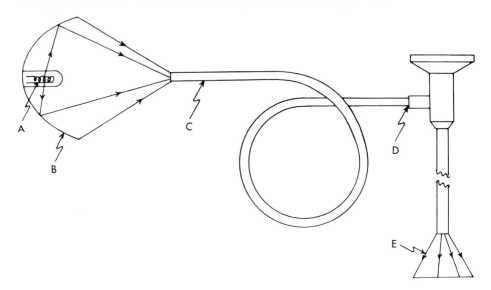

Fig. 3-9. Fiber optic light guide, *C*, is illuminated by light of tungsten halogen (or arc) lamp, *A*, which is concentrated on one of its ends by reflector, *B*. Transmitted light is coupled into fiber optic light guide of endoscope at *D* and emitted at *E* to illuminate field of view of endoscope. (From Prescott, R.: J. Med. Primatol. **5:**133-147, 1976.)

carries the illuminating light from a connection with the above light guide to the tip of the endoscope. The separate light guide, although less efficient, as the loss of light at a light guide–to–light guide connection is about one third, allows the light guide itself, which is exposed to much abuse and is relatively cheap, to be replaced when damaged.

It can be shown that the intensity of a fiber optic light guide as a source is proportional to the intrinsic brightness, not the total intensity, of the prime light source, to the effective area of the light guide, and to the product of the effective transmissivities of each of the elements of the system. In the system shown in Fig. 3-9 the primary light source is an electric arc discharge or a coiled tungsten filament. In the latter case the average brightness over the source area is considered first, then the reflectance of the reflector, the effective area of all the fiber cores as compared to the total area of the fiber optic bundle, the transmission of the individual fiber core (the loss due to reflectance is about 5% or 6%), the transmission of the light guide (about .85 per meter), the loss at the connection to the endoscope due to reflectance and mismatch of the core-to-core ends, and the losses in the fiber optics of the endoscope itself and its termination. It is particularly important that the area of the source image at the fiber optic bundle be amply large to fully illuminate all the fibers and that the light guide be somewhat larger than the fiber optic bundle of the endoscope at the connector so that each fiber in the endoscope is also fully illuminated.

Summary. For maximum illumination, as in photography, a source of high intrinsic brightness such as an arc lamp should be used. It must be imaged on the end of the fiber optic light guide by a suitable reflector or lens system. The light guide should not be excessively long, the glass bundle itself must be of a larger diameter than the input to the light guide on the endoscope, and no unnecessary joints or couplings should be used.

References

1. International Correspondence, Society of Obstetricians and Gynecologists: Ob-Gyn Collected Letters, Series XIV, pp. 73-77, May 1, 1973.
2. Johnson, L. L., Schneider, D., Goodman, F., Bullock, J. M., and DeBruin, J. A., Jr.: Cold sterilization method for arthroscopes using activated dialdehyde, Orthop. Rev. 6(9):75-77, 1977.
3. Prescott, R.: Optical principles of endoscopy, J. Med. Primatol. 5:133-147, 1976.
4. U.S. Patent 3,257,902 "Optical system having cylindrical rod-like lenses," Harold H. Hopkins, June 28, 1966.

4. Instrumentation in arthroscopy

Watanabe arthroscopes

Robert W. Jackson

Following in Prof. Takagi's footsteps, Dr. Watanabe continued with the development of instrumentation for the visualization of the interior of the knee joint. Numerous models were made, each numbered consecutively. Variations of widths, lengths, lenses, and lights were tested and rejected or revised.

The Watanabe no. 19 was the first arthroscope to be used extensively, but as this had a 90° side-viewing lens, considerable experience and expertise were required to keep it oriented. The boom in optical and electronic technology in the 1950s in Japan led to rapid improvements, and in 1960 the Watanabe no. 21 was perfected (Fig. 4-1). This instrument has remained in common use until the present day. It deserves its reputation as the first instrument to be widely accepted and used throughout the world and is in large part responsible for the sudden appreciation of the possibilities that arthroscopy offers.

The instrument basically consists, as all arthroscopes do, of an optical system, an irrigation system, and a lighting system. The optical system is encased in a rigid tube with a series of magnifying lenses providing an angle of vision of 102° (in air) and a depth of focus from 0.5 mm to infinity. The direction of vision is 0° or straight ahead. Magnification varies inversely with the distance of the lens from the object and is approximately 1:1 at 1 cm distance and ten times larger at 1 mm distance.

The lighting system consists of a tungsten bulb that is offset at the distal end of a light carrier so that it lies beside the optical system. It also extends just beyond the tip of the lens to avoid shadowing (Fig. 4-2). The light carrier and the telescope are both nested within the sheath, which is 6.5 mm in diameter. The light carrier is powered by a transformer, which is connected to the electric mains. The transformer provides an output of 7 V for visualization purposes and has a second built-in circuit, which doubles the intensity to 15 V for photographic purposes. There is space between the light carrier, the telescope, and the encasing sheath for the irrigation fluid to flow from the distal end of the instrument. The irrigation system is designed for continuous irrigation with a pressure head provided by elevating a bottle of saline at room temperature to a height of approximately 1 m above the knee. An outflow tube is inserted into the knee, usually into the suprapatellar pouch region. Any blood or debris is washed away from the lens and out the outflow tube. Thus excellent visualization is facilitated.

26

One of the major advantages of the Watanabe system is the light bulb, which, because it is offset, can be used as a tool for retracting synovial fronds or for pulling back the anterior capsule and fat pad in order to obtain a better and almost panoramic view of the compartment that is being examined. Unfortunately the offset light bulb, while an advantage in this respect, has also been a source of difficulty for inexperienced examiners. It is possible to bend the light bulb away from the underlying telescope when sweeping the instrument through the joint (Fig. 4-3). Repeated bending weakens the junction between the light bulb and the light carrier, and breakage of this light bulb has been reported. Moreover heat is produced by the

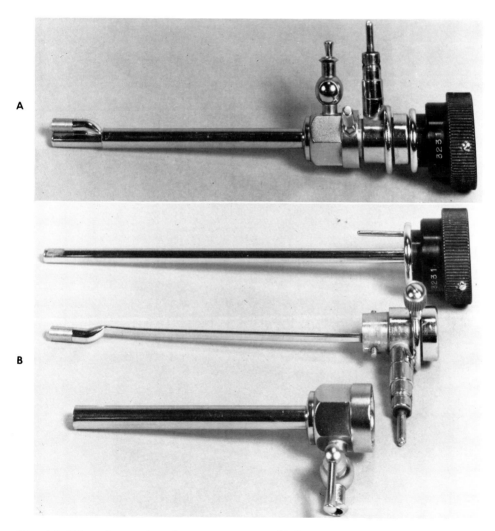

Fig. 4-1. Watanabe no. 21 arthroscope. **A,** Assembled. **B,** Component parts. Top: optical system; middle: light carrier; bottom: sheath. (From Recent Adv. Orthop. no. 2, pp. 217-234, 1975.)

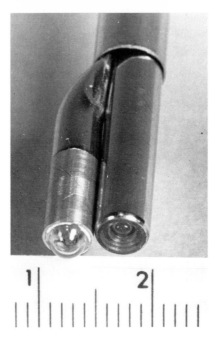

Fig. 4-2. Tungsten light bulb is offset and extends slightly beyond end of optical system to avoid shadowing. (From Jackson, R. W., and Dandy, D. J.: Arthroscopy of the knee: modern orthopedic monographs, New York, 1976, Grune & Stratton.)

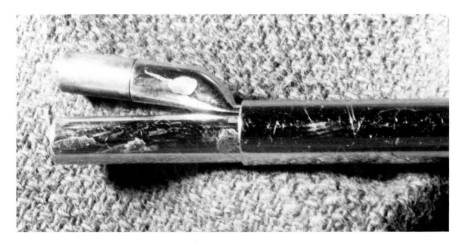

Fig. 4-3. With rough handling, light bulb may be bent away from lens. Breakage may then follow. (From Jackson, R. W., and Dandy, D. J.: Arthroscopy of the knee: modern orthopedic monographs, New York, 1976, Grune & Stratton.)

bulb, which conceivably could harm intraarticular structures, and there is an occasional electrical short circuit, which produces a strong and sustained contraction of the quadriceps.

Photography, both still and cine, is possible using high-speed film that has been adjusted for artificial light (tungsten light). Due to the wide field of vision, the depth of focus, and the offset light bulb, excellent pictures are obtained with good contrast of any irregular surfaces on the femoral condyle or on the menisci.

Operating tools can be used "blindly" through the sheath (upon removal of the telescope and light carrier) or under direct vision by inserting an auxiliary sheath through a second portal of entry (Fig. 4-4). In this latter instance the operating tools, consisting of scissors or biopsy forceps, are visualized, and under direct vision a meniscus or loose body can be removed, a plica transected, or a biopsy of a synovial frond done (Fig. 4-5).

Recent advances include the Watanabe no. 22, which encircles the lens with fiber light (Fig. 4-6). The telescope with its attached fiber light can be inserted through the 6.5 mm sheath. However, the addition of fiber light in a ring around the tip of the telescope necessitated some reduction in the field of vision, from 102° to 88° (in air).

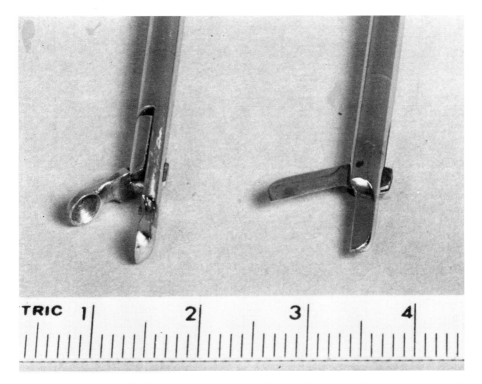

Fig. 4-4. Operating tools for endoscopic surgery. Biopsy forceps *(left)* and scissors *(right)*. (From Jackson, R. W., and Dandy, D. J.: Arthroscopy of the knee: modern orthopedic monographs, New York, 1976, Grune & Stratton.)

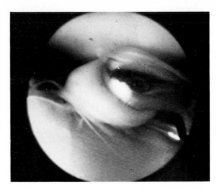

Fig. 4-5. Removal of small loose body, using biopsy forceps. (From Jackson, R. W., and Dandy, D. J.: Arthroscopy of the knee: modern orthopedic monographs, New York, 1976, Grune & Stratton.)

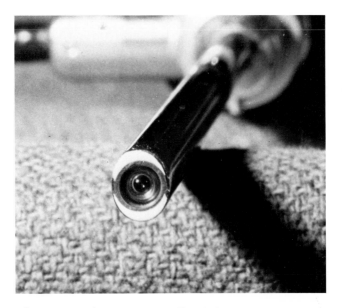

Fig. 4-6. Watanabe no. 22 arthroscope. Note fiber light crescents on either side of optical system. (From Jackson, R. W., and Dandy, D. J.: Arthroscopy of the knee: modern orthopedic monographs, New York, 1976, Grune & Stratton.)

    The Watanabe no. 24 is an arthroscope that uses the 2 mm diameter Selfoc fiber developed in Japan for visualization and fiber light for illumination. The no. 25 is also a small-diameter arthroscope, using a series of lenses for visualization. Nos. 26 to 31, mostly small-diameter arthroscopes, are currently in the developmental stage.

    One instrument that may prove specially useful is the Watanabe no. 21 CL. This instrument has fiber light ringing the telescope (with some reduction in the field of vision) plus a solid, unbreakable, offset "retractor" shaped like the Watanabe no. 21 light carrier.

Undoubtedly, other major technical advances will be realized in the years to come, but the Watanabe no. 21 will always be regarded as the "Model T" of arthroscopy.

Fiber optic arthroscopes

John J. Joyce III

Illumination and image clarity pose two of the most difficult problems in arthroscopy. Lack of a lens system and scant illumination of the area to be observed limited the progress of the early nineteenth century investigators. Edison's incandescent lamp and the addition of an optical system to his instrument made Nitze's endoscope the original model after which subsequent ones were patterned.

OPTICAL SYSTEMS

The development of the rod-lens system by Hopkins provided a significant advance in the evolution of the endoscope. Instead of using small widely separated lenses within the instrument, Hopkins used long, rodlike lenses separated by small spaces (Fig. 4-7). This innovation has resulted in a clearer and brighter image due to less aberration and light loss. Furthermore these lenses could be made in a smaller diameter. The result has been a narrower instrument, which not only can be introduced into smaller joints but also into a sheath along with operating accessories. Surgery within the knee joint through a small incision is thus possible.

The Selfoc arthroscope was devised by Watanabe in conjunction with the Nippon

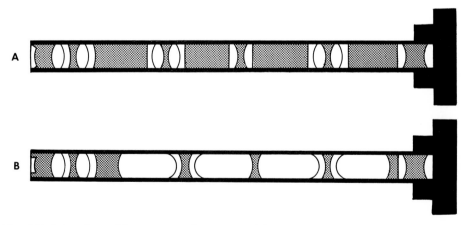

Fig. 4-7. A, Traditional lens system, showing small lenses with wide separation. **B,** Hopkins rod-lens system, showing elongated lenses with minimal separation.

Glass Company. This ingenious instrument consists of a specially treated single-image transmitting fiber thread. It is produced in 1.7 and 2.2 mm diameters (Fig. 4-8). Such a device has already opened new frontiers in arthroscopy. Not only are the hip and shoulder joints able to be inspected, but the elbow, wrist, ankle, and metacarpophalangeal articulations can also be viewed.

The flexible fiber optic endoscope is currently used only to explore other organs. The instrument consists of a bundle of optical glass fibers, each of which transmits a portion of the visible field. Unfortunately, this system has not as yet been developed to the point where it can be made into a flexible arthroscope because of size constraints, though in this era of rapid technical advancement the future possibility appears to be only a matter of time. At the present time the so-called fiber optic arthroscopes generally consist of a rod-lens system surrounded by multiple light-conducting glass fibrils. These two systems are enclosed in a specially treated rigid metallic sheath (Fig. 4-9).

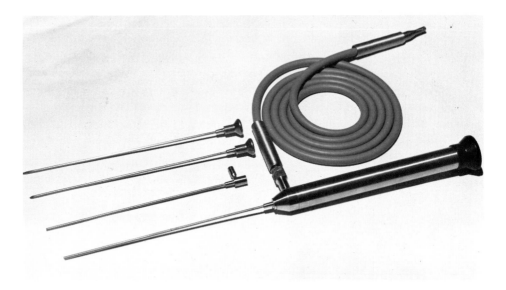

Fig. 4-8. Needlescope. This remarkable instrument is made in diameters of 2.2 and 1.7 mm. Its minute size allows visualization of smaller joints. (Courtesy Dyonics, Inc., Woburn, Mass.)

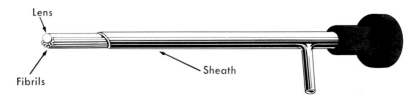

Lens

Fibrils

Sheath

Fig. 4-9. Fiber optic arthroscope. Note light-conducting fibrils surrounding Hopkins rod-lens system.

DIRECTION OF VIEW AND VIEWING ANGLE

The *direction of view* refers to the line of sight in relation to the horizontal axis of the arthroscope. Although a large variety of instruments is available, the usual ones vary between a direct (0°), forward-oblique (30°), and a 90° direction. Probably the most frequently used arthroscope is the forward-oblique one. By rotating the instrument around its longitudinal axis a larger area of the joint may be observed. Because the direction of view remains essentially forward, orientation may easily be maintained. On the other hand the 90° arthroscope, such as that available with the Watanabe no. 21 instrument, is useful in seeing around corners as well as some obstructions. This device has the disadvantage of making orientation difficult.

The *viewing angle* refers to the field encompassed by the lens (Fig. 4-10). The visible area varies according to the design of the optical system. For example, the

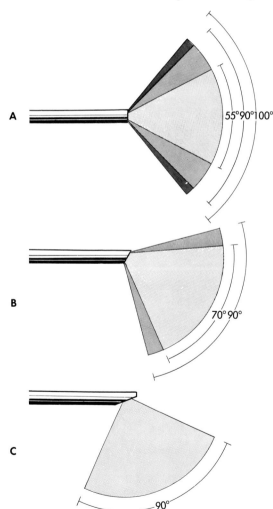

Fig. 4-10. Direction of view and viewing angle. **A,** Direction of view is 0° or straight ahead. Viewing angle is represented by various designs. Darkest (100°) is viewing of Watanabe arthroscope; lightest (55°) is viewing angle of direct-view Needlescope; intermediate shade (90°) is viewing angle of Storz and Wolf instruments. **B,** Foreward-oblique arthroscopes have direction of view of 30°. Viewing angle of Storz and Wolf instruments is 90° (*darker area*) while that of foreward-oblique Needlescope is 70° (*lighter area*). **C,** Direction of view is 70°. Viewing angle of 90° (*stippled area*) enables observer to maintain orientation and also affords wide field of vision.

viewing angle of the Watanabe no. 21 direct-view arthroscope is 100° in air, while that of the Selfoc arthroscope is 70°. Wider viewing angle facilitates orientation of the observer.

FIBER OPTIC LIGHT SOURCES

The development of fiber optic lighting eliminated many problems associated with older methods. The fiber optic cable consists of a bundle of specially prepared glass fibers encased in a protective sheath. One end of the bundle is attached to a light source that is remote from the operative field. The other end of the cable is attached to the arthroscope, which is surrounded by fiber optic fibrils.

The intensity of illumination of the observed field is governed by several factors. Since the light reaching an area varies with the square of the distance, it is desirable to have as short a cable as feasible. The intensity at the source of illumination is controlled by means of a rheostat. The amount of light reaching the area is directly related to the number of glass fibers in the cable extending between the light source and the instrument as well as the quantity surrounding the arthroscope. Since the glass fibers inside the cable are fragile, care must be taken to avoid tight bends or undue pressure on it. Fiber destruction causes loss of ability to conduct light. Instrument manufacturers have cables that can be adapted to the various available light sources.

For general inspection of a joint a simple 150 W tungsten bulb is usually sufficient for most arthroscopes. Since photography and video recording require more light, additional powerful sources are available. Since the light intensity in both the tungsten and xenon systems is adjustable, they can be used for diagnostic, operative, and photographic purposes.

Electronic strobe flash units are available from various manufacturers and can be adapted to most arthroscopes. Excellent still photographs can be produced by this equipment. Movies and video recordings of course are unavailable with flash lighting.

ACCESSORIES

The small diameter of the fiber optic arthroscopes has afforded significant advances in the accessories available to the surgeon. Not only are various operating instruments available that can be introduced through a separate incision, but more recently operating arthroscopes enable one to pass such items as scissors, biopsy forceps, knives, and grasping instruments through the sheath containing the lens system (Fig. 4-11). The latter arrangement has the advantage of having the tip of the instrument directly in the field of vision. Not only can it be frustratingly difficult to locate visually the instrument passed through a separate incision from that used for the arthroscope, but the operator then must have three hands. One hand is needed for the arthroscope, a second is required to maneuver the instrument, and the third is used to manipulate the extremity. An able and interested assistant is therefore desirable.

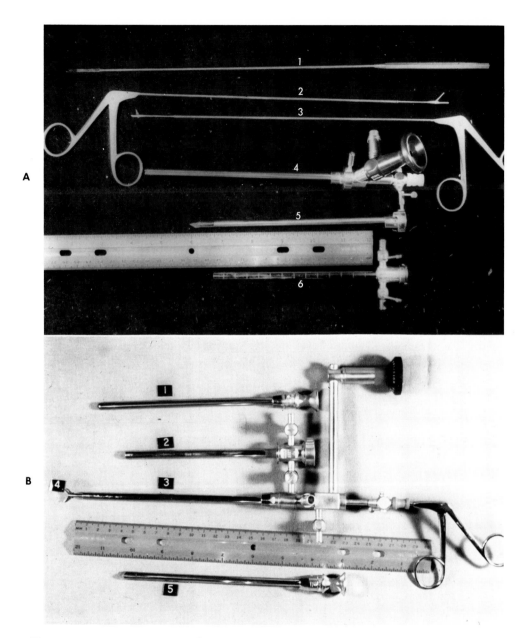

Fig. 4-11. A, Storz operating arthroscope. *1,* Knife for division of tissues. *2,* Grasping forceps. *3,* Scissors. *4,* Arthroscope. *5,* Trocar. *6,* Sheath. **B,** Wolf operating arthroscope. *1,* Obturator. *2,* Sheath for arthroscope. *3,* Operating arthroscope. *4,* Scissors in arthroscope. *5,* Trocar.

The use of a beam splitter enables an assistant or observer to visualize the same area as the surgeon. Operative procedures are thereby facilitated. The teaching attachment may be rigid or flexible. A prism mechanism may also be attached to a small television camera, which provides an excellent method of teaching. The arthroscopic findings may be recorded on tape, or a resident may be supervised by means of a monitor. This same type of apparatus can be used with a movie camera.

STERILIZATION OF THE FIBER OPTIC ARTHROSCOPE

Sterilization of the instruments is by gas through a 4-hour cycle or by other methods. They can be immersed in an antiseptic solution (such as Cidex) for an appropriate period of time. Formalin vapor is still used in Japan. Some fiber optic arthroscopes can be autoclaved under carefully controlled conditions. If the manufacturer's instructions are not rigidly followed, steam sterilization will damage the arthroscope.

Needlescope *

Lanny L. Johnson

The Needlescope is the smallest endoscope available. It comes in two sizes: 1.7 and 2.2 mm outside diameters. It consists of a 1 mm diameter graduated refractory index (GRIN) lens surrounded by the small bundle of fiber optic light and housed in a metallic cannula (Fig. 4-12).

*Dyonics, Inc., Woburn, Mass.

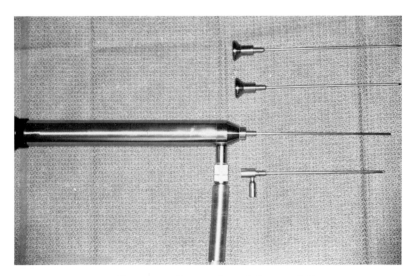

Fig. 4-12. Needlescope with cannula and sharp and blunt trocars.

The Watanabe no. 24 arthroscope has a similar GRIN lens in the "needle portion" but has a different series of corrective lenses. It does not have the same handle design.

The Needlescope was introduced in North America in 1973. It was hoped that it would be advantageous for probing small cavities of the body. Initially it was antici-pated that it would be valuable in the areas of ear, nose, and throat, obstetrics, and gynecology.

The Japanese had utilized the Watanabe no. 24 arthroscope for visualization of small joints,[1] but Watanabe stated that this diameter arthroscope was not useful in the knee joint.[10] The original GRIN lens was treated with a thallium salt, and its optical quality was not excellent. The change to cesium for the curing salt ionizing process improved the optical clarity by a factor of two.

The small-diameter endoscope provided a means of inspecting the knee joint under local anesthesia.[4] By virtue of its small diameter, access to the posteromedial and posterolateral compartments, heretofore not visualized with the larger-diameter endoscopes and techniques, became a reality. It was also possible to pass the endo-scope into Baker cysts and also under the menisci. The value of the Needlescope in other joints, that is, shoulder, elbow, and ankle, had fewer clinical applications than for the knee joint at that time.

Arthroscopy with the Needlescope is well accepted in North America, and there are hundreds of orthopedic surgeons regularly utilizing the instrument for arthros-copy of the knee and other joints with the patient under local anesthesia.[2,6,7,9] My personal, clinical experience exceeds 2,000 cases.[4] There are several other men who have performed over 1,000 arthroscopies with this instrument.[3,5]

CONSTRUCTION

The optical properties of the arthroscope were discussed in Chapter 3.

The endoscope comes in both straight (35°) and forward-oblique views (70°). The former has somewhat better optical clarity. The degree of angle of view in air is approximately double that in saline. That is true for any endoscope. The Model III Needlescope has 100° view in air, plus improved optical clarity. The advantages of the Needlescope are its small diameter and the well-balanced instrument in the hand (Fig. 4-13).

A smaller-diameter instrument injures less tissue and is virtually imperceptible to the patient undergoing the arthroscopy, even when he is under only local anesthesia. When multiple punctures are necessary in order to establish a diagnosis, there is no leakage from the previous puncture site. The leakage created by larger endoscopes results in deflation of the knee joint and increased difficulty in subsequent access to other compartments. The containment of a sterile field is of paramount importance to an orthopedic surgeon. The construction of the Needlescope with the ocular at a distance from the hand and the patient's body offers maximal protection from con-tamination. It is not necessary that the surgeon wear a sterilized mask or shield and redraping is rarely necessary when the arthroscopy immediately precedes an open arthrotomy.

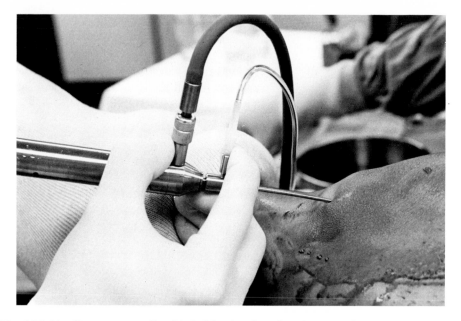

Fig. 4-13. Needlescope is comfortably held in hand, and ocular is sagely away from contamination.

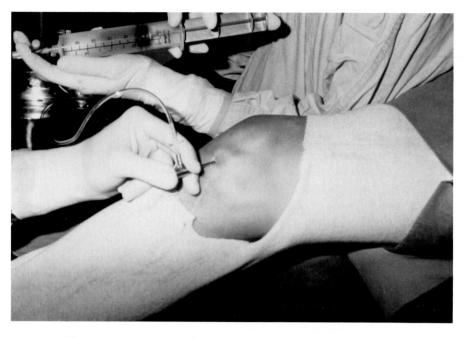

Fig. 4-14. Distension with 60 ml saline provides maximal viewing.

The Needlescope is accompanied by sharp and blunt trocars as well as a cannula (see Fig. 4-12). The Needlescope system does not have a luer lock or clumsy gadgetry adjacent to the ocular as seen in other endoscopes. Therefore, the risk of contamination while touching and manipulating these gadgets is eliminated. The cannula is tapered to the Needlescope and the trocar so that there is automatic locking and release with a simple twist. Yet the fit is so carefully engineered that there is no fluid leakage. The other advantage to the cannula is that it provides opportunity for vacuuming of the joint, cleansing, and reinstillation of saline (Fig. 4-14). It is possible under pressure to force saline adjacent to the endoscope when it is assembled and the arthroscopist is viewing.

The Needlescope housing is finely tapered at the end. This, plus the small diameter, reduces the risk of abrasion of the articular cartilage.

DISADVANTAGES

The alleged disadvantage of the Needlescope is that it is more fragile than other endoscopes. In the hands of certain endoscopists, that has been so. I have not experienced any breakage in over 4½ years in more than 2,000 cases. I attribute this to the fact that I purchased the equipment; therefore, I had a vested interest. Also, I was the only surgeon using the instrument. Only one surgical nurse handles and stores the equipment and unpacks it. It is sent in the packaged state to the central supply area for ethylene oxide sterilization. By tradition and training, orthopedic surgeons have been used to handling tools and not instruments. An arthroscope is an instrument; it must be handled as a fine instrument. It also is constructed of glass and should be handled as such. If one has at least average eye-hand coordination, sensitivity, and proprioception, he should be able to avoid breakage during the performance of the procedure. An endoscope is not a crowbar or a substitute for mechanical leverage. It is a viewing instrument. One should also become aware of the optical sign of bending; when an elliptic image occurs, the stress on the endoscope should be reduced.

TECHNIQUE

Arthroscopy is basically photography with the physician's retina as the film. As with any photography, the quality image is predominantly dependent upon the amount of light thrown on the object and the amount of light that can be transmitted to the film. The smaller-diameter lens transmits less light than does a larger-diameter lens. Also the volume of light bundles is less in a smaller-diameter endoscope. Therefore, the best viewing with the Needlescope, or for that matter with any other endoscope, is with the maximal light potential. The Dyonics Model 500 and the Storz xenon light sources would be the choice of the serious arthroscopist.

The technique with the Needlescope differs from the traditional methods of Watanabe and Jackson. First, for diagnosing problems, arthroscopy can easily be done with the patient under local anesthesia. Second, this technique enters medial to the patellar tendon and a finger breadth above the tibial plateau. The medial

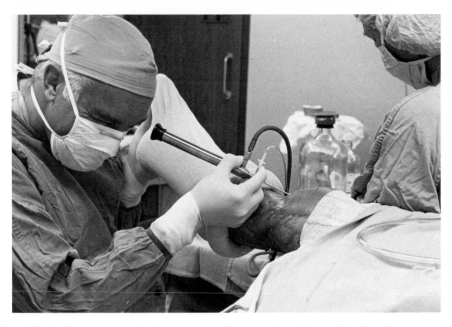

Fig. 4-15. Arthroscopist is viewing suprapatellar area from below. The Needlescope ocular provides safe distance between the arthroscopist's hand and his contaminated head and eye.

puncture is central in the knee compared to the eccentric lateral entry. Also the technique allows the arthroscopist to sit in front of the patient's knee, reducing the contortions and necessity for genuflecting in order to carry out the procedure. In addition, the Needlescope ocular is at a distance from the position of the arthroscopist's hand, reducing the chance of contamination (Fig. 4-15). This technique also affords entry into the posterolateral and posteromedial compartments in those patients in whom there is a normal examination from the anterior inspection.

The posteromedial puncture is performed in any patient in whom arthroscopic inspection of that compartment from the anterior position proves normal. If there is a potential surgical lesion identified from the anterior inspection, and the posterior compartment will be opened at the time of surgery, then a posterior arthroscopic inspection would not be necessary. This posteromedial puncture is performed at a point posterior to the tibial collateral ligament, inferior to the femoral condyle, and superior to the posterior horn of the meniscus. Loose bodies and meniscal tears not possibly seen from the anterior inspection are visualized by this route.

Posterolateral inspection is carried out for similar reasons (Fig. 4-16). Entry is at a point where a line drawn along the lateral muscular septum intersects with a line drawn up from the posterior aspect of the fibula. The knee must be maximally distended and the trocar enters pointing sightly inferior and anterior. This allows one to view in the posterolateral compartment, posterior and superior to the meniscus, and inferior to the femoral condyle. In many patients access to the

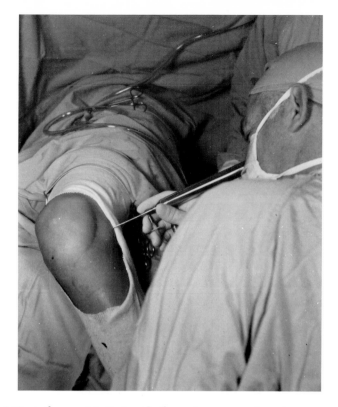

Fig. 4-16. Arthroscopist sits to side to see into posterolateral compartment.

popliteal tendon sheath is possible. Lesions of the meniscus or loose bodies in the posterior compartment or popliteal tendon sheath or both can be identified.

This technique, with a small-diameter puncture, allows one to carry out arthroscopy either immediately prior to an anticipated arthrotomy, or when performed diagnostically, the arthrotomy can be performed safely without risk of infection any day thereafter.

DOCUMENTATION

The 1.7 mm Needlescope has one fourth the illumination capacity of the 2.2 mm–diameter Needlescope. Therefore documentation with the 1.7 mm–diameter Needlescope is only good on a modified black and white video system.*

The 2.2 mm Needlescope provides adequate documentation with 35 mm color slides, super 8 and 16 mm movie film, or video. The color slide is best achieved by photoflash methods (Figs. 4-17 to 4-20). The Beauleiu 40082M4 super 8 camera with

---

*Sony Surveillance Camera AVC-1400, modified by Cruse Communications, East Lansing, Mich.

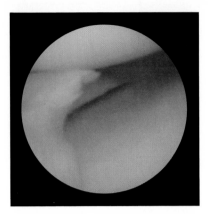

Fig. 4-17. Torn medial meniscus to right, and femoral condyle above. There is methylene blue dye in joint.

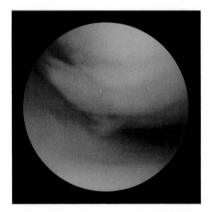

Fig. 4-18. Osteochondritis dissecans is best seen with contrasting dye.

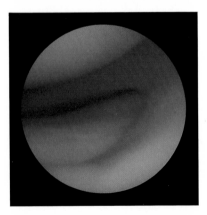

Fig. 4-19. Entire medial compartment is seen at a glance. Note good view of anterior horn.

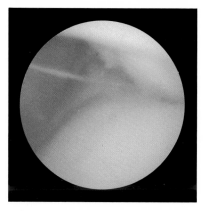

Fig. 4-20. Posteromedial compartment shows condyle to right and meniscus below.

a C-mount adapter (Dyonics) provides a simple method with cassette-loading capacity. Most 16 mm color movie cameras are reel-to-reel loading but offer excellent material for professional showing. Both the Hitachi and Sony video systems have excellent quality images. The video document is immediately secured and also may be edited. Video provides a means of facilitating operative arthroscopy.

References

1. Cheng, Y.: Arthroscopy of the ankle joint, Int. Rev. Rheumatol. (Special Issue), L'Arthroscopie, 1976.
2. Ewing, J. W.: Personal communication.
3. James, P.: Personal communication.
4. Johnson, L. L.: Comprehensive arthroscopy of the knee, St. Louis, 1977, The C. V. Mosby Co.
5. McGuire, G.: Personal communication.
6. Pickering, L.: Personal communication.
7. Poehling, G.: Personal communication.
8. Prescott, R.: Optical principles of endoscopy, J. Med. Prin. 133-147, 1976.
9. Shneider, D. A.: Personal communication.
10. Watanabe, M.: Arthroscope, present and future, Surg. Ther. **26:**73, 1972.

5. Anatomy of the knee

Arthroscopic anatomy

Michael Harty

Arthroscopy and arthrography have opened up a new diagnostic and investigative field that allows visualization of the living joint cavity under a wide range of motions, strains, and stresses, both normal and abnormal. The basic intrinsic structures have not changed, but a new emphasis has appeared. The close-up view combined with a two to ten magnification obtained by the arthroscope introduces a new dimension in what may have been considered previously as trivial minutiae. Small, early, pathologic changes in cartilage, synovium, and intraarticular structures are now noticed and examined in precise detail. The direct view allows the arthroscopist to inspect, palpate, photograph, do a biopsy of, or excise the area under consideration. We must realize that the arthroscopist obtains a direct view of the area in question, while the arthrographer, with great skill, interprets a silhouette of the same region. A clear mental picture of the anatomic changes found during the normal range of joint motion forms an indispensable adjunct to an accurate evaluation of symptomatology.[5] Needless to add, the synovial membrane and other visualized intraarticular structures, such as the cruciate ligaments, also present that same changing picture, which must be ever appreciated.

Today the arthroscopist can inspect (1) the articular cartilage on the patella, the femoral condyles, and the central areas of the tibial plateau; (2) the synovial membrane and suprapatellar pouch, and (3) the patellar ligament, the popliteal tendon, the menisci, the anterior cruciate ligament, and most of the posterior cruciate ligament.

SURFACE ANATOMY

The bony features at the knee joint are readily palpable on the anterior and collateral aspects, but muscles, fat, and the neurovascular bundle to the leg and foot hide the posterior bony prominences (Fig. 5-1). The medial and lateral tibial plateaus, the femoral condyles, the patella, and the fibular head form the major orientation features for the arthroscopist. In full extension of the joint the infrapatellar fat pad protrudes slightly on both sides of the patellar ligament. In the flexed

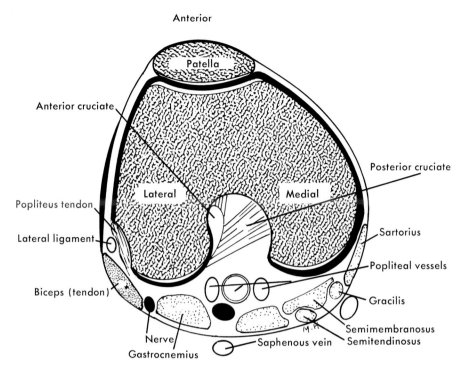

Fig. 5-1. Transverse section of left knee at level of femoral condyles. Distended joint cavity is shown in black.

position the femoral condyles, the tibial plateau, and the patellar ligament outline a medial and lateral triangular depression, which provides the commoner approaches utilized by the arthroscopist to reach the joint cavity, but the posteromedial, posterolateral, and suprapatellar routes are also used.[3] While the knee is flexed to about 90,° the level of the posterior joint line must correspond to the joint depression at each side of the patellar ligament (Fig. 5-2). The interests of the arthroscopist and arthrographer are centered on the structures as visualized from the distended articular cavity, but a working knowledge of some basic anatomy and biomechanics is essential to provide a clear picture of that cavity. Flexion from 30° to 60° allows the maximal distension and relaxation of the ligaments and capsule. Varus strains will open the lateral joint compartment 5 to 10 mm.[2] However, a valgus strain produces much less separation of the medial compartment except under pathologic conditions. Selective compression of the distended joint capsule often elucidates a confused arthroscopic feature and may produce a striking movie. As in all endoscopic examinations the magnified image provided by the arthroscope naturally restricts the area of inspection so the final picture must be made up of a conglomerate of the individual views.

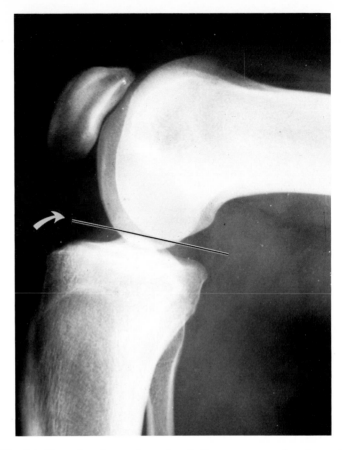

Fig. 5-2. Knee flexed to indicate level of posterior joint line *(arrow)*.

JOINT ANATOMY

The knee joint has the largest and most distensible cavity in the human body. It is lined and limited by articular cartilage and synovial membrane.

Cartilage

The articular cartilage, bonded to the underlying bone ends by a layer of calcified cartilage, forms a firm, resilient, smooth, avascular wall. It is commonly of the hyaline variety except where it encloses articular bone ends developed from membrane that are covered by fibrous tissue, for example, at the mandibular head. It contains no nerves, lymph, or blood vessels and derives its nutrition from the vascular loops in the underlying bone, from the vascular anastomoses at its peripheral margins, and from the synovial fluid. The general contours of the articular surfaces are well known and have been described in great detail, yet in synovial joints every single joint surface has an individual contour that will not fit accurately into any other

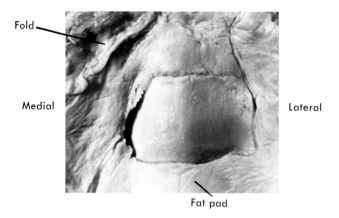

Fold

Medial

Lateral

Fat pad

Fig. 5-3. Peripatellar synovial-covered cushion of fat. Note additional synovial fold.

matching bone except its original mate. This property has been termed "joint privacy" and presents one of the many problems in partial joint replacement. The nonarticulating peripheral margin of joint cartilage is overlapped by 2 to 4 mm of synovial membrane, which covers the vascular articular anastomoses. This transitional zone between the fixed avascular cartilage and the mobile synovium is of particular interest to the clinician because it often demonstrates the late and even the early stages of villi, lipping, and osteophytic changes (locus minoris resistentiae).

Synovium

The normal synovial membrane forms a thin, yielding, multiridged lining of the joint capsule. It appears smooth, glistening, almost transparent, and of a pale pink color tinted by the red striations of the subsynovial blood vessels. Even minor irritations, chemical, physical, or traumatic, increase the vascularity and will produce bleeding from the subsynovial vessels. The synovial membrane lines the capsule, covers the intracapsular ligaments and tendons, overlaps the peripheral margins of the articular cartilage for 2 to 4 mm, and may become continuous with the lining of adjacent bursas but does not cover the surfaces of the menisci. Synovial membrane has been classified as fibrous, fatty, or areolar, depending on the nature of its subsynovial tissue. The *fibrous type* is thin and grayish pink in color. It is adherent to the popliteal tendon, the medial collateral ligament, the patellar ligament, and the anterior wall of the suprapatellar bursa.

The mobile *fatty type* of synovium has a yellow hue and covers the intracapsular fat cushions. The extensor mechanism, made up of the quadriceps tendon, the medial and lateral retinacula, and the patellar ligament, converges onto the anterior aspect of the patella. The dead space underneath this fibrous aponeurosis is occupied by a fimbriated, continuous, peripatellar, synovial-covered wreath of fat (Fig. 5-3). This includes the infrapatellar fat pad so commonly encountered by the arthroscopist. It continues in a proximal direction at both sides of the patella, and these two folds join superiorly to complete the circle. Another small fat pad conceals the femoral attachment of the posterior cruciate ligament, and a third covers the posterior surface of the suprapatellar pouch. Serosa-covered fat cushions occupy many small body areas, especially where motion must be accomodated—the larger branches of the coronary arteries float in a fatty bed. The fat pads are made up of soft fat lobules suspended in a fibroelastic stroma, which allows rapid adaptation and recovery of their ever changing shape and contour enforced by joint motion. MacConaill[7] and Freeman and Wyke[1] emphasized the large concentration of pain receptors and the high sensitivity of the intracapsular fat pads.

The *infrapatellar fat pad* filling the irregular space between the patella, the femoral condyles, and the tibia undergoes an extraordinary array of shapes and sizes during normal joint motion. The mucosal fold or dorsal expansion of synovium stretching to the intercondylar notch ranges from a thin strand to a persistence of the total septum. Commonly it is a fenestrated partition that may obstruct arthroscopic movements and the field of view.

The *alar folds* extend bilaterally between the femoral condyles and the superior surface of the anterior horns of the menisci (Fig. 5-4). At the medial and lateral ends, these alar folds either blend imperceptibly with the medial and lateral synovial lining or continue in a proximal direction, covering the parapatellar fat folds. Small, very mobile, pedunculated synovial villi are a constant finding in normal knee joints, and their number increases with advancing age, even without accompanying pathologic changes. They are found typically at the chondrosynovial junctions on synovial folds and along the course of the cruciate ligaments.

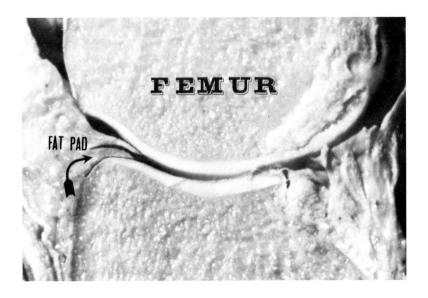

Fig. 5-4. Alar fold of infrapatellar fat pad situated between medial femoral condyle and medial meniscus (*arrow*).

The *areolar type* of synovial membrane floats freely on the deep aspect of the capsule. It has numerous folds, ridges, and recesses, some of which have acquired names, while others remain nameless. These folds change, not only in number, size, and tension but also in direction, shape, and position during the normal range of knee joint motions. The more common synovial folds or plicae encountered in the knee joint are (1) plica synovialis suprapatellaris, (2) plica synovialis mediopatellaris (the shelf), (3) chordae obliquae synovialis, and (4) the synovial fringes on the infrapatellar fat pad, as mentioned above. Smaller or larger synovial folds, some covering fat lobules, are a common finding in the knee joint.

Plica synovialis suprapatellaris. The plica synovialis suprapatellaris is simply a peripheral remnant of the complete septum of embryonic life that separated the suprapatellar bursa from the knee joint cavity and still persists in 10% of joints. The plica or peripheral remnant occurs in 70% of knees; it has a crescentic outline and is larger and more commonly found on the medial side (Fig. 5-5). In the extended position the plica or septum is directed horizontally backward from the upper pole of the patella, but when the knee is flexed it lies vertically and follows the contour of the underlying medial femoral condyle, where it often imprints a vertical groove (Fig. 5-6, *white arrow*).

Shelf. The shelf is a vertically directed synovial fold medial to the parapatellar fat pad. It varies in size and extent. When fully developed it extends from the medial and superior corner of the infrapatellar fat pad to the undersurface of the suprapatel-

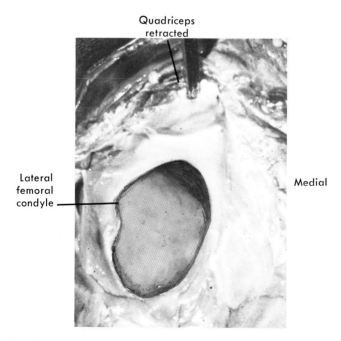

Quadriceps
retracted

Lateral
femoral
condyle

Medial

Fig. 5-5. Annular plica synovialis suprapatellaris. (From Harty, M., and Joyce, J. J.: Orthop. Rev. **6:**10, 1977.)

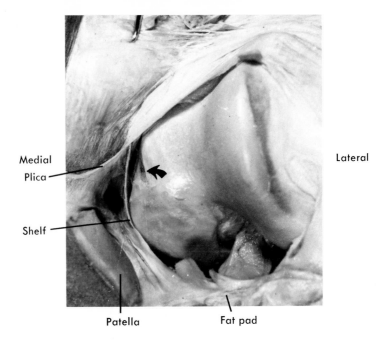

Medial
Plica

Lateral

Shelf

Patella   Fat pad

Fig. 5-6. Patella split of left knee. Shelf drops from plica to infrapatellar fat pad. Note groove on anterior margin of medial femoral condyle *(arrow)*.

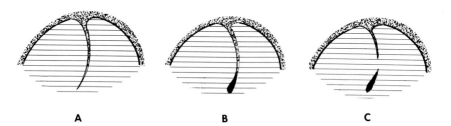

A   **B**   **C**

Fig. 5-7. A, Synovial fold. **B,** Fold with fibrosed free margin. **C,** Fold with detached fibrosed free margin.

lar plica (Fig. 5-6). This has received many titles, from its original one, "chorda cavi articularis genu mediopatellaris" in 1918, to "Iino's band" in 1939, or simply "the shelf" in 1948.[6,8,9] It ranges from a small vertical synovial fold (1 to 2 cm in length) passing proximally from the fat pad, to the fold of the fully formed shelf shown in Fig. 5-6. In the distended and extended knee joint the well-formed shelf is perpendicular to the suprapatellar plica (Fig. 5-6), but in the flexed position both lie parallel and are commonly stretched or even tensed over the anterior margin of the medial femoral condyle. Sakakibara (1976)[10] gave an excellent detailed description of the shelf. Practically all these so-called chordae are simply folds or plicae projecting from the synovial membrane. Some may develop a fibrosed, thickened, inelastic edge and more rarely a fenestrated plica will have a separate, free, cordlike border similar to a bucket-handle tear (Fig. 5-7).

Chordae obliquae synovialis.[11] Chordae obliquae synovialis or oblique synovial folds are noticed only during full extension when the medial and lateral retinacula are under tension, and the fat pad is compressed. They diverge from the collateral margins of the patella distally to the tibiofemoral joint line and delineate the medial and lateral margins of the infrapatellar fat pad. The clinical manifestations of the plicae, folds, and shelf are discussed in later chapters.

The semimembranosisgastrocnemius bursa, when it is present, may communicate with the posteromedial joint compartment adjacent to the posterior margin of the medial meniscus, but more commonly the bursal opening is found high on the posterior capsule close to the origin of the medial head of the gastrocnemius. While using the posteromedial arthroscopic approach, with the joint flexed and distended, this bursa may be entered and cause some orientation problems, because the communication to the joint cavity is hidden at the superior end of the anterior bursal wall. Arthrograms have illustrated the extensive ramifications of many of these periarticular bursas in the knee region.

Menisci

The medial and lateral menisci, made up predominantly of dense, fibrous tissue, occupy the incongruous areas on the articular facets of the tibiofemoral joint. They are semilunar in outline and cover the peripheral articular margins of the medial and lateral tibial plateaus. They are almost flat on their inferior surface, where they allow sliding and some rotation on the tibial surfaces. However, they are distinctly concave on their superior aspect to fit the convex medial and lateral femoral condyles. The menisci are thick on their peripheral margins where they blend with the adjacent synovial membrane. The inner margins always thin out to a sharp edge, but the width of the disks varies considerably. At the anterior horn, the medial meniscus measures from 6 to 8 mm; deep to the medial collateral ligament, it ranges from 5 to 12 mm; and posteriorly it stretches from 12 to 20 mm on the tibial aspect. The lateral meniscus measures from 10 to 15 mm in each area, except where it is indented by the popliteal tendon. A synovial recess is always found on the superior junction of meniscus and tendon, but that recess may or may not open on the inferior aspect of the meniscus. The horns of the lateral meniscus are close to each other at their tibial attachments (Fig. 5-8), whereas the horns of the medial meniscus are more widely separated. In full extension of the knee joint the anterior ends of the menisci are forced apart by the femoral condyles. When the femoral pressure is released by flexion, the elastic transverse ligament stretching from the anterior horn of the medial meniscus to the peripheral margin of the lateral meniscus approximates both anterior margins. The meniscosynovial junction may present a varying and confusing picture to both the arthroscopist and arthrographer. Depending on the position of the joint, the synovium stretches as a smooth or pleated sheet from the meniscal margins, or it may be so slack as to allow a shallow recess or gutter. This is often

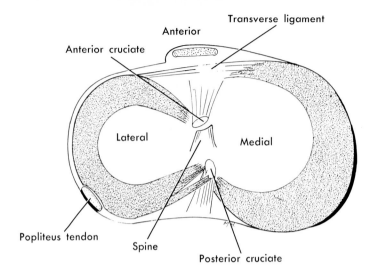

Fig. 5-8. Medial and lateral menisci in left knee.

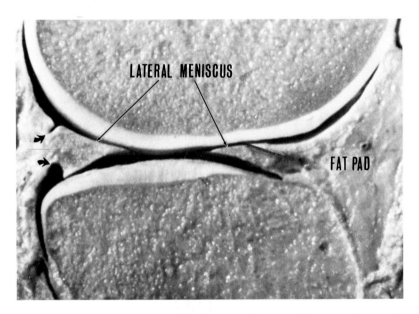

Fig. 5-9. Posterior, superior, and inferior meniscosynovial gutters (*arrows*).

found at the posterior margin of the medial and lateral menisci, especially when the knee is flexed (Fig. 5-9).

The anatomy of the knee joint cavity as seen through an arthroscope is not as straightforward as that seen in the anatomy laboratory, but practice, perseverance, and patience again will eventually pay their reward of anatomic orientation and identification.

References

1. Freeman, M. A. R., and Wyke, B.: The innervation of the knee joint, J. Anat. **101:**505-532, 1967.
2. Harty, M.: Anatomical features of the lateral aspect of the knee joint, Surg. Gynecol. Obstet. **130:**11, 1970.
3. Harty, M.: Knee joint anatomy, Orthop. Rev. **5**(9):23-25, 1976.
4. Harty, M., and Joyce, J. J.: Synovial folds in the knee joint, Orthop. Rev. **6**(10):91-92, 1977.
5. Harty, M., and Joyce, J. J.: Surgical anatomy and exposures of the knee joint. In American Academy of Orthopaedic Surgeons Instructional Course Lectures, vol. XX, St. Louis, 1971, The C. V. Mosby Co., p. 206.
6. Iino, S.: Normal arthroscopic findings of the knee joint in the adult cadaver, J. Jpn. Orthop. Assoc. **14:**467-523, 1939.
7. MacConaill, M. A.: The movements of bones and joints. III. The synovial fluid and its assistants, J. Bone Joint Surg. [Br.] **32:**244-252, 1950.
8. Mayeda, T.: Ueber das strangartige Gebilde in der Kniegelenkhoehle (Choda cavi articularis genu), Mitt. Med. Fakult. Univ. Tokyo, **21:**507-553, 1918.
9. Mizumachi, S., et al.: So-called synovial shelf in the knee joint, J. Jpn. Orthop. Assoc. **22:**1-5, 1948.
10. Sakakibara, J.: Arthroscopic study on Iino's band, J. Jpn. Orthop. Assoc. **50:**513, 1976.
11. Watanabe, M.: The development and present status of the arthroscope, J. Jpn. Med. Instr. **25:**11, 1954.

Arthrographic anatomy

Murray K. Dalinka

MEDIAL MENISCUS

The medial meniscus is C-shaped in configuration. It is triangular in cross section with its free border shaped like an isosceles triangle. It is normally largest in its posterior portion and decreases in size from posterior to anterior[1] although occasionally the mid portion is smaller than the anterior horn[12] (Fig. 5-10).

The medial meniscus is firmly adherent to the deep fibers of the medial collateral ligament and the joint capsule throughout.[2] Lindblom[10] measured arthrographic images of the medial meniscus and found the posterior horn to average about 14 mm in width and the anterior horn 6 mm; both horns were 3 to 5 mm thick at the base. A small, posterior, superior recess is frequently present,[2,3] and a posterior inferior recess is not uncommon (Fig. 5-11). These recesses may project over the posterior horn of the medial meniscus and simulate a tear; with careful evaluation they can be traced to the meniscosynovial junction. The medial meniscus is a biconcave structure with the greater curvature usually on the femoral surface.

The base of the infrapatellar fat pad and its lateral extensions are frequently projected over the anterior horn of the medial meniscus and may be a cause for confusion.[2,7] Careful fluoroscopy generally differentiates this from a torn cartilage.

The medial meniscus is smooth and regular throughout with a triangular free edge and an attached base. Any deviation from this appearance is abnormal.

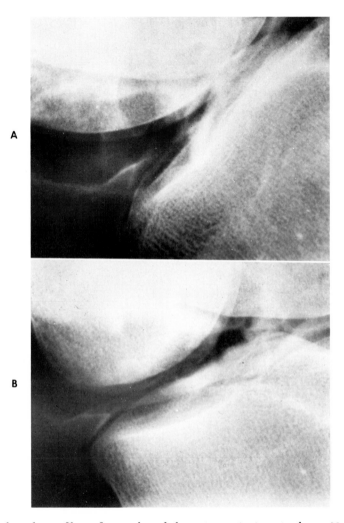

Fig. 5-10. Selected spot films of normal medial meniscus. **A,** Anterior horn. Note sharp triangular appearance of normal meniscus. Condyles are close together, indicating that film is very anterior. Suprapatella bursa is well seen. **B,** Mid anterior horn. Suprapatella bursa is well seen as is triangular-appearing, normal medial meniscus.

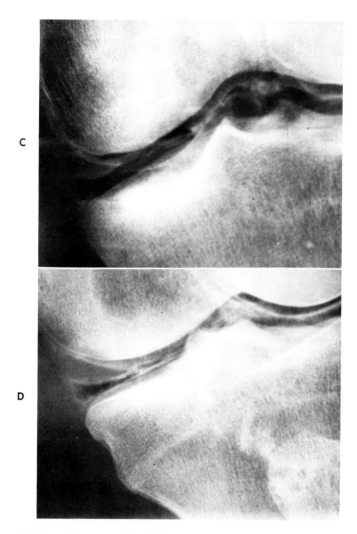

Fig. 5-10, cont'd. C, Mid portion of medial meniscus. Meniscus is well defined. Suprapatella bursa is no longer identified, and condyles are not overlapped. Projection is almost directly posteroanterior. **D,** Posterior horn of medial meniscus. Condyles are overlapped. Meniscus appears larger than in other films. Articular cartilage over femur and tibia is well defined. (From Dalinka, M. K., Coren, G. S., and Wershba, M.: CRC Crit. Rev. Clin. Radiol. Nucl. Med. **4:**1-59, 1973, © 1973 CRC Press, Inc. Used by permission of CRC Press, Inc.)

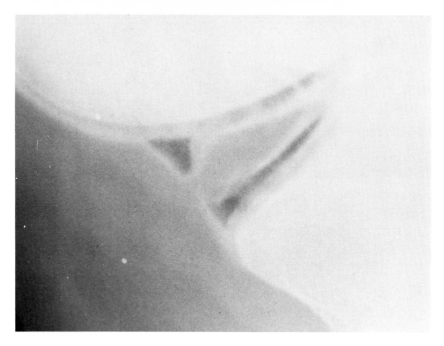

Fig. 5-11. Posterior horn of medial meniscus. Note superior and inferior recesses posteriorly. Articular cartilage over femur and tibia is well demonstrated.

LATERAL MENISCUS

The lateral meniscus is nearly circular in configuration and covers a larger portion of the tibial surface than does the medial meniscus. Its free edge is also shaped like an isosceles triangle. The lateral meniscus changes only slightly in size from the anterior to the posterior horn with an average width of 10 mm[8] (Fig. 5-12). The surfaces of the lateral meniscus are slightly concave.[4]

The anterior horn of the lateral meniscus is attached to the anterior intercondylar area of the tibia, posterior and lateral to the anterior cruciate[4] ligament attachment. A large recess is frequently present anterior inferiorly (Fig. 5-13). The posterior horn inserts into the intercondylar fossa, anterior to the medial meniscal attachment.

The posterior horn is separated from the joint capsule where the popliteal tendon communicates with the posterior portion of the joint. Two thin synovial attachments run from the posterior horn of the meniscus to the joint capsule.[4,11] McIntyre[11] has called these "struts," and Jelaso[6] refers to them as "fascicles." Jelaso's[6] dissections show them to be thin, synovial, lined ligaments. A superior defect in the attachment is a constant finding. There is frequently an inferior opening as well through which the popliteal muscle exists (Fig. 5-14), but sometimes the muscle and outer bursal lining combine with the muscle re-forming beneath it.[9] A communication of the popliteal bursa with the tibiofibula joint is present in approximately 35% of pa-

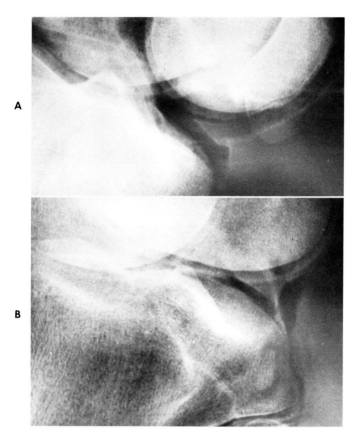

Fig. 5-12. A, Anterior horn of lateral meniscus. Note triangular shape. Patella and supra-patella bursae are evident. Articular cartilage is well defined. **B,** Posterior horn of lateral meniscus. Popliteal fossa is well demonstrated as are attachments of posterior horn of meniscus to joint capsule. (From Dalinka, M. K., Coren, G. S., and Wershba, M.: CRC Crit. Rev. Clin. Radiol. Nucl. Med. 4:1-59, 1973, © 1973 CRC Press, Inc. Used by permission of CRC Press, Inc.)

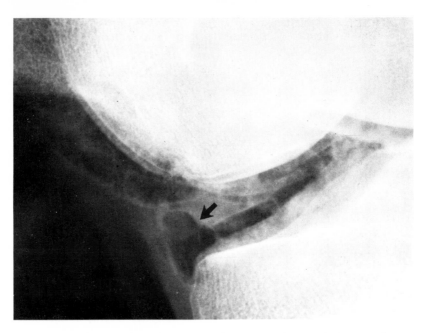

Fig. 5-13. Anterior horn of lateral meniscus demonstrated normal, large, inferior recess. (From Dalinka, M. K., and Brennan, R. E.: Radiation Science Update Series 3, 1976.)

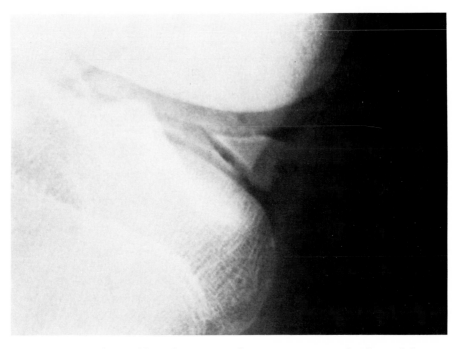

Fig. 5-14. Posterior horn of lateral meniscus, demonstrating normal inferior defect in attachment between meniscus and joint capsule.

tients. The posterior horn of the lateral meniscus is mobile, and its bursal separation may give it a detached appearance.[3,4,11]

The capsular attachments and the bursal openings are responsible for the mobility of the lateral meniscus, which moves upward and centrally with stress. The thin capsular attachments can usually be seen as can the defects in them for the popliteal muscle.

ARTICULAR CARTILAGE

The articular cartilage, particularly that portion over the femoral condyle, can be well seen and parallels the articular cortex. The cartilage is smooth and regular throughout. The intercondylar fossa and spines are free of articular cartilage.

ANTERIOR CRUCIATE LIGAMENT

The anterior cruciate ligament is intracapsular but extrasynovial, being partially covered by synovial reflections throughout most of its course. It inserts anterior to the intercondylar spines on a rough, nonarticular surface of the tibia. It extends obliquely in a cephalad and posterior direction to its proximal attachment to the lateral femoral condyle. It appears taut on lateral films, particularly when performing the anterior drawer maneuver.[2,5,11]

The normal infrapatellar synovial fold has a similar course but inserts more anteriorly on the tibia and in front of the anterior cruciate ligament on the anterior aspect of the intracondylar notch.[5]

JOINT CAPSULE

The joint capsule and its synovial lining is smooth throughout; septa are occasionally present within it. The menisci divide the joint into superior and inferior capsular spaces. The synovium covering the cruciate and the infrapatella fold divides the joint into medial and lateral compartments.[12] A small, regular, posterior compartment is normal and best seen on flexion. Extension films distend the suprapatella bursa, which is continuous with the joint and extends approximately 7 cm above the patella.

References

1. Butt, W. P., and McIntyre, J. L.: Double contrast arthrography of the knee, Radiology 92:487-499, 1969.
2. Dalinka, M. K., Coren, G. S., and Wershba, M.: Knee arthrography, CRC Crit. Rev. Clin. Radiol. Nucl. Med. 4:1-59, 1973.
3. Dalinka, M. K., and Brennan, R. E.: The technique, evaluation and significance of knee arthrography, Radiation Science Update Series 3, 1976.
4. Dalinka, M. K., Lally, J. F., and Gohel, V. K.: Arthrography of the lateral meniscus, Am. J. Roentgenol. Radium Ther. Nucl. Med. 121:79-85, 1974.
5. Dalinka, M. K., and Garofola, J.: The infrapatellar synovial fold: a cause for confusion in the evaluation of the anterior cruciate ligament, Am. J. Roentgenol. Radium Ther. Nucl. Med. 127:589-591, 1976.
6. Jelaso, D. V.: The fascicles of the lateral meniscus: an anatomic-arthrographic correlation, Radiology 114:335-339, 1975.

7. Hall, F. M.: Pitfalls in knee arthrography, Radiology **118:**55-62, 1976.

8. Heiser, S., LaBriola, J. H., and Meyers, M. H.: Arthrography of the knee, Radiology **79:**822-828, 1962.

9. Kaye, J. J.: Personal communication.

10. Lindblom, K.: Arthrography of knee: roentgenographic and anatomic study, Acta Radiol. [Suppl.] (Stockh.) **74:**1-112, 1948.

11. McIntyre, J. L.: Arthrography of the lateral meniscus, Radiology **105:**531-536, 1972.

12. Ricklin, P., Ruttimann, A., and Del Buono, M. S.: Meniscus lesions. Practical problems of clinical diagnosis, arthrography and therapy (American translation by K. Muller), New York, 1971, Grune & Stratton.

6. Technique of arthroscopy

John B. McGinty

To become a proficient arthroscopist a surgeon must master two separate but obviously related skills: the psychomotor technique of using the instrument reliably, safely, and skillfully, sufficient to attain a complete and thorough examination of the joint; and the interpretive skill of accurately recognizing the normal from the abnormal.

Most experienced arthroscopists think that a minimum of 50 examinations is necessary for the average orthopedic surgeon to gain sufficient self-confidence to approach arthroscopy with diagnostic reliability. Certainly the more procedures a surgeon does, the more accurate he will become. One of the truly satisfying aspects of this procedure is that even after hundreds of examinations, the endoscopist is frequently encountering new situations that challenge his interpretive skills. However, he must completely master the technique first. It is axiomatic that one must learn to drive an automobile before he can tour the countryside.

There are many different approaches to the arthroscopic examination of the knee. A surgeon must learn one technique well before he modifies it in developing his own style. Watanabe and Jackson perform the examination with the patient supine on the operating table and flex the knee without breaking the foot of the table. Casscells breaks the foot of the operating table, allowing the knee to flex to 90%. Johnson uses a multiple-puncture technique with the Needlescope and the knee flexed 90° over the end of the table. He also requires the aid of an assistant. The technique illustrated in this chapter will be with a single puncture, except in specific clinical circumstances, with the patient supine, and with the manipulations performed on the fully extended operating table.

INDICATIONS FOR ARTHROSCOPY

As experience has increased, the indications for arthroscopy, similar to any diagnostic procedure, have become less rigid.

Patient selection

If the procedure is to be done under local anesthesia, it must be fully explained to the patient in explicit detail before he is brought to the operating room. Time must be spent in gaining the patient's full confidence, or the procedure will be unsatisfactory. There are a few patients who are too apprehensive or have too low a pain threshold to tolerate the procedure with local anesthesia. If there is a medical contraindication to general anesthesia, the procedure cannot be done. In general, patient selection is similar to myelography for a suspected ruptured, lumbar, intervertebral disc; namely, if surgery is not contemplated, do not do an arthroscopy.

Diagnosis

There is no better way to establish a diagnosis in a questionable clinical situation than to see the lesion. Arthroscopy, however, does not replace a good history, a thorough physical examination, and an adequate radiographic study. These steps are necessary prerequisites to any special diagnostic study and must not be bypassed or abbreviated. When a patient is referred to me for arthroscopy, even when the referral is from another orthopedic surgeon, I first see the patient in my office for a history, physical examination, and review of x-ray films. Once the lesion is seen, it is a simple matter to obtain tissue for histologic study with the arthroscope, either blindly or under direct vision.

Even after he has considerable experience, it is amazing how often a surgeon is surprised when he thinks that he is certain of the clinical diagnosis prior to the arthroscopic examination. It is not a rare event to find two lesions, such as tears of both the medial and the lateral meniscus, or to find a mechanical derangement superimposed on synovial disease. One patient, presenting with a locked knee, arthroscopically showed the suspected displaced bucket-handle tear of the medial meniscus, plus a large, fragmented tear of the posterior horn of the lateral meniscus. I no longer do an arthrotomy for meniscal pathology without first doing a preliminary arthroscopy.

Arthroscopy has eliminated the need for arthrotomy for synovial biopsy. With the arthroscope the surgeon can far more efficiently seek out the lesion and examine it directly.

Documentation and education

There are certain knees with vague symptomatology that can be defined photographically through the arthroscope for medicolegal problems, for compensation-liability cases, or simply for future reference. There is no better way to follow a patient's clinical course, with changing symptoms or a new injury, than to refer to photographs taken at an earlier time. Certainly for teaching arthroscopy or the pathogenesis of joint disease, photographs through the endoscope are essential.

Follow-up

Arthroscopy provides an excellent method for sequentially following the evolution of disease. For example, the lesions of osteochondritis dissecans can be periodically inspected to assess the status of articular cartilage which is not apparent on roentgenograms. If the lesion is followed, surgery can be properly timed or non-surgical management planned with greater assurance.

Intraarticular surgery

Some lesions can be definitively managed arthroscopically, such as loose bodies, synovial bands (medial shelf or hypertrophic suprapatellar plicae), and intraarticular fractures with small, loose fragments. Some arthroscopists are becoming proficient at partial meniscectomy with the operating arthroscope. Preliminary work is being done on endoscopic chondroplasty for chondromalacia.

Research

The arthroscope provides an excellent opportunity to study the pathogenesis of intraarticular disease, such as the evolution of the various stages of osteoarthritis and rheumatoid arthritis. The interior of the joint can be easily examined periodically with minimal morbidity.

CONTRAINDICATIONS
Infection

Systemic infection with actual or potential bacteremia is an absolute contraindication to arthroscopy. The possibility of seeding bacteria in the joint, particularly with a possible hemarthrosis, is certainly far too great a risk to justify diagnostic examination. The infection must first be treated and eliminated before the integrity of the joint is violated. Also infection of the skin around the involved joint must be treated and eliminated prior to arthroscopy to prevent direct inoculation of the joint. On the other hand, septic arthritis can be inspected, cultured, and irrigated with the arthroscope.

Limited range of motion

Arthroscopy is a bimanual examination, requiring manipulation of the knee synchronized with manipulation of the instrument. It is desirable to have a range of motion from 15° to 90° of flexion to get a satisfactory examination. With less motion, the reasons must be quite compelling to justify arthroscopy.

Coagulation defect

Clotting problems represent only a relative contraindication to arthroscopy. As with any surgical procedure, the defect must be identified and corrected before an incision is made.

ANESTHESIA

Originally arthroscopy was developed using general or spinal anesthesia. As experience was gained, it became apparent that the procedure could be satisfactorily carried out with local anesthesia under most circumstances. In a purely diagnostic situation, I prefer local anesthesia because of lower morbidity, decreased cost, and the ability to study the dynamic anatomy of the knee.

General and spinal anesthesia

The young child, probably under the age of 10, will not cooperate sufficiently to justify local anesthesia. He is usually too frightened, presenting the risk of sudden movement with consequent intraarticular breakage of the instrument or at least damage to articular cartilage. Also the risk of psychic trauma exists in the young child who does not understand the procedure or the goals of the surgeon.

If an arthrotomy will probably be needed, I use general or spinal anesthesia, being prepared to reprepare and redrape the extremity and proceed with an arthrotomy immediately after the arthroscopy.

In patients with extreme, unrelenting anxiety, general or spinal anesthesia should probably be used. The chance of sudden movement when local anesthesia is used results in too high a risk of intraarticular damage.

Finally local anesthesia should not be used when a surgeon is learning the technique of arthroscopy. Perhaps this situation could be referred to as the "surgeon with extreme anxiety." It is difficult enough to learn the technique of arthroscopy without having to worry about the patient's anxiety or comfort. I recommend that the surgeon learning arthroscopy should plan for an arthrotomy based on his usual clinical criteria. He then may precede each arthrotomy with an arthroscopy, giving himself a finite period of time to accomplish the arthroscopy (30 minutes is a good average). At the end of this time he concludes the arthroscopy, whether he has accomplished a complete examination or not, reprepares, and redrapes for the arthrotomy. If he does not utilize a definite period of time, he will become discouraged if he is having trouble with visualization. One day, when he completes a satisfactory arthroscopic examination without seeing any lesion, he will cancel the arthrotomy. He will then have crossed the first hurdle in gaining self-confidence.

Local anesthesia

The use of local anesthesia represents a significant advance in making arthroscopy a simple, outpatient diagnostic procedure, with no more risk than arthrography. The patient does not require admission to the hospital, preoperative anesthetic evaluation with laboratory studies and chest x-ray films, or postanesthetic recovery. He is brought directly to the operating room without premedication, undergoes the procedure, and goes directly home without time in the recovery room. He rarely has pain or significant effusion and can usually return to his employment or school on the following day. The result is lower morbidity, less risk, and lower cost. Local anesthesia also allows the surgeon to study the dynamics of the knee, for example, the relationship of the patellofemoral joint can be observed during quadriceps contraction with active knee extension (Fig. 6-1).

In the operating room the knee is fully scrubbed, prepared with povidone-iodine (Betadine), and draped. The draping *must* be as complete as for an arthrotomy. The skin, subcutaneous tissue, and capsule are infiltrated with 5 ml of 0.5% lidocaine (Xylocaine) (Fig. 6-2). The joint is not distended with saline; some experience is necessary to prevent penetrating the synovium with the sharp trocar and damaging

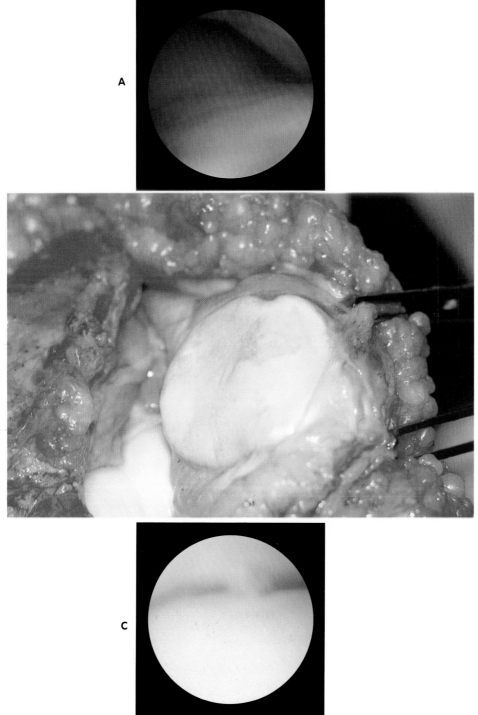

Fig. 6-1. A, Gap in medial side of patella when this 15-year-old girl with subluxation of patella actively extends her knee during arthroscopy done with patient under local anesthesia. **B,** Chondromalacia on medial facet of patella, corresponding to area failing to articulate normally. **C,** Arthroscopy 1 year after lateral release and vastus medialis advancement, demonstrating correction of gap with active knee extension.

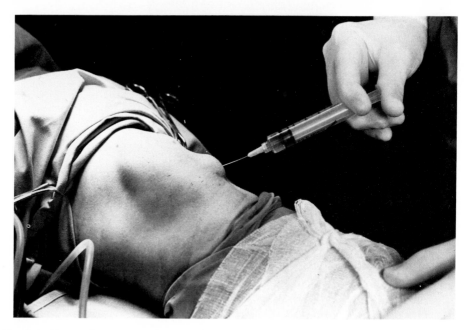

Fig. 6-2. Skin, subcutaneous tissue, and capsule are infiltrated with 5 ml of 0.5% lidocaine, and 5 ml is instilled directly into joint. Delay of 3 minutes is essential prior to inserting sheath and arthroscope.

the articular cartilage. An additional 5 ml of 0.5% lidocaine is injected directly into the joint. A delay of at least 3 minutes is essential before further steps are taken. This delay allows the anesthesia to set and the surgeon to reassure the patient. After a minimum of 3 minutes, the incision is made, and the sheath is inserted into the knee in the usual way (see "Technique and Procedure") and finally sealed with the arthroscope. Ten milliliters of 0.5% bupivacaine (Marcaine) is then instilled directly into the joint through the sheath. The total dose of local anesthetic is 50 mg lidocaine and 50 mg bupivacaine, well within toxic limits. The procedure is then carried out in the usual way with intermittent saline irrigation. I have worked for as long as 1 hour with this dosage without discomfort to the patient. If the patient becomes apprehensive or complains of pain, an additional 10 ml of 0.5% lidocaine is injected directly into the sheath. Lidocaine is used for its rapid onset and bupivacaine for its prolonged action.

TECHNIQUE AND PROCEDURE

The technique for arthroscopy will be described as if the patient is under general anesthesia. The extremity is shaved prior to the patient's arrival in the operating room. The patient is placed in the supine position on the operating table. A tourniquet is not applied unless a subsequent arthrotomy is planned. If a tourniquet is applied it is not inflated during the arthroscopy. Bleeding has not interfered with

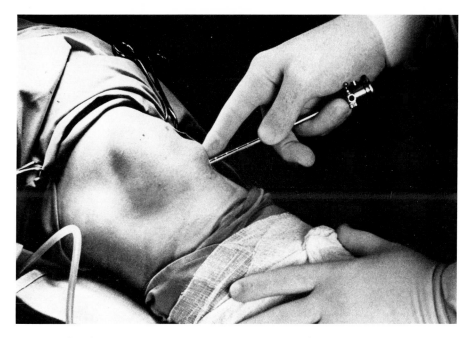

Fig. 6-3. Index finger acting as a guard to prevent overpenetration with sharp trocar and subsequent damage to articular cartilage. Motion during insertion is rotatory until penetration of capsule is felt.

adequate visualization, and avascularity produced by a tourniquet interferes with the normal appearance of synovium. The extremity is thoroughly scrubbed with povidone-iodine (Betadine) soap and prepared with povidone-iodine solution in the same way and for the same length of time as in preparation for an arthrotomy. Similarly a complete draping is performed.

The knee joint is distended with 75 to 125 ml of normal saline to push the synovium away from the articular cartilage and to minimize the risk of damage during penetration. A 1 cm transverse incision is made one finger breadth above the tibial margin at the lateral border of the patellar tendon in a small triangular depression that can readily be identified with the handle of a scalpel. The sheath with the sharp trocar is directed, at a 45° angle in all planes, at the intercondylar notch until the capsule is penetrated—there is a definite sudden release felt as the capsule is penetrated. The index finger of the hand holding the sheath is extended to act as a guard and to prevent overpenetration (Fig. 6-3). When the sheath is through the capsule but has not entered the synovial cavity, the sharp trocar is exchanged for the blunt trocar. The sheath is then passed through the synovium superiorly under the patella into the suprapatellar pouch. The trocar is then exchanged for the telescope. The examiner must not forget to attach the bridge to the sheath prior to locking the arthroscope into place, or the tip of the optical instrument will be protruding beyond the end of the sheath and therefore be subject to damage. I have seen an x-ray film of

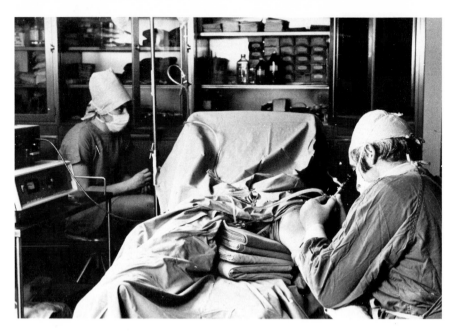

Fig. 6-4. Closed system of sterile saline is 1 m above table and connected to inflow system by Y-tube. Note light source is on opposite side of table from examiner. Complete sterile draping is essential. Padding is placed under knee to facilitate flexion.

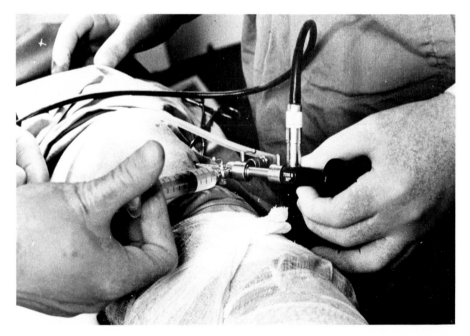

Fig. 6-5. Ten milliliters of 0.5% bupivacaine (Marcaine) is instilled directly into joint at beginning of procedure, through inflow valve. Outflow valve is connected to wall suction and used intermittently.

a knee with the tip of an arthroscope embedded in the femoral condyle. A liter of normal saline in a closed system is connected to the inflow valve of the sheath, and the valve is opened (Fig. 6-4). The plastic reservoir of saline is hanging on a pole about 1 m above the table and therefore maintaining a constant head of hydrostatic pressure, a factor that seems to help control capillary bleeding. The outflow tube is connected to the other valve on the sheath and to wall suction (Fig. 6-5). This valve is kept closed except during intermittent irrigation. It is good practice to connect the inflow and outflow tubes to the same sides of the sheath during each procedure so that the surgeon can reflexly know which valves to open and close to irrigate the joint.

The procedure is divided into four parts and should always be carried out in the same manner to establish a routine, making it less likely to overlook abnormalities. It is a simple matter to return to an area of the joint for further study or to take photographs. The examination is bimanual, manipulation of the knee occurring simultaneously with manipulation of the arthroscope. This technique permits the surgeon to conduct all manipulations without assistance while looking through the instrument, an advantage in some operating rooms.

Suprapatellar pouch and patellofemoral joint (Fig. 6-6)

Examination of the area starts in the suprapatellar recess. The quality of the synovium can be easily inspected. It is an excellent location for synovial biopsy. The arthroscope is withdrawn and the quality of the plica noted. Withdrawal is continued until the patella and adjacent femur are visualized. The patella is scanned from medial to lateral while moving it from side to side with the free hand. By moving the arthroscope back and forth in a pistonlike motion the patellar surface from the superior to inferior poles is inspected. The knee should be fully extended and then flexed to 90° to observe the patellofemoral relationship.

Medial compartment (Fig. 6-7)

The knee is flexed to 45° and the foot allowed to drop off the side of the table. By pressing on the lateral side of the knee, the examiner can readily apply a valgus stress. The arthroscope is moved over the condyle to the medial compartment, keeping the condylar horizon and medial retinaculum in view until the coronary ligament is seen. The instrument must be deep enough so that visualization is not obscured by the infrapatellar fat pad. The free edge of the medial meniscus is identified and the meniscus examined, first anteriorly, then posteriorly under the femoral condyle. The degree of visualization of the posterior horn will vary, depending on the laxity of the knee; about 50% of the posterior horn of the medial meniscus cannot be seen in the average knee.

Intercondylar notch (Fig. 6-8)

The foot is brought back onto the table, allowing the knee to assume its resting position in 30° to 40° of flexion. The arthroscope is directed into the intercondylar

Text continued on p. 74.

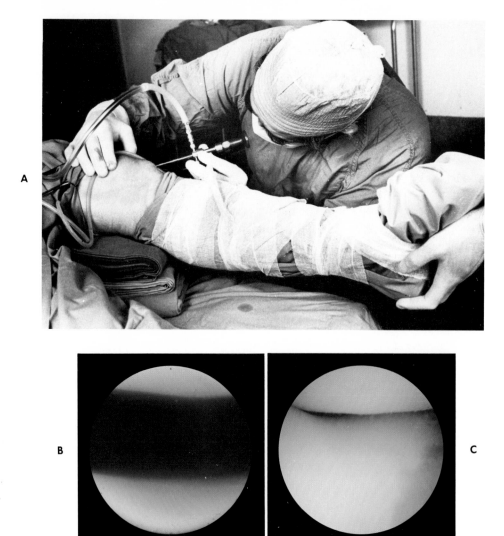

Fig. 6-6. A, Knee is extended and arthroscope placed under patella to scan articular surface while opposite hand manipulates patella. **B,** Patellofemoral joint: midportion patella above and femoral groove below. **C,** Patellofemoral joint, showing normal articulation during active extension.

Fig. 6-7. Medial compartment. **A,** Foot is dropped over side of table to allow flexion of knee and apply valgus strain to open medial compartment. **B,** Anterior horn of medial meniscus: top surface visualized with femoral condyle above. **C,** Middle third of medial meniscus: femoral condyle above and coronary ligament to right, just out of field. **D,** Posterior horn of medial meniscus visualized under femoral condyle as valgus strain is applied. **E,** Posterior attachment of medial meniscus as intercondylar notch is approached on right.

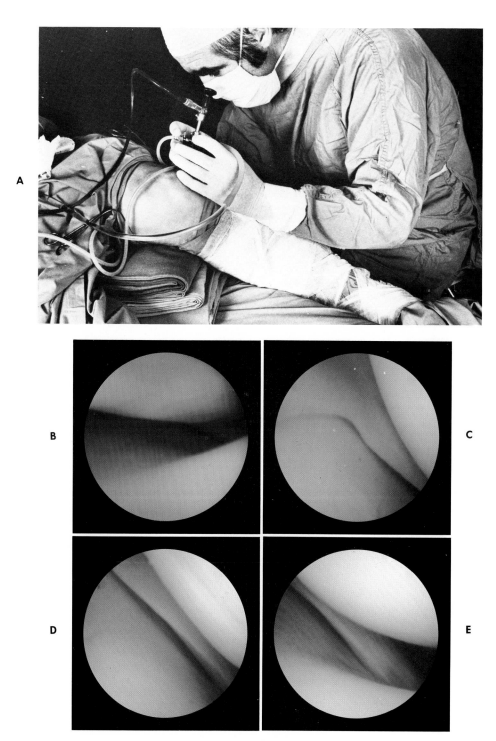

Fig. 6-7. For legend see opposite page.

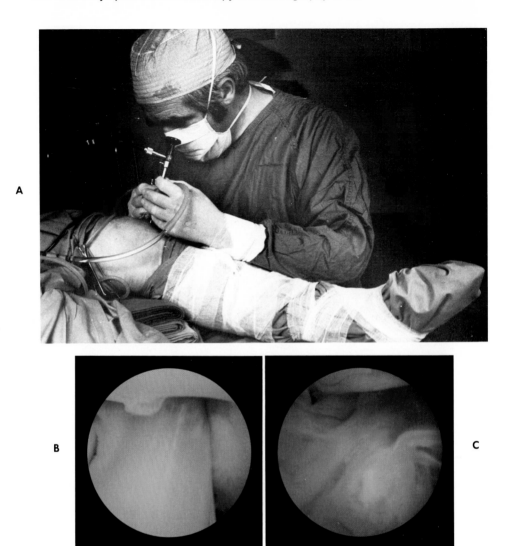

Fig. 6-8. Intercondylar notch. **A,** Foot is brought back up onto table in about 30° of flexion to visualize intercondylar notch. Arthroscope is moved from deep to superficial to avoid fat pad. **B,** Proximal attachment of anterior cruciate ligament. **C,** Anterior cruciate ligament, showing vascular pattern of synovium overlying ligament.

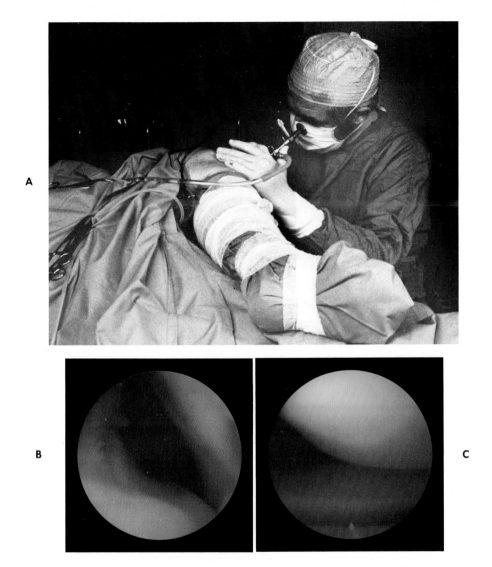

Fig. 6-9. Lateral compartment. **A,** Involved extremity is flexed to 90° and allowed to rest on opposite proximal tibia, with knee dropping into varus by gravity and opening up lateral compartment. **B,** Posterior attachment of lateral meniscus in lower portion of field under lateral femoral condyle, with attachment of anterior cruciate on medial surface of lateral condyle in upper field. **C,** Posterior horn of lateral meniscus under lateral femoral condyle.

Continued.

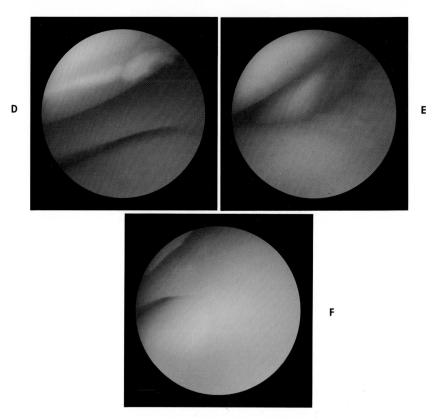

Fig. 6-9, cont'd. D, Junction of posterior and middle thirds of lateral meniscus under lateral femoral condyle. **E,** Popliteal tendon in posterolateral corner. Note junction of meniscus and synovium on right. **F,** Middle and anterior thirds of lateral meniscus.

notch. It still must be deep enough to avoid the fat pad. Occasionally the ligamentum mucosum will present an obstruction, and the instrument must be directed superiorly to get around it. The anterior cruciate ligament is identified at its proximal insertion and followed distally. In the presence of an intact anterior cruciate ligament the posterior cruciate ligament cannot be visualized.

Lateral compartment (Fig. 6-9)

The leg is now crossed over the other extremity with the lateral malleolus of the involved extremity resting on the tibial tubercle of the uninvolved extremity, thereby allowing the knee to drop into a varus position by gravity. If this maneuver is carried out properly, the tip of the arthroscope will drop off the anterior cruciate ligament into the posterolateral compartment. If more varus is desired at any time, the examiner need only lean on the flexed knee. The free edge of the posterior horn of the lateral meniscus is first seen at its attachment, and is then followed laterally to its middle third and finally to the anterior horn while simultaneously extending the knee. In 90° of flexion the popliteal tendon may be seen in the

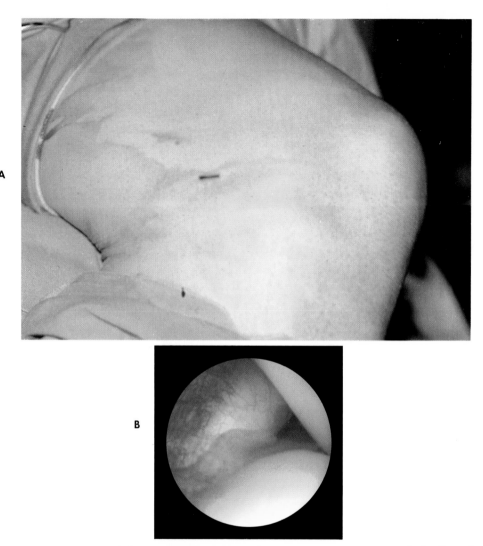

Fig. 6-10. Posteromedial compartment. **A,** Site of incision just posterior to medial collateral ligament. **B,** Posterior surface of femoral condyle on right, posterior cruciate ligament on left, and posterior surface of medial mensicus below.

posterolateral corner. The arthroscope is withdrawn and the joint thoroughly irrigated through the sheath. A single suture is placed in the wound and a pressure dressing applied. When the patient has recovered from the anesthesia he is allowed to go home fully ambulatory.

Posteromedial compartment (Fig. 6-10)

The peripheral margin of the posterior horn of the medial meniscus cannot be visualized from an anterior approach. If a lesion is suspected in this area, the posteromedial compartment can be examined independently. The joint is distended with saline, and a transverse 1 cm incision is made at the joint line just posterior to the medial collateral ligament. The extremity is crossed as in the examination of the lateral compartment to allow the popliteal structures to drop away from the posterior capsule. The sheath is inserted with the blunt trocar only. The surgeon uses the curve of the condyle as a guide to enter the joint. When the sheath is in the joint, saline will gush forth. If saline is not forthcoming, the joint has not been entered, and a second attempt must be made. Once the joint has been entered, the trocar is replaced with the bridge and the telescope. The entire peripheral attachment and the superior surface of the posterior horn of the medial meniscus are readily seen. The distal attachment of the posterior cruciate ligament can also be examined.

If further detail in the lateral compartment is desired, it may be examined from an additional puncture made one finger breadth above the tibial plateau at the medial border of the patellar tendon. In this way some lesions of the lateral meniscus may be better defined.

PROBLEMS IN ARTHROSCOPY
Hemarthrosis

Extensive bleeding in the joint can obscure adequate visualization. When the surgeon is examining the knee, he should allow 24 hours to elapse between injury and arthroscopy, or a tourniquet should probably be used. Bleeding can usually be controlled with intermittent irrigation, leaving the inflow valve open with a head of hydrostatic pressure. I do not believe a two-puncture technique is necessary for irrigation.

Red-out

The field of view may suddenly change to a completely red field. This usually means that the objective lens of the instrument is extrasynovial. Usually deeper penetration will solve this problem. It is better to work from deep to superficial rather than vice versa.

Fat pad

If the field becomes yellow or orange, usually the fat pad is obstructing the view. By deeper penetration, manipulation of the arthroscope, and flexion of the knee, the problem can usually be solved.

Hypertrophic synovium

In the presence of a proliferative synovitis, injected, edematous, hypertrophic synovial fronds may block visualization. This situation presents a difficult problem, which requires increasing irrigation and patient manipulation of the instrument and the knee.

Adhesions

Fibrous adhesions may present a formidable barrier to the arthroscope. One author has shown a bent sheath from trying to lyse adhesions. It is probably better to abandon an examination rather than to try to break up adhesions if the surgeon is unsuccessful in steering his way around them.

Orientation

Because of the extreme proximity and magnification of the objects in the knee, when viewed with the arthroscope, it is quite easy to become disoriented. The examiner must then return to a landmark, such as the patella, the condylar horizon, or the meniscus, and replot his course to the area in which he is interested.

Magnification (Fig. 6-11)

At 1 mm distance between the object to be visualized and the objective lens of the arthroscope, magnification approaches ten times. With this much magnification, it is

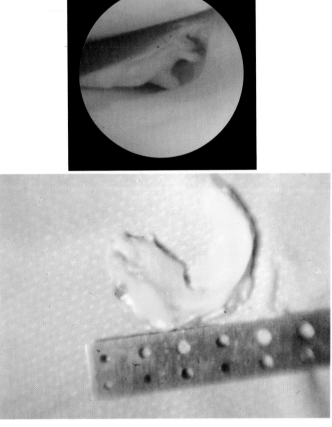

Fig. 6-11. Note size of vertical tear in arthroscopic view of lateral meniscus compared to size of tear in specimen. Magnification must be considered in interpreting observations of lesions.

not difficult to overinterpret a lesion, such as a small tear of the meniscus. This problem decreases somewhat with increasing experience. However, by returning to a familiar object viewed at the same distance, the problem is obviated.

Illumination

In some areas of the knee, such as articular cartilage when viewed directly, the brightness may be too great. By changing the rheostat on the light source, the brightness can be varied at any time during the examination.

SUMMARY

A method of technique, a look at a normal examination, and discussion of some problems have been presented. As the orthopedic surgeon increases his experience with arthroscopy he will modify technique to satisfy his own needs. Arthroscopy should be learned with a great deal of patience and with the realization that there will be moments of frustration. When the frustration becomes too great, stop the examination and try again on another day. The examination should always be gentle; vigorous manipulation of the instrument is never necessary. With these principles a thorough examination can be accomplished, allowing the surgeon the opportunity to view and study the inside of a joint with a different eye and from a different point of view. It could be said that with his visual organ inside the joint, he becomes an inside observer.

Suggested readings

Burman, M. S.: Arthroscopy or the direct visualization of joints, J. Bone Joint Surg. **13**:669, 1931.

Burman, M. S., Finkelstein, H., and Mayer, L.: Arthroscopy of the knee joint, J. Bone Joint Surg. **16**:225, 1934.

Butt, W. P., and McIntyre, M. B.: Double contrast arthrography of the knee, Radiology **92**:487, 1969.

Casscells, S. W.: Arthroscopy of the knee joint, J. Bone Joint Surg. [Am.] **53**:287, 1971.

Dandy, D. J., and Jackson, R. W.: The impact of arthroscopy in the management of disorders of the knee, J. Bone Joint Surg. [Br.] **57**:346, 1975.

DeHaven, K. B., and Collins, H. R.: Diagnosis of internal derangement of the knee. The role of arthroscopy, J. Bone Joint Surg. [Am.] **57**:802, 1975.

Jackson, R. W., and Abe, I.: The role of arthroscopy in the management of disorders of the knee, J. Bone Joint Surg. [Br.] **54**:310, 1972.

Jackson, R. W.: The role of arthroscopy in the management of the arthritic knee, Clin. Orthop. **101**:28, 1974.

Jackson, R. W., and Dandy, D. J.: Arthroscopy of the knee, New York, 1976, Grune & Stratton.

Johnson, L. L., and Becker, R. L.: Arthroscopy, technique, and role of the assistant, Orthop. Rev. **5**(9):31, 1976.

McGinty, J. B., and Freedman, P. A.: Arthroscopy of the knee, Clin. Orthop. **121**:171, 1976.

McGinty, J. B., and Mapza, R. A.: Arthroscopy of the knee, evaluation of an out-patient procedure under local anesthesia, J. Bone Joint Surg. [Am.] **60**:787, 1978.

Nicholas, J. A., Freiberger, R. H., and Killoran, P. J.: Double contrast arthrography of the knee, J. Bone Joint Surg. [Am.] **52**:203, 1970.

O'Connor, R. L.: The arthroscope in the management of crystal-induced synovitis of the knee, J. Bone Joint Surg. [Am.] **55**:1443, 1973.

O'Connor, R. L.: Arthroscopy in the diagnosis and treatment of acute ligament injuries of the knee, J. Bone Joint Surg. [Am.] **56**:333, 1974.

Takagi, K.: Practical experiences using Takagi's arthroscope, J. Jpn. Orthop. Assoc. **8**:132, 1933.

Watanabe, M., Takeda, S., and Ikeuchi, H.: Atlas of arthroscopy, Tokyo, 1957, Igaku Shoin Ltd.

Watanabe, M., Takeda, S., and Ikeuchi, H.: Atlas of arthroscopy, ed. 2, Tokyo, 1969, Igaku Shoin Ltd.

7. Technique of arthrography

Harry J. Griffiths

The arthrographer must understand the normal anatomy of the knee before embarking on arthrography. The interested reader is referred to chapter 5 for a discussion of arthroscopic anatomy.

INDICATIONS FOR ARTHROGRAPHY

1. To evaluate the knee symptoms that do not have obvious causes—with or without previous trauma
2. To evaluate possible or probable meniscal tears and to identify the tear and ascertain its size and significance
3. To evaluate other abnormalities, either involving the contralateral meniscus, the collateral ligaments, or the cruciate ligaments
4. To evaluate the locked knee
5. To evaluate the knee with recurrent effusions
6. To evaluate the status of the articular cartilage (covering both the femoral and tibial articular surfaces as well as in the patellofemoral joint)
7. To evaluate the status of the knee after meniscectomy
8. To evaluate the status of any internal derangement prior to proposed surgery
9. To evaluate patients with presumed disability for workmen's compensation insurance
10. To evaluate the size and ramifications of Baker (popliteal) cysts
11. To evaluate synovial tumors and other soft tissue masses related to the knee joint

SURGICAL METHOD AND PREPARATION

The following materials are required for arthrography:
1. Povidone-iodine (Betadine) and gauze pads for cleaning the skin
2. One 2 ml syringe for 1% local anesthetic
3. One 5 ml syringe for contrast medium
4. One 50 ml syringe for air (or carbon dioxide)
5. An interconnecting tube so that once the needle is in place the syringe may be used away from it without jogging the needle tip and coming out of the synovial space

6. Various needles although a 22-gauge 1½ inch needle is the one most frequently used for actually entering the knee joint itself

Choice of contrast agent

Basically there is a choice between a single-contrast and a double-contrast technique. Most experienced arthrographers are now using double-contrast arthrography for most joints in the body but particularly for the knee. Four milliliters of positive-contrast medium and 40 to 80 ml of air or carbon dioxide are usually used, but the actual amounts will vary from place to place. If more than 4 ml of positive-contrast medium is used, puddling of the contrast occurs posteriorly in the popliteal bursa or anteriorly in the dependent part, possibly obscuring the underlying lesion. In fact some authorities are now using only 3 ml of positive-contrast medium. With respect to the type of positive-contrast agent most arthrographers are using meglumine diatrizoate (Renografin-60 or Renografin-76), but recently a number of articles have appeared[3,8,9,14] that advocate using newer contrast agents such as methyl glucamine iocarmate (Dimer X) and a nonionic contrast agent, metrizamide (Amipaque). The rationale for finding new contrast agents is that meglumine diatrizoate is absorbed very rapidly, and although this process can be slowed down somewhat by the use of epinephrine, some of the newer contrast agents are absorbed much more slowly and produce less focal inflammatory reaction.

For the negative-contrast agent, oxygen was initially used, but because this was absorbed too rapidly most arthrographers now use either room air or carbon dioxide or a mixture of the two. In the collected experience of a number of authorities there has been no case reported of an air embolus occurring in double-contrast arthrography. Pure carbon dioxide has the disadvantage of being absorbed fairly rapidly, and room air is far better in this respect and is of course more readily obtainable. In a collected series of over 30,000 arthrograms performed with room air only one infection of the knee joint has been seen.

Initially arthrography was mainly single contrast, either negative contrast (air or oxygen) or single positive contrast. Nowadays double-contrast techniques have largely replaced single-contrast arthrography in most situations. Single positive contrast techniques are useful in the delineation of Baker cysts and in looking for loose bodies. A single-contrast arthrogram may be readily converted to a double-contrast arthrogram by removing as much contrast as possible and then adding air as a secondary procedure. Single-contrast air arthrography has no real indication except in one very rare situation. I once had to perform an arthrogram on a patient who had had a cardiac arrest during an intravenous pyelogram and it was considered judicious not to use any positive-contrast material for the knee arthrogram. A meniscal tear was adequately demonstrated in this patient by the use of air alone.

TECHNIQUE AND PROCEDURE

Once the indications for the procedure are understood by the arthrographer, the patient is examined and a clinical history obtained. The choice of contrast medium is made, and the procedure is explained to the patient. The patient is placed supine with the affected leg on the side of the table toward the examiner. Scout films are taken if none are available. These should include a fluoroscopic scout film and anteroposterior, lateral, and tunnel views of the knee. The skin of the knee is prepared by a sterile technique; the arthrographer wears sterile gloves and scrubs his hands beforehand. The patella is moved laterally by the fingers of the left hand, and the infrapatellar surface is palpated. The junction of the upper one third and the lower two thirds of the patella is the entry point of choice. The skin is punctured and some local anesthetic run in as the needle is advanced running parallel to the patella through the subcutaneous tissues and the joint capsule. If more local anesthetic is then injected and the tip of the needle lies within the knee joint, little or no resistance to the injection is experienced (Fig. 7-1). If a joint effusion is present, as much of this should be aspirated as possible before continuing, because excess fluid will dilute the contrast agent. Some 30 to 50 ml of air or carbon dioxide is then injected, and if the needle is correctly placed within the knee joint, the dimple on the medial side of the joint will bulge almost immediately. Following the injection of air, the positive contrast is injected; this is done after the radiologist initially ascertains, by aspirating some air out first, that the tip of the needle still lies within the knee joint. Because the contrast is rather viscous it is more difficult to inject than is the air, and once the 4 ml of positive-contrast medium is injected, a "chaser" of 5 to 10 ml of air precedes the removal of the needle. Upon removal, the puncture site is rubbed to prevent escape of air, and the patient is encouraged to move his knee himself or the

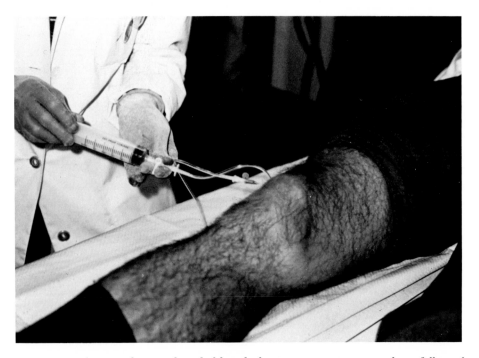

Fig. 7-1. Lateral approach is used, and although this is an outpatient procedure, full sterile technique is employed (sterile drape has been removed for clarity).

examiner may move the knee joint passively. This is normally performed with the patient still in the supine position, but many arthrographers get the patient to walk around the x-ray room to admix the air and contrast material to coat the synovial and articular surfaces more adequately. The patient is warned that the knee will make squelching and popping sounds and be slightly distended for 2 to 4 days, but that he is able to do anything on that leg which he did prior to the arthrogram.

Use of epinephrine

It is well known that meglumine diatrizoate is resorbed very rapidly from the knee, and to get adequate radiographs it is necessary to work quickly; in fact Staple[15] recommends that 15 minutes is the maximum time allowable before the definition of the articular surfaces becomes so poor as to be useless. Moreover in a teaching hospital situation where the training of residents is an integral part of the procedure, 15 minutes is not an adequate length of time to complete the arthrogram. Hall[6] advocated the use of epinephrine in a dosage of 0.35 mg (0.35 ml of a 1:1,000 solution) to be mixed with the contrast agent. This not only resulted in an initial improvement in the sharpness of the contrast-outlined intraarticular structures but also produced a marked persistence of this enhanced detail, presumably due to the vasoconstrictive effects of epinephrine. Several other authors have advocated the routine use of epinephrine with the diatrizoate salts, and no side effects have been reported to date.[2,3,14]

Filming technique

The use of fluoroscopy and a vertical beam has made the radiographic evaluation of the contrast-filled knee joint extremely simple to perform.[1,2,4,13] Arthrography is best performed using a small focal spot (preferably 0.3 mm) without either automatic collimation or an Iontomat (automatic exposure) device. For relatively little expense it is possible to short-circuit the Iontomat and then to take a sequence of fluoroscopic scout films to ascertain the correct kilovoltage required to adequately visualize the knee. The correct kilovoltage usually lies between 50 and 60 kV for women and 55 to 70 kV for men. The patient is placed prone and some form of a strap or board put around the lower thighs, on which either a valgus or a varus stress may be applied to the knee joint.

A "scout" film in the anteroposterior plane is taken to provide an overview of the knee joint, the cartilage, the menisci, and the joint capsule. Then the patient is placed on one side or the other. If it is the left knee that is being examined, the patient faces left (lying on his right side), and the band is placed on the left side of the table. If it is the right leg, then the patient lies on the left side facing right, with the band attached to the right side of the table.

A lateral film is then taken. This may be a stress view in order to show the synovial tent that covers the cruciate ligaments. This view will also demonstrate the presence of a Baker cyst.

Then under fluoroscopic control, 12 views of each meniscus should be taken from anterior to posterior, with the examiner making sure that the femoral condyles

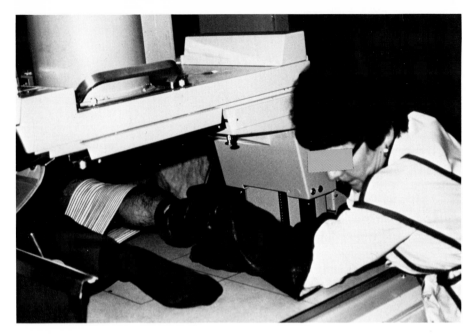

Fig. 7-2. Patient is prone and lying on his left side. Band is attached to left of table, and operator pulls to right to open medial compartment for view of posterior horn medial meniscus.

overlap almost totally front and back to ensure adequate coverage of the whole meniscus arthrographically. If the left leg is being examined, keep the patient in the position outlined above, and put traction on the leg both downward and against the band (varus stress) in order to open out the joint laterally to see the lateral meniscus anteriorly. Also make sure that the tibial plateau is vertical as well so that the meniscus is seen in profile (see "Frequent Pitfalls"). The patient is rotated slowly through 180°, first onto his face and then up onto his left side with the examiner taking radiographs every 15° or so in order to demonstrate as much of the meniscus as possible. If it is the right leg, the patient begins on the left side and rotates 180° to lie eventually on his right side.

To cover the whole of the other meniscus it is only necessary to reverse this process, taking 12 views of the medial meniscus with valgus stress on the lower leg (Fig. 7-2). Many marking devices have been described to differentiate the medial meniscus from the lateral one, and the left leg from the right. The more sophisticated ones also include markers to denote the anterior, middle, and posterior horns. However, it frequently takes more time to set up the marker than to take the films, and many experienced arthrographers identify the views when the procedure is completed.

Additional views may be necessary to delineate a Baker cyst, loose body, cruciate tear, or synovial tumor. These include delayed films (up to 3 hours) and tomography (for cruciate tears).

Single-contrast technique

The surgical preparation and approach for the single-contrast technique is identical to that used in double-contrast arthrography, but instead of air, 35 ml of positive-contrast agent is used. A greater volume than this may be painful for the patient although the pain can be alleviated to some extent by the use of 1% local anesthetic mixed with the contrast. Single-contrast arthrography is indicated in the evaluation of Baker cysts, loose bodies, and possibly in the evaluation of cruciate ligament tears. These indications will be discussed in more detail in later chapters.

INTERPRETATION
Normal arthrogram

On a normal arthrogram the joint capsule and its bursae should be demonstrated (Fig. 7-3). The synovial lining should be intact, and the synovial "tent" lying over the cruciate ligaments should be visible (Fig. 7-4). The articular cartilage should be

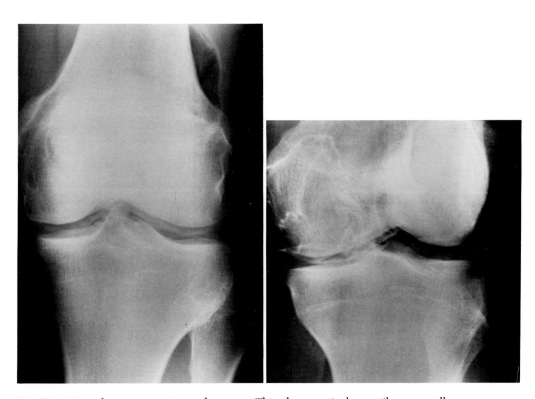

Fig. 7-3. Normal anteroposterior arthrogram. This shows articular cartilage as well as any gross abnormalities in joint, **A**, and often will demonstrate a discoid meniscus if present on lateral aspect, **B**.

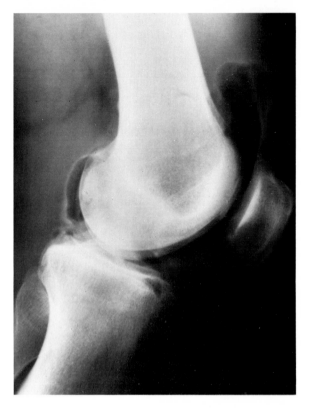

Fig. 7-4. Normal lateral arthrogram. This view delineates extent of joint and its bursae, as well as shows synovial tent overlying cruciates and will often demonstrate loose bodies or popliteal cyst if present.

evaluated, and the menisci should be present throughout their normal length and not absent, torn, or truncated unless there has been a history of previous surgery (Figs. 7-5 to 7-7).

Abnormal arthrogram

The abnormal arthrogram will be discussed more fully in the following chapters, but tears of the menisci constitute by far the largest group of lesions seen at arthrography. Discoid menisci, bucket-handle tears of menisci, postmenisectomy-retained posterior horns, loose bodies, ligamentous tears, Baker cysts, synovial lesions, articular infractions, arthritis, and developmental abnormalities constitute other findings that are apparent on an abnormal arthrogram.

FREQUENT PITFALLS

There are three classic errors in performing and in interpreting arthrograms.[4,6,10-14] The first error concerns the correct angle that the meniscus subtends to

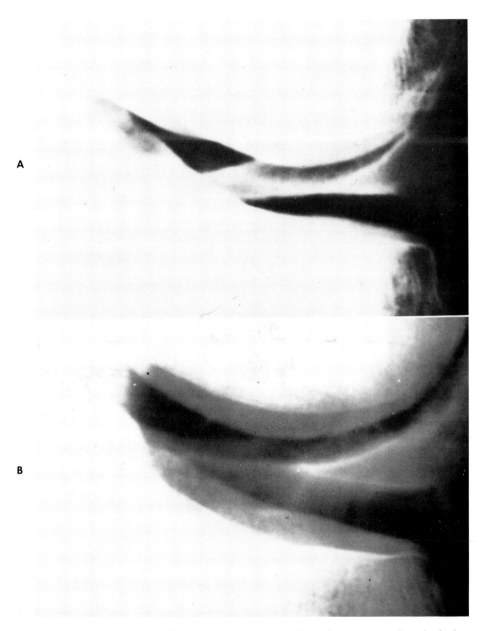

Fig. 7-5. Three views of normal lateral meniscus in an orthograde position with air both above and below triangular shadow caused by meniscus. **A,** Anterior horn. **B,** Middle horn.

Continued.

C

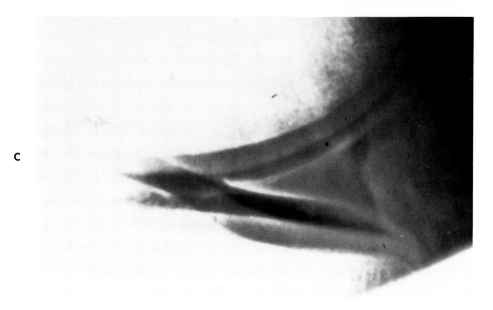

Fig. 7-5, cont'd. C, Posterior horn.

the x-ray beam. The meniscus should be orthograde when visualized on the fluoro-scopic screen; this means that the longitudinal axis of the meniscus should lie in the plane of the x-ray beam. If this is not true, double images, overlapping lines, and confusing shadows (pseudotears) become obvious (Fig. 7-8).

The second error in arthrography concerns a fat pad that is usually seen in the region of the anterior horn of the medial meniscus (Hoffa fat pad) and that may be confused with a tear or irregularity of the anterior horn of either meniscus (Fig. 7-9). This fat pad is usually seen overlapping the anterior horn of the medial meniscus, but it may appear on the lateral side where the same confusion can arise.

The third error is that problems in interpretation may occur in the region of the popliteal bursa (or hiatus popliteus), which represents the tendon sheath of the pop-liteal muscle and which runs obliquely through the insertion of the posterior horn of the lateral meniscus. This is a difficult region to interpret, and an exact knowledge of its anatomy and radiographic appearances is essential. Since the tendon runs through the meniscus obliquely, it will initially appear as a superior "recess" on the meniscus; then it appears as a rhomboid-shaped lucency within the meniscus with superior and inferior struts of normal tissue connecting the meniscus to the synovium. Finally and most posteriorly it appears as an inferior "recess" before leaving the joint space. This is a confusing area, and if the meniscus is not visualized in an exactly orthograde fashion, then interpretation becomes more difficult than it should be (Fig. 7-10).

With respect to recesses, most patients have small inferior and superior recesses
Text continued on p. 93.

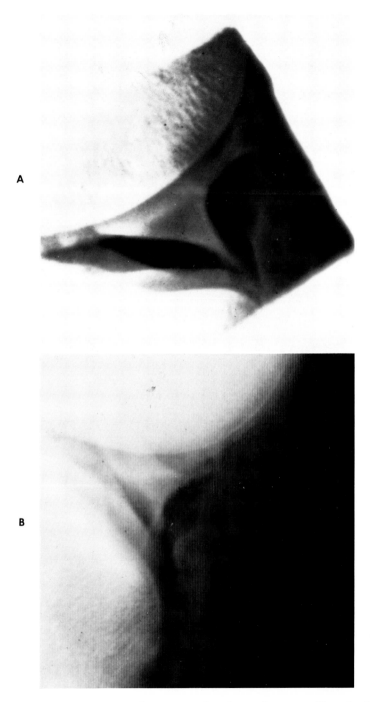

Fig. 7-6. Normal popliteal bursa. These views show bursa that runs obliquely through posterior horn of lateral meniscus in two planes. **A** is at central portion of this bursa and shows both struts to be intact. **B,** More posterior view of popliteal bursa with defect through inferior surface as popliteal tendon exits from meniscus. Superior strut is intact in this normal arthrogram.

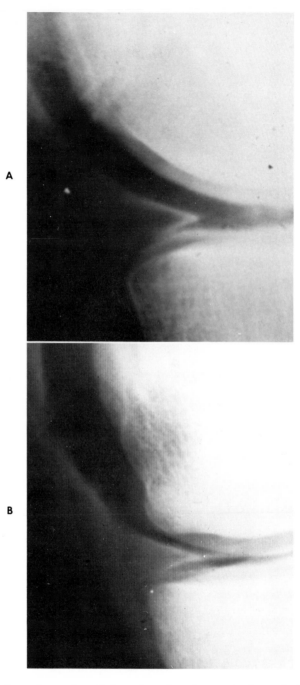

Fig. 7-7. Three views of normal medial meniscus from its anterior horn, **A,** through its middle horn, **B,** to its posterior horn, **C.**

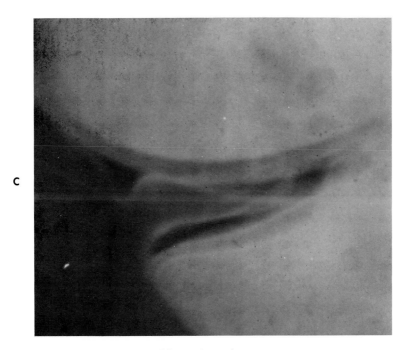

C

Fig. 7-7, cont'd. For legend see opposite page.

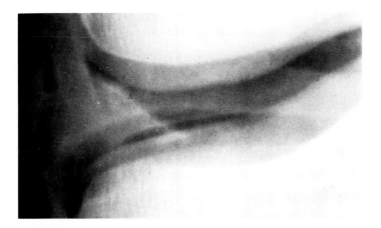

Fig. 7-8. Source of error: nonorthograde projection. This results in several shadows being seen, and no clear-cut view of meniscus can be obtained.

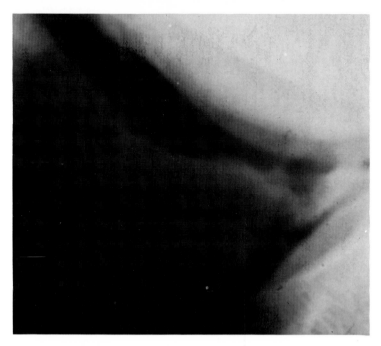

Fig. 7-9. Source of error: Hoffa fat pad. This view of anterior horn medial meniscus shows many confusing shadows that may be interpreted as representing a tear. However, this is normal appearance of Hoffa fat pad.

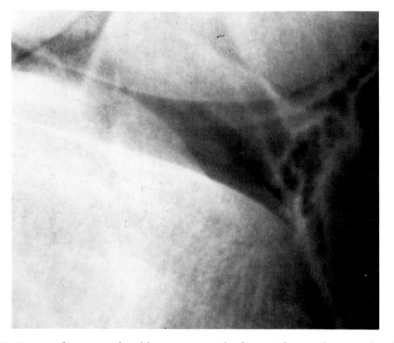

Fig. 7-10. Source of error: popliteal bursa improperly shown. This results in confused image of posterior horn lateral meniscus, often simulating tear.

in the posterior horn of the lateral meniscus. The radiographic hint as to whether a true tear is present or not is the fact that damaged cartilage "imbibes" contrast (or absorbs it abnormally rapidly) so that if a delayed film (15 to 30 minutes) is taken, then a tear will appear blurred and denser than surrounding tissues, whereas a pseudotear or pseudorecess will appear normal.

Other errors in technique include failure to inject the liquid contrast medium into the joint. In this situation it is usually injected into the fat between the anterior surface of the femur and the suprapatellar bursa, but this should be immediately recognizable under fluoroscopy. Also super imposition of a bursa, Baker cyst, or recess may cause problems in interpretation by obscuring the menisci, particularly in their posterior aspects.

COMPLICATIONS AND DANGERS

In a collected series of over 30,000 arthrograms, there have been no fatalities. Allergic reactions to the iodinated contrast medium are rare, although a few cases of hives have been reported. Sympathetic effusions will occasionally occur, and pain is not common after arthrography. There has been one proven case of infection and two other possible cases, but one should anticipate that infection will be rare if the proper aseptic technique is carefully followed. The radiation exposure to the gonads is extremely low.[11] The procedure is justified in almost all patients, although on general principles, arthrography should not be performed on pregnant women.

ACCURACY RATES

Some arthrographers claim a 100% accuracy rate, but they must be remarkable. Most authorities claim an accuracy rate of 90% to 95% for the medial meniscus and an 80% to 90% accuracy rate for the lateral meniscus.*

False-positive results are common in the posterior horns of both menisci, and false-negative results commonly occur when there are simple, horizontal, cleavage tears present. Loose bodies and tears of the cruciate ligaments are frequently missed on arthrography unless the examiner has been alerted beforehand. Also most experienced arthrographers do not attempt either to describe the tear (i.e., horizontal, oblique, vertical, or complex) or its exact position, because at operation the tear will often extend far beyond the area seen on the radiographs and may be a far more complex lesion than the arthrographers were able to diagnose. So a simple report of "tear of the posterior horn medial meniscus" should suffice.

Recently a number of studies have been reported[7,14] in which the overall accuracy rates of arthrography and arthroscopy are compared. Although these have been discussed elsewhere in this book, it is worth mentioning that a true accuracy rate of between 65% and 75% has been found for arthrography when everything is taken into account, such as ligamentous injuries, capsular tears, minimal degenerative changes, chondromalacia patellae, loose bodies, and early fibrillation of the menis-

---

*References 1, 2, 4, 5, 7, 12-14.

cus. This does not alter the fact that arthrography is a safe, simple, widely available method to confirm the presence of meniscal tears prior to surgery and to delineate internal derangements of the knee and other joints.

SUMMARY

Arthrography of the knee is a procedure that is widely available, simple to perform, safe, and has a high diagnostic accuracy rate with respect to meniscal injuries. Our technique is briefly outlined; it essentially uses vertical beam fluoroscopy with 12 spot films taken of each meniscus. Variations of this technique are mentioned, as are the pitfalls of interpretation, dangers to the patient, and overall accuracy rate. In my opinion arthrography is still the procedure of choice in meniscal injuries to the knee.

References

1. Butt, W. P., and McIntyre, J. L.: Double-contrast arthrography of the knee, Radiology **92**:487-499, 1969.
2. Dalinka, M. K., Coren, G. S., and Wershba, M.: Knee arthrography, CRC Crit. Rev. Clin. Radiol. Nucl. Med. **4**:1-59, 1973.
3. Foote, G. A.: Arthrographic contrast media. In Miller, R. E., and Skucas, J., editor: Radiographic contrast agents, Baltimore, 1977, University Park Press, pp. 451-462.
4. Freiberger, R. H., Killoran, P. J., and Cordona, G.: Arthrography of the knee by double contrast method, Am. J. Roentgenol. Radium Ther. Nucl. Med. **97**:736, 1966.
5. Hall, F. M.: Epinephrine-enhanced knee arthrography, Radiology **111**:215, 1974.
6. Hall, F. M.: Pitfalls in knee arthrography, Radiology **118**:55-62, 1976.
7. Hirschowitz, D.: Clinical assessment, arthrography, arthroscopy and arthrotomy in the diagnosis of internal derangement of the knee, J. Bone Joint Surg. **58**:367, 1976.
8. Johansen, J. G., and Berner, A.: Arthrography with amipaque (Metrizamide) and other contrast media, Invest. Radiol. **11**:534-540, 1976.
9. Katzberg, R. W., Burgener, F. A., and Fischer, H. W.: Evaluation of various contrast agents for improved arthrography, Invest. Radiol. **11**:528-533, 1976.
10. Kessler, I., Silberman, Z., and Nissim, F.: Arthrography of the knee. A critical study of errors and their sources, Am. J. Roentgenol. Radium Ther. Nucl. Med. **86**:359, 1961.
11. Larson, L. E.: Quoted by Ricklin, P., Ruttiman, A., and Del Buono, M. S.: Meniscus lesions. Practical problems of clinical diagnosis, arthrography and therapy, New York, 1971, Grune & Stratton.
12. Lindblom, K.: Arthrography of the knee: a roentgenographic and anatomical study, Acta Radiol. [Suppl.] (Stockh.) 74, 1948.
13. Ricklin, P., Ruttiman, A., Del Buono, M. S.: Meniscus lesions. Practical problems of clinical diagnosis, arthrography and therapy, New York, 1971, Grune & Stratton.
14. Roebuck, E. J.: Double contrast knee arthrography. Some new points of technique including the use of Dimer X, Clin. Radiol. **28**:247-257, 1977.
15. Staple, T. W.: Extra meniscal lesions demonstrated by double contrast arthrography of the knee, Radiology **102**:311-319, 1972.

8. Lesions of the synovium

Arthroscopy

Alan L. Bass

The twentieth century has seen great strides forward in the investigation and treatment of joint disease both from the medical and the surgical viewpoint. The development of replacement prostheses has been paralleled by the use of isotope scans and thermography in investigation and by the plethora of antiinflammatory drugs that now exists in the modern pharmacopoeia.

However, one of the great innovations, namely arthroscopy, has not yet been fully exploited by investigative physicians interested in synovial lesions. Pioneers in arthroscopy have been overwhelmingly surgical in their background, and much of our information on endoscopy in arthritis is derived from Watanabe, Jackson, Casscells, and others.

In the field of internal medicine, workers such as Robles-Gil and Katona in Mexico unfolded the wonders of medical arthroscopy as late as 1968, while in Europe Jayson and Aignan among others have been most intimately involved with this technique over the past decade.

Such neglect by physicians interested in synovial lesions has been unfortunate in many respects, and we have been unable to equal the achievements of respirologists and gastroenterologists, who have grasped endoscopy as a method of more clearly identifying and recording the extent of a lesion and following the natural history of a particular disease. With arthroscopy, biopsy and serial assessments become easy, and it is only in the last few years that some rheumatologists have shown a serious interest in this technique.

The indications for arthroscopy are well delineated elsewhere in this book. Those indications of particular importance for physicians are unexplained monarticular swelling, contradictory objective findings, persistent complaints of pain, and those situations less common to a physician, where compensation or litigation are involved. The procedure is, of course, most helpful where an accurate prognosis is required.

The technique of synovial arthroscopy is very similar to that used generally when seeking information on predominantly orthopedic conditions, but a few minor alterations can considerably facilitate the ability of the arthroscopist to view, do a biopsy of, and photographically record synovial abnormalities.

First, one should consider the type of instrument that could be most helpful. In the early 1970s, virtually all those interested in arthroscopy used the Watanabe no. 21 arthroscope with its tungsten light source. The "double-barreled" presence in the joint of both bulb and telescope side by side was very helpful when used skillfully to push away large fat pads and exuberant proliferative synovium. Good photography was possible, and through a separate incision it was possible to perform a biopsy of synovial membrane. The light intensity, however, was limited, and this caused occasional difficulty when viewing the relatively nonreflective synovium, a problem not encountered when looking at highly reflective surfaces such as hyaline cartilage. Some difficulties, however, were encountered in those knees where the capacity to maneuver was limited, such as the joints of small children and the tight adult knees where osteoarthritic osteophytes protruded from the bone edges. The advent of fiber optic light and introduction of the more modern rod-lens system into arthroscopy produced considerable changes. The arthroscope became more versatile, and instruments from 2 to 6 mm in diameter were developed. This facilitated their use not only in the knee but also in other joints. Direct vision biopsy was facilitated by the appearance of angled telescopes and biopsy forceps that could fit together with the telescopes into the same sheath. With the use of intense light with a color temperature of 5,200 degrees kelvin, a value just below that of natural daylight. Photography became easier, and along with it there was the possibility of better intraarticular movies, and for the first time a color television camera could be clipped onto the arthroscope in order to obtain permanent video records.

GUIDELINES IN SYNOVIAL ARTHROSCOPY OF THE KNEE

When performing arthroscopy for various synovial conditions, it soon becomes apparent that problems other than those encountered in meniscal, cartilaginous, and bony lesions can cause difficulty. Very frequently there is an effusion into the joint, which is rarely clear but more frequently serosanguineous and almost always slightly opalescent. This can cause a great deal of difficulty in target visualization for the unwary arthroscopist. In addition there can be a profusion of loose bodies, varying in size from chondral "snow" to sizeable chunks of cartilage and excessive fibrin, all of which can obscure the field of the instrument; similarly, tight joints due to adhesions limit the maneuverability of the instrument itself. The greatest problem, however, comes from the synovium itself, which in many conditions can be extremely friable; even the most gentle arthroscopist will find his field obscured by oozing of blood within the joint.

Adequate distension of the joint immediately prior to making the arthroscopic incision undoubtedly helps, and one sometimes feels the popping of small intraarticular adhesions during this process. Full distension of the joint will also reduce the risk of traumatizing friable synovium as the arthroscope is initially inserted and passed into the suprapatellar pouch. Various approaches are suggested, but the examiner cannot really improve on the one most frequently used, namely, the inferolateral approach as described by Watanabe. With the straight, forward-oblique, and right-angle telescopes now available, all that is necessary can be seen through an incision in the Harty-Joyce triangle.

The *flow of saline* in synovial arthroscopy should be the reverse of that used in routine inspection of menisci. The presence of fibrinous debris, exudate, and blood requires a more adequate and less easily clogged exit than a simple no. 16 needle. If the flow is one of high volume and pressure, which can be achieved easily by raising the level of the reservoir 2 feet above the level of the patient, an adequate "washing" effect can be obtained, and any debris that cannot pass around the telescope during the procedure can be removed by simple withdrawal of this part of the instrument from its sheath. While it is true that an inflated tourniquet will reduce the oozing that occurs, the bleaching of the synovium gives a false picture using this method. One should also remember that saline flowing through the joint should be approximately at body temperature because synovial vessel dilatation is obtained if the saline used is either overheated or insufficiently warmed.

The usual no. 16 or even no. 14 needle through which the joint is irrigated is frequently unsatisfactory, as the sharp bevel on the tip can traumatize the synovium and increase the oozing; alternatively it may become blocked by thickened synovium when the knee is moved during the procedure so the examiner can visualize the medial and lateral compartments. Therefore a blunt multidirectional needle, such as a no. 15 antral cannula with small holes on its sides at fixed distances serves not only to reduce the problem of trauma once the central trocar is removed, but the side ports allow for free access of saline with less danger of blockage. If the drilled holes are a measured distance apart, they can also be used to determine more accurately the size of any lesion alongside which the cannula can be placed within the joint. Since the common site for the cannula is in the upper part of the patellofemoral compartment, its value in measurement is restricted to lesions of the suprapatellar pouch and the patella itself.

Adequate lighting and good lens resolution have been stressed earlier, but the use of the newer fiber optic light source has really obviated the necessity for further comment in this respect.

Slow movement of the arthroscope within the joint is of paramount importance if the trauma to already friable tissue is to be reduced to a minimum. Careful maneuvering of the instrument as it passes into the various compartments will reduce considerably the cloudiness that can accompany even comparatively minor trauma to hyperemic synovium. Once the procedure is under way, and the cloudiness has disappeared, it is often possible for the examiner to improve his view of the synovium by closing the outflow and allowing the joint to distend fully from the reservoir. This not only causes distension of the joint, thus allowing better visualization of the suprapatellar pouch, but it also allows for a better view of the synovial villi. When the joint is fully distended, these tend to stand erect from the synovium, making their visualization and recognition easier.

After completion of the procedure and closure of the incision, a *modified form of compression* should be applied, using cotton wadding and a tensor bandage for 12 to 18 hours. This reduces the frequency of postarthroscopy effusions, which can be troublesome, especially in those cases where tissue biopsy has been taken. The presence of a relatively bulky dressing will serve also to restrict the patient's activity for a critical period of time, after which the wadding can be removed, and a simple tensor bandage will then provide adequate support.

Any postarthroscopic inflammatory reaction can be reduced by the use of *non-steroidal antiinflammatory drugs*, if these are not already being used for the condition itself. If it is deemed advisable to use them, they should be administered in full therapeutic doses for a limited period, 4 to 5 days.

CLINICAL INTERPRETATION IN ARTHROSCOPY

Interpretation in synovial arthroscopy is dependent on the ability to recognize normal synovium and nonpathologic villi that can be seen in any knee. When the examiner is looking at synovial membrane itself, it is important to remember that it may vary from one area to another within the knee, but undoubtedly it is best seen in the suprapatellar pouch. Its color will depend to a certain extent on the light source, but generally speaking it is pinkish red in color, and the fine reticular network of blood vessels crossing through it can be seen in most cases (Fig. 8-1).

Certain folds in the synovium have been described; unless these folds are identified at an early stage, some confusion may arise. The plica semilunaris (Fig. 8-2) is a transverse fold in the suprapatellar pouch; it forms an arch of varying size with its base on the posterior aspect of the pouch, the fold itself being suspended from the anterior and side walls. It is seen when the joint is fully distended. The plica synovialis mediopatellaris (Iino's band) is a longitudinal fold on the medial aspect of the pouch; it varies from a slim pleat (Fig. 8-3) to the hyperemic edematous ridge seen in Fig. 8-4 en route to its insertion in the region of the infrapatellar fat pad. This particular band was the cause here of a painful snapping sensation felt over the anteromedial aspect of the knee as the joint was flexed and extended; it followed a direct blow to this region.

Fig. 8-1 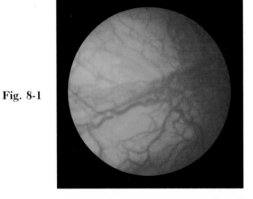 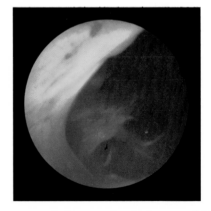 Fig. 8-2

Fig. 8-1. Normal synovium. Note color of synovium and clarity with which synovial blood supply can be seen.

Fig. 8-2. Plica semilunaris. Medial half of this fold is seen here from below. Upper part of suprapatellar pouch is seen extending beyond fold.

Various types of synovial villi can soon be recognized; these have been well described by Watanabe in his *Atlas of Arthroscopy*. Normal villi may be threadlike or may appear as thin membranes but can always be distinguished by the fact that their blood vessels are clearly visible, and they are always translucent. They are most frequently recognized in the suprapatellar pouch on the posterior wall just above the femoral condyles and are frequently present around the lower pole of the patella (Fig. 8-5). They are rarely if ever seen in the synovium of a normal medial or lateral compartment.

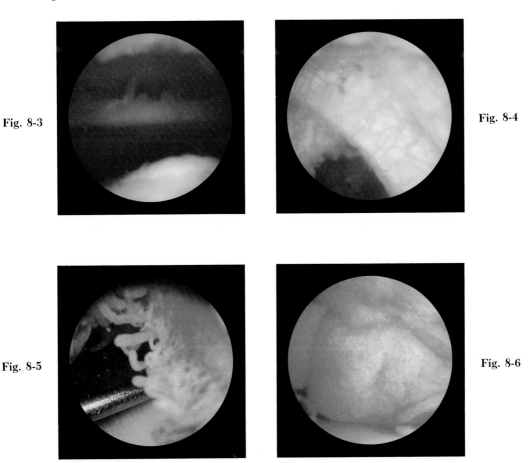

Fig. 8-3

Fig. 8-4

Fig. 8-5

Fig. 8-6

Fig. 8-3. Plica semilunaris mediopatellaris (Iino's band). From its origin high on medial wall of suprapatellar pouch, upper part of band appears as a fold or pleat as it courses downward.
Fig. 8-4. Plica semilunaris mediopatellaris (lower half of band seen in Fig. 8-3). As it passes to its insertion in region of infrapatellar fat pad, this particular band becomes edematous and hyperemic. Snapping symptoms were relieved by division and partial resection of plica.
Fig. 8-5. Normal villi. Note translucency and facility with which their blood supply can be seen.
Fig. 8-6. Acute synovitis. Edematous synovial folds with loss of normal vascular pattern are characteristic of this condition.

Once the appearance of normal synovium is recognized, there is little difficulty in appreciating that the reddened, edematous, and thickened synovial folds seen in (Fig. 8-6) represent acute inflammation. This photograph (Fig. 8-6) was taken in a case of traumatic synovitis. Suppurative synovitis in its early stage presents a very similar picture, but in addition there is a fibrinous exudate and at a later stage fibrinous adhesions.

Fig. 8-7 is from a rather unusual case of recurrent effusion in a knee for 6 months after surgery. Once again the thickened synovium can be appreciated, but in addition there were discrete raised yellow areas, two or three of which can be seen in the

Fig. 8-7 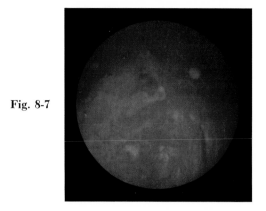 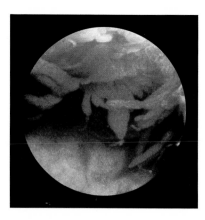 Fig. 8-8

Fig. 8-7. Chronic synovitis, may be due to talc. Note small discrete yellow "tubercles," containing granules.
Fig. 8-8. Chronic hypertrophic synovitis in rheumatoid arthritis. Villi are fleshy and discrete, with no vascular pattern. Note adjacent normal synovium.

Fig. 8-9 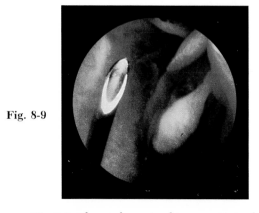 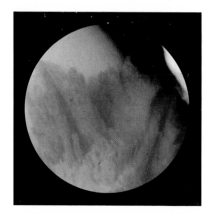 Fig. 8-10

Fig. 8-9. Chronic hypertrophic synovitis in rheumatoid arthritis. Enlargement shows some of club-shaped villi alongside a no. 16 needle within joint. Club-shaped villi are suggestive but not diagnostic of rheumatoid arthritis.
Fig. 8-10. Rheumatoid pannus. Thickened abnormal synovium is seen here creeping over edge of femoral condyle.

illustration. These were not unlike the tubercles described by Watanabe, and the presence of giant cells on section plus the gross quads wasting suggest tuberculous infection. Guinea pig culture was negative, and close study of the section showed a granular central area in each tubercle, which was finally diagnosed as talc.

Chronic synovitis is most frequently seen in those patients suffering from rheumatoid disease (Figs. 8-8 to 8-10). Fig. 8-8 shows the thickened synovium and fleshy edematous villi of chronic inflammation, but as is frequently seen in rheumatoid disease there is an area in the lower part of the picture where the synovium is totally normal. Here is yet one more reason for the preference of visual over blind punch biopsy when the diagnosis is in doubt. An enlargement of the individual club-shaped chronic villi (Fig. 8-9) is typical of that which is seen in chronic synovitis; the size of the villi can be judged by the adjacent no. 16 needle. The final picture in this series (Fig. 8-10) demonstrates rheumatoid pannus creeping over the edge of the medial femoral condyle in a case of rheumatoid arthritis. In addition to these findings, one can sometimes find detached necrotic villi, which frequently appear as large amounts of debris within the joint itself. The picture in osteoarthritis is similar to that seen in rheumatoid disease except that the inflammatory areas are usually localized to parts of the synovium adjacent to articular cartilage, and there is very rarely, if ever, a generalized inflammatory reaction in the region of the suprapatellar pouch.

Pigmented villonodular synovitis with its colorful, hemosiderin-stained, thick, membranous villi is shown in Fig. 8-11.

Hemophilic arthritis, with its recurrent hemarthroses, presents a similar picture (Fig. 8-12) except that there is frequently staining of the femoral condyles, and a

Fig. 8-11 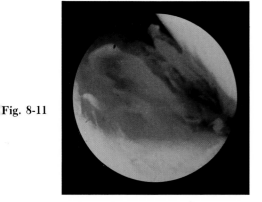 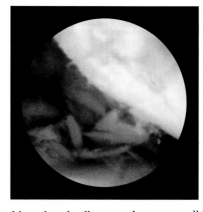 Fig. 8-12

Fig. 8-11. Pigmented villonodular synovitis. Highly colored villi are rather seaweedlike in conformation and hemosiderin stained. (Courtesy Dr. Robert W. Jackson.)

Fig. 8-12. Hemophilic arthritis. Note similarity with Fig. 8-11 except that there is also staining of femoral condyle, and synovitis involves whole joint.

glance into the suprapatellar pouch (Fig. 8-13) demonstrates the general nature of the synovial reaction in addition to the almost diagnostic color of the villi. The presence of necrotic debris and fibrinous deposits should also be noted.

Crystal synovitis in the form of gout (Fig. 8-14) can be diagnosed arthroscopically by the edematous, chronic inflammatory villi, but here one notes also the somewhat glazed appearance and the fact that in the walls of the villi there appear many highly reflective areas, representing crystalline deposition. A glance at the femoral condyles of the same patient (Fig. 8-15) shows plaques that are further crystal aggregations.

Miscellaneous conditions that can be clearly demonstrated on arthroscopy in-

Fig. 8-13
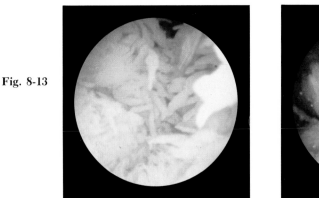
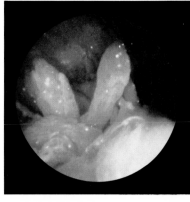
Fig. 8-14

Fig. 8-13. Hemophilic arthritis. Suprapatellar pouch of case shown in Fig. 8-12. In addition to characteristic staining of villi, necrotic debris and fibrin can be seen.
Fig. 8-14. Crystal synovitis (gout). Glazed, thickened villi with crystalline deposition can be clearly seen.

Fig. 8-15
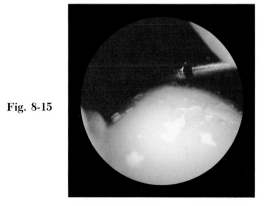
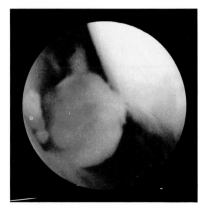
Fig. 8-16

Fig. 8-15. Crystal synovitis (gout). "Cheesy" raised crystalline deposits on femoral condyle from case shown in Fig. 8-14.
Fig. 8-16. Osteochondroma. This solitary osteochondroma, trapped in medial compartment, was the cause of recurrent symptoms and probably the cause of lesion on femoral condyle seen on right.

clude the solitary osteochondroma. Fig. 8-16 shows a solitary osteochondroma with a feathery cover of synovium. This particular osteochondroma was trapped in the medial compartment and partially attached to synovium there.

Multiple osteochondromas can be seen in the suprapatellar pouch (Fig. 8-17), and here they are adherent to synovium and surrounded by a widespread synovial inflammatory reaction with edema and the presence of chronic inflammatory villi.

Tumors of synovium are rarely seen by physicians, but the final illustration, Fig. 8-18, was taken through a Watanabe no. 21 arthroscope. The patient had a thickened area in the suprapatellar pouch with recurrent effusion, and inspection revealed a hemorrhagic mass, which is shown here and which on biopsy revealed itself to be a synovioma.

The rate of *complications* of arthroscopy for synovial lesions is just fractionally higher than that seen in simple orthopedic conditions. Part of this may be due to the age group in which many of the patients suffering from arthritis fall. Also one has to be aware of the recurrent effusion, the possibility of infection, and in those cases where varicose veins are present, the remote possibility of venous thrombosis.

The *advantages* of synovial arthroscopy include the facts that it is an accurate and fast procedure, it is simple and relatively atraumatic, it is inexpensive and painless, and finally it is acceptably repeatable as far as the patient is concerned. Since it can be performed under either local or general anesthesia, the use of the former method permits it to be done in an outpatient setting, thus reducing the financial burden on the patient and the Medicare system.

There is much that still has to be achieved in the field of synovial arthroscopy. Better lighting with lenses of even greater resolution will further improve our visual conception of arthritides. Faster films will improve our records until perhaps we reach the stage when routine serial arthroscopy in arthritis will become a reality. At

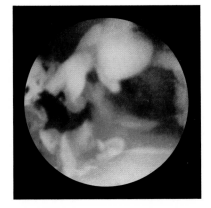
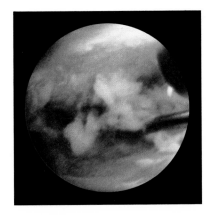

Fig. 8-17

Fig. 8-18

Fig. 8-17. Multiple osteochondromas. View of suprapatellar pouch showing an appearance not unlike stalagmites and stalactites surrounded by inflammatory change.

Fig. 8-18. Synovioma. Unsuspected friable mass in suprapatellar pouch. Note hemorrhagic appearance of area around tumor.

that time we will be able to evaluate and observe patients through the natural history of their disease with small cost and minimal discomfort and will be able to better understand that disease.

Suggested readings

Casscells, W. W.: Arthroscopy of the knee joint, J. Bone Joint Surg. [Am.] **53**:287, 1971.

Delbarre, Aignan, and Ghozlan: L'arthroscopie du genou, Institute of Rheumatology, Faculty of Medicine, Paris, 1976, Cochin.

Jackson, R. W., and Abe, I.: Role of arthroscopy in the management of disorders of the knee, J. Bone Joint Surg. [Br.] **54**:310, 1972.

Jayson, M. S. and Dixon, A. S.: Arthroscopy of the knee in rheumatic diseases, Ann. Rheum. Dis. **27**:503, 1968.

Robles-Gil, J., and Katona, G.: Arthroscopy as a means of diagnosis and investigation, Exerpta Medico Foundation, International Congress Series **145**:16, 1968.

Robles-Gil, J., and Katona, G.: Arthroscopy as a means of diagnosis and research, Proceeding of the Fourth Panama Congress on Rheumatology, Amsterdam, 1969, Exerpta Medica Foundation, p. 209.

Sakakibara: Arthroscopic study on Iino's band (plica synovialis medicopatellaris), J. Jpn. Orthop. Assoc. **50**(7):513, 1976.

Takeda: Relationship Between arthroscopic findings and histological change of the synovial membrane, J. Jpn. Orthop. Assoc. 34, 1960.

Watanabe, M., Takeda, S., and Ikeuchi, H.: Atlas of arthroscopy, ed. 2, Tokyo, 1969, Igaku Shoin Ltd.

Arthrography

Harry J. Griffiths

DISEASES OF THE SYNOVIUM

Many of the diseases that involve the synovium have characteristic, plain-film roentgenographic features. These include chondrocalcinosis, which occurs in hyperparathyroidism, gout, and pseudogout; juxtaarticular erosions and osteoporosis, which occur in rheumatoid arthritis; and destruction or invasion of bone, which occurs in synovial tumors. However, there are three situations in which arthrography is of proven use: in the diagnosis of Baker cysts, to define the degree of damage caused by synovial proliferation in rheumatoid arthritis, and to define the exact extent of tumors and more specifically to diagnose villonodular synovitis.

BAKER CYSTS

Many different terms are used to describe posterior outpouchings of the capsule of the knee joint: popliteal bursa, semimembranosogastrocnemial bursa, popliteal cyst, and Baker cyst. The small posterior outpouching frequently seen in a knee joint adequately distended with air at arthrography is normal and is properly called the "popliteal bursa." All other cystic connections to the posterior knee joint are abnormal and will be described in this chapter using the generic term "Baker cysts" because this is the phrase most commonly used throughout the world.*

---

*References 1, 2, 6, 9, 10, and 12.

Baker cysts occur in three situations. First, there are some congenital Baker cysts that lie under the tibial head of the gastrocnemius muscle or the semimembranosus muscle and represent accessory bursae.[9] These are usually of no significance and will not be considered further here. Second, in patients with long-standing rheumatoid arthritis, large Baker cysts with multiple ramifications and synovial proliferation are often seen.[3,7,11] Third, Baker cysts can occur after trauma in which there is a direct association with meniscal tears.[6]

The roentgenographic diagnosis of Baker cysts is based on the arthrographic findings. Two factors must be taken into consideration: first, that if double-contrast arthrography is used, frequently only air or gas will enter the cyst, and the diagnosis thus becomes unnecessarily difficult. Second, in order to outline the true contours of

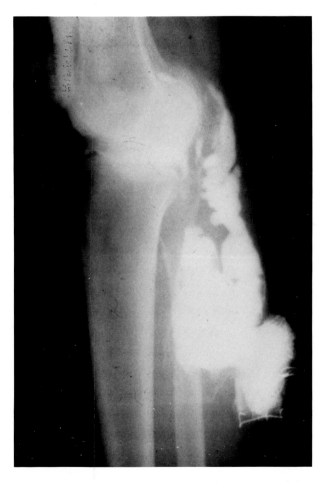

Fig. 8-19. Delayed film of rheumatoid popliteal cyst. In this patient with long-standing rheumatoid arthritis a single-contrast arthrogram demonstrated a multilocular cyst with many ramifications. Previous surgical removal had been attempted. (Courtesy Dr. Leland Sosmand.)

the cyst it is often necessary to take delayed films. Hence the correct radiologic approach is to inject 35 ml of iodinated contrast material into the joint and to get the patient to gently exercise the leg (by walking up and down the room for example) and to take lateral or oblique films or both at 15, 30, and 60 minutes and occasionally if necessary at 1½, 2, and 3 hours. Should a double-contrast study be considered necessary, it is easy to replace the needle into the knee joint, to remove as much positive-contrast material as possible, and to inject air as a secondary procedure.[4]

With the overgrowth of the synovium that occurs in rheumatoid arthritis, the intraarticular pressure rises, and Baker cysts are common. Moreover they often have multiple ramifications down the back of the calf, and, of course, parts of the cyst may become disconnected from the knee joint itself.[1,2,8,11,12] Some patients with rheumatoid Baker cysts have enormous cysts (Fig. 8-19), and with others the cysts become so full of synovial mucus that it often proves impossible to delineate the whole extent of the cyst (Fig. 8-20). Finally with respect to rheumatoid Baker cysts, in an acute exacerbation of the rheumatoid arthritis the cyst may rupture, and it is then possible to demonstrate the rupture arthrographically[1,2,5,7] (Fig. 8-21), which is important because the differential diagnosis includes deep-vein thrombosis, which has a very different form of therapy.

Traumatic Baker cysts are associated with meniscal injuries in the majority of

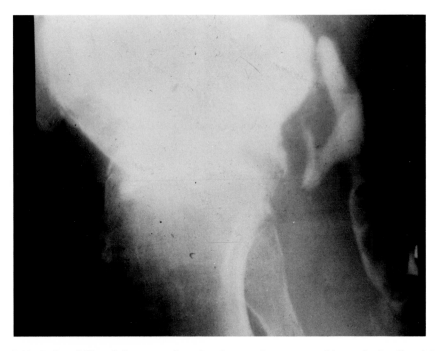

Fig. 8-20. Delayed film of rheumatoid popliteal cyst. This 63-year-old man had suffered from rheumatoid arthritis for 30 years and had multiple cysts removed from his calf at different times. This single-contrast arthrogram demonstrates one cyst, packed full of mucous material.

cases. If the congenital and rheumatoid cysts are excluded, and a Baker cyst is found arthrographically, it behooves the radiologist to search for a meniscal injury. Classically a posttraumatic Baker cyst is associated with a tear of the posterior horn of the medial meniscus, but any part of either meniscus may be torn. In most arthrographers' experience, some 85% of posttraumatic Baker cysts are associated with tears, although Lindblom[6] in an autopsy study found all the Baker cysts were associated with meniscal tears. It is important for the arthrographer to demonstrate the connection between the knee joint and the cyst and to show how many interconnecting channels are present and how large the cyst itself has become (Fig. 8-22). These are best visualized using single positive–contrast arthrography as stated earlier.[4]

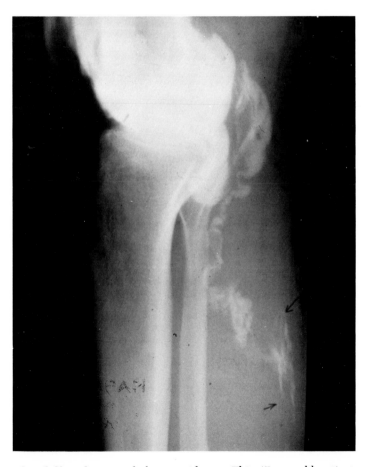

Fig. 8-21. Delayed film of ruptured rheumatoid cyst. This 45-year-old patient complained of calf pain. A single-contrast arthrogram demonstrated a multilocular popliteal cyst with serpiginous ramifications. Delayed film illustrated the contrast leaking out into soft tissues (*arrows*) at site of rupture. (From Griffiths, H. J.: Orthop. Rev. **5**(9):71, 1976.)

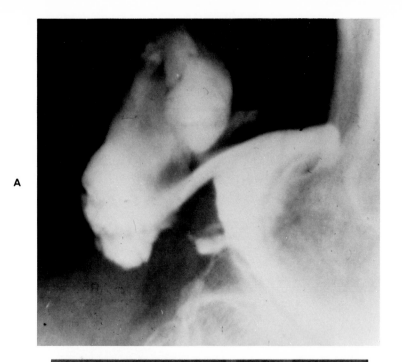

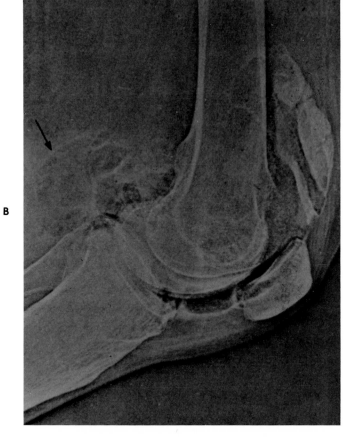

Fig. 8-22. For legend see opposite page.

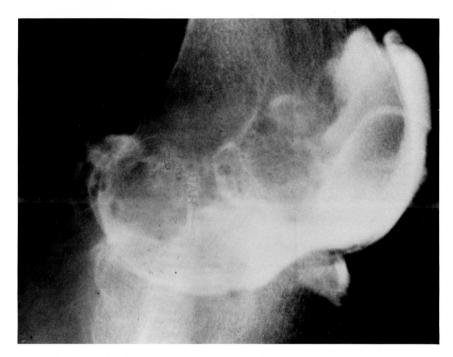

Fig. 8-23. Rheumatoid arthritis. A single-contrast arthrogram demonstrates multiple smooth filling defects in knee of 47-year-old woman with long-standing rheumatoid arthritis. (From Griffiths, H. J.: Orthop. Rev. **5**(9):71, 1976.)

SYNOVIAL PROLIFERATIVE DISEASES: RHEUMATOID ARTHRITIS

The diagnosis of rheumatoid arthritis is often a clinical one in association with characteristic changes seen in the hands, wrists, and feet: juxtaarticular erosions, osteoporosis, narrowing of articular cartilage space, and effusions, all seen best in the larger joints. With respect to the knee, the diagnosis of small effusions is discussed elsewhere in this book, and the demonstration of Baker cysts is discussed above. Apart from these, the arthrographic picture is one of synovial overgrowth with multiple fronds and filling defects (Fig. 8-23). In conjunction with the clinical picture and the roentgenographic picture, the diagnosis of rheumatoid arthritis is simple.[5,11,12]

Fig. 8-22. Posttraumatic popliteal cysts. **A,** In this 40-year-old man who had a recent injury to his knee, apart from a posterior horn medial meniscus tear, there was a popliteal cyst. Single-contrast arthrography demonstrated connection between cyst and knee joint. **B,** This 26-year-old woman who had fallen off a horse had a posttraumatic popliteal cyst, here demonstrated using xeroradiography at termination of a double-contrast arthrogram. Tear of anterior horn of medial meniscus is also demonstrated. (**A** from Griffiths, H. J.: Orthop. Rev. **5**(9):71, 1976.)

SYNOVIAL TUMORS: VILLONODULAR SYNOVITIS

There are many synovial tumors, both benign and malignant, including synovial chondrosarcomas, synoviomas, and fibromas, but the only one in which arthrography is useful is in the diagnosis of villonodular synovitis.[4,10,13] This tumor is usually benign and is associated with extensive synovial overgrowth. It may involve any joint in the body, although it is relatively common in the knee. In the early stages there are no plain-film findings apart from a soft tissue mass. In the later stages, villonodular synovitis may cause pressure defects and produce cysts in adjacent bone,[13] and should it become malignant (usually turning into a fibrosarcoma) then direct invasion and destruction of bone will occur.

The arthrographic appearances of villonodular synovitis are characteristic, with marked proliferation of synovium, the appearance of multiple fronds often localized

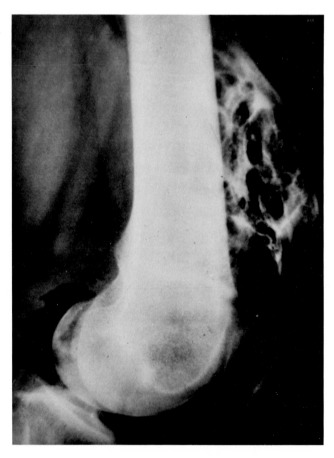

Fig. 8-24. Villonodular synovitis. A double-contrast arthrogram demonstrated a large multi-nodular filling defect in superior patella bursa, which was shown to be villonodular synovitis at surgery (Courtesy Dr. Murray Dalinka.)

to one part of the knee joint, and loss of volume of the joint itself[4,19,13] (Fig. 8-24). Presumably other synovial tumors would appear similar, although fibromas, myxomas, and lipomas are usually unilocular and appear as single, well-circumscribed, filling defects, frequently in the suprapatellar bursa.

SUMMARY

Arthrography is useful in the delineation of Baker cysts, both with respect to their connection to the knee joint as well as their ramifications down the leg. Arthrographically the appearance of rheumatoid arthritis is that of a synovial proliferative disease, and an arthrogram can also demonstrate concomitant Baker cysts, articular damage, and meniscal degeneration. In villonodular synovitis and other synovial tumors arthrography will delineate the extent of the tumor and often confirm the diagnosis.

References

1. Clark, J. M.: Arthrography diagnosis of synovial cysts of the knee, Radiology 115:480-481, 1975.
2. Dixon, A. S., and Grant, C.: Acute synovial rupture in rheumatoid arthritis. Clinical and experimental observations, Lancet 1:742-745, 1964.
3. Hall, A. P., and Scott, J. T.: Synovial cysts and rupture of the knee joint in rheumatoid arthritis. An arthrographic study, Ann. Rheum. Dis. 25:32-40, 1966.
4. Horns, J. W.: Single contrast knee arthrography in abnormalities of the articular cartilage, Radiology 105:537-540, 1972.
5. Lapayowker, M. D., Cliff, M. M., and Tourtellotte, C. D.: Arthrography in the diagnosis of calf pain, Radiology 95:319-323, 1970.
6. Lindblom, K.: Arthrography of the knee joint, Acta Radiol. [Suppl.] (Stockh.) 7, 1948.
7. Myles, A. B.: Posterior synovial leaks in arthritis of the knee, Proc. R. Soc. Med. 64:262-264, 1971.
8. Perri, J. A., Rodnan, G. P., and Mankin, H. J.: Giant synovial cysts of the calf in patients with rheumatoid arthritis, J. Bone Joint Surg. [Am.] 50:709-718, 1968.
9. Ricklin, P., Rüttiman, A., and Del Buono, M. S.: Meniscus lesions, New York, 1971, Grune & Stratton.
10. Staple, T. W.: Extrameniscal lesions demonstrated by double-contrast arthrography of the knee, Radiology 102:311-319, 1972.
11. Taylor, A. R.: Arthrography of the knee in rheumatoid arthritis, Br. J. Radiol. 42:493-497, 1969.
12. Weissman, B. N. W., and Sosman, J. L.: The radiology of rheumatoid arthritis, Orthop. Clin. North Am. 6:653-674, 1975.
13. Wolfe, R. D., and Giuliano, V. J.: Double-contrast arthrography in the diagnosis of pigmented villonodular synovitis of the knee, Am. J. Roentgenol. Radium Ther. Nucl. Med. 110:793-799, 1970.

9. Lesions of articular cartilage

Arthroscopic classification

Ralph T. Lidge

Lesions of the articular or hyaline cartilage as visualized by arthroscopy may be classified as to origin, location, and cause.

ORIGIN

Dechondral	From the surface
Intrachondral	From within
Subchondral	From below
Osteochondral	From both bone and cartilage

Dechondral lesions

The dechondral lesion, or a lesion from the cartilaginous surface, is invisible to the naked eye. It manifests itself in the synovial fluid as specks of cartilage and has been given the descriptive term "cartilage snow" by Johnson (Fig. 9-1).

Larger particles, several millimeters in size, that can be visualized on careful examination in the aspiration from the knee joint, are commonly seen in the supra-patellar pouch wedged between the femur and tibia (Fig. 9-2) or lying free in the

Fig. 9-1 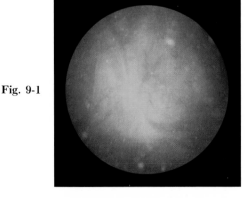 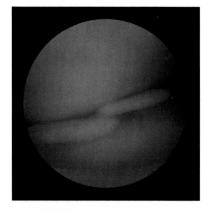 Fig. 9-2

Fig. 9-1. Chondral snow. Specks of cartilage invisible to naked eye.
Fig. 9-2. Particles of cartilage trapped between femoral and tibial condyle.

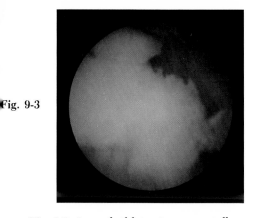

Fig. 9-3

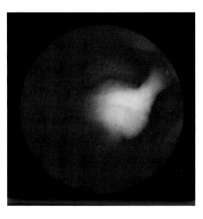

Fig. 9-4

Fig. 9-3. Large hail lying in suprapatellar pouch.
Fig. 9-4. Small hail in gutter being engulfed by synovia.

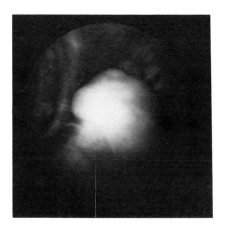

Fig. 9-5

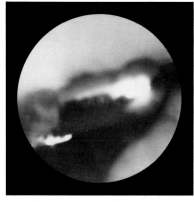

Fig. 9-6

Fig. 9-5. Hail adherent to synovia and being absorbed by same.
Fig. 9-6. Probing of undersurface of patella with a Verres needle to determine presence of soft, yielding, surface chondromalacia grade I.

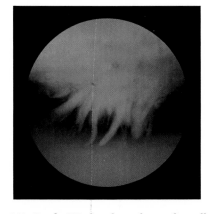

Fig. 9-7

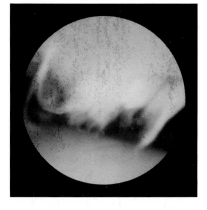

Fig. 9-8

Fig. 9-7. Grade III chondromalacia of patella. Example of recurrent subluxation.
Fig. 9-8. Grade III chondromalacia of patella; patella compression syndrome. Note patellar facies of lower femur appears intact.

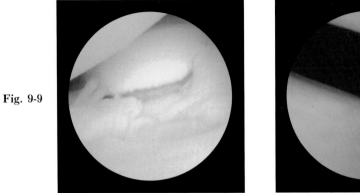

Fig. 9-9

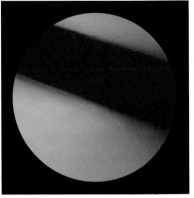

Fig. 9-1

Fig. 9-9. Grade IV chondromalacia: ulceration, chondrolysis, patellar facies of lower femur.
Fig. 9-10. Normal patellofemoral joint. Note color, contour, and continuity.

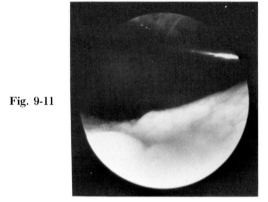

Fig. 9-11

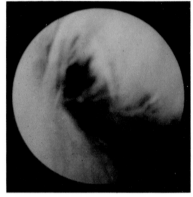

Fig. 9-12

Fig. 9-11. Degenerative changes involving both patella, grade II, and femur, grade IV.
Fig. 9-12. Degenerative osteoarthrosis: grade III of patella, grade II of femur.

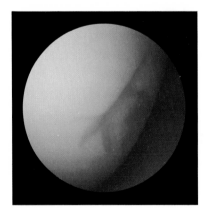

Fig. 9-13. Chondral crater or ulcer, site of previous trauma. Note stellatelike fissuring of medial femoral condyle, an intrachondral lesion.

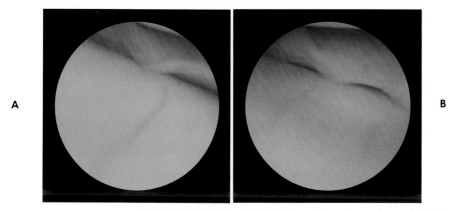

Fig. 9-14. A, Intrachondral lesion. Note vertical fracture line through cartilage of tibial plateau. **B,** Same area after methylene blue staining. Parallel tracking is now revealed with fracture lines through cartilage.

gutter (Figs. 9-3 to 9-5). The term "chondral hail" is appropriate in describing this condition. During arthrotomy, however, these particles are commonly not visualized.

Intrachondral lesions

The intrachondral form of articular cartilage change is usually termed "chondromalacia," or "softening of the cartilage," and can be divided into four types.

Grade I	Grossly normal but soft and yielding on probing
Grade II	Irregular with evidence of fibrillation
Grade III	Roughened, shaggy, and furlike
Grade IV	Fragmented, ulcerated, with evidence of chondrolysis

Lesions of the intrachondral cartilage, namely, chondromalacia, may be classified according to location and cause.

Patella. The patella is a common site of chondromalacia (Fig. 9-6). Changes may be more common secondary to congenital causes, such as increased mobility associated with subluxating or dislocating tendency (Fig. 9-7), compression syndrome (Fig. 9-8), trauma, degeneration, and iatrogenesis.

Lower anterior femur. The patellar facies of the lower femur may show an isolated lesion, and the surface of the patella may be free of change (Fig. 9-9). This condition is relatively uncommon and appears to be due, in great part, to local trauma or degenerative phenomena.

Patellofemoral joint. The patellofemoral articulation involving both patella and patellar facies of the lower femur (Fig. 9-10) often shows a combined lesion, which in most instances is more advanced in the patella than in the femur (Figs. 9-11 and 9-12).

Condyles. The condylar surface of the femur and tibia are commonly associated

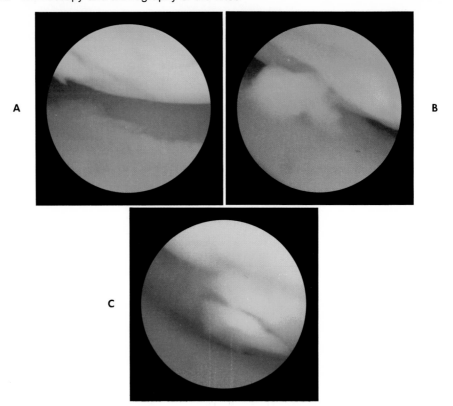

Fig. 9-15. **A,** Football player sustained an injury to lateral aspect of knee and was unable to bear full weight on same. Arthroscopy revealed a partial transverse tear of lateral meniscus, middle third, with adjoining intrachondral fracture of lateral femoral condyle. **B,** Fallout of portion of cartilage of lateral femoral condyle. **C,** Close-up of adjacent chondral fracture next to fallout.

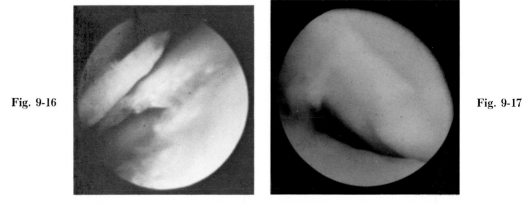

Fig. 9-16. Tear of medial meniscus with adjoining loose piece of hyaline cartilage from neighboring medial femoral condyle.

Fig. 9-17. Grade IV chondromalacia of lateral femoral condyle after old fracture of lateral tibial condyle.

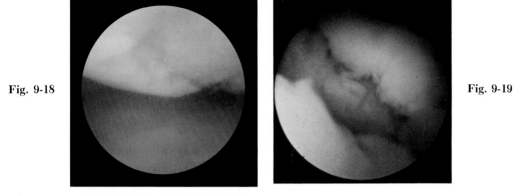

Fig. 9-18

Fig. 9-19

Fig. 9-18. Grade IV advanced chondromalacia of medial femoral condyle after surgical medial meniscectomy. Note area of ulceration. Tibia shows grade II chondromalacia.

Fig. 9-19. Grade IV chondromalacia of medial femoral condyle. Severe chondrolysis with exposed subchondral bone after surgical meniscectomy.

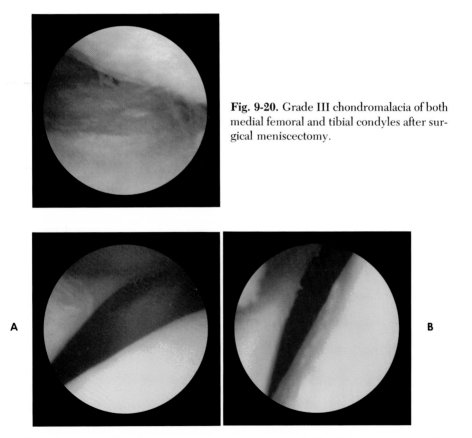

Fig. 9-20. Grade III chondromalacia of both medial femoral and tibial condyles after surgical meniscectomy.

A

B

Fig. 9-21. A, Medial shelf with knee in extension. **B,** Medial shelf with knee in flexion. Note area of reactive chondromalacia, cartilage change manifested by irregularity of surface of cartilage of medial femoral condyle with flattening at site of impingement.

with chondromalacia. Trauma is a leading cause, whether primary (Figs. 9-13 and 9-14) or secondary to lesions associated with meniscal injury (Figs. 9-15 to 9-17).

Degenerative changes (Figs. 9-18 to 9-20) can be secondary to wear and tear. Chondromalacia may exist before and after meniscectomy. Compression and impingement are also responsible. The compression may be congenital and caused by a dislocating or subluxating patella, and the impingement caused by a medial shelf against the medial femoral condyle (Fig. 9-21). Iatrogenic causes associated with surgical attempts to correct the patellar abnormalities can cause chondromalacia (Fig. 9-22).

Subchondral lesions

The subchondral lesion, below the cartilage, resulting in changes in the articular surface, is exemplified by subchondrolysis and manifested by elevation of the cartilaginous surface. When a subchondral lesion is found, it is usually in the tibial condyles (Figs. 9-23 and 9-24). The exact cause is not known and may be secondary to trauma or to a degenerative phenomena. It appears to represent a cleavage through the cartilage-bone junction site.

Osteochondral lesions

The osteochondral lesion is the combined form of lesion, involving both bone and cartilage. The joint location may be peripheral or central. The usual site of change is at the peripheral cartilage, is thought to be degenerative, and is commonly called "osteoarthritis." It is characterized by so-called marginal lipping or spurring (Figs. 9-25 to 9-27). The central area of change is best manifested by osteochondritis dissecans. This condition can be divided into four categories.

Fig. 9-22   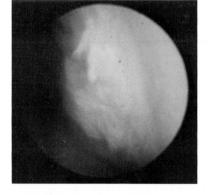 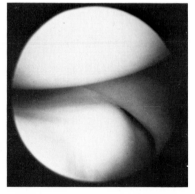   Fig. 9-23

Fig. 9-22. Iatrogenic grade III chondromalacia of medial aspect of medial femoral condyle following Hauser procedure secondary to patella compression.
Fig. 9-23. Subchondrolysis. Subchondral lesion with elevation of articular surface of tibial condyle, forming either a slight bulge or a peaking.

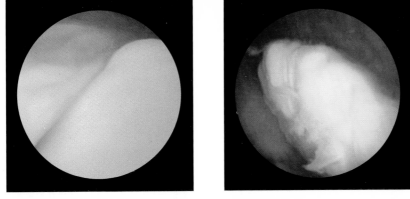

Fig. 9-24

Fig. 9-25

Fig. 9-24. Another case of subchondrolysis with similar findings. Note adjacent meniscus.
Fig. 9-25. Osteochondral lesion with marginal osteochondral proliferation of the medial femoral condyle.

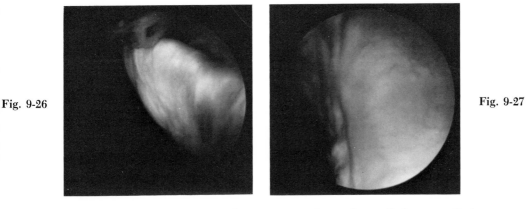

Fig. 9-26

Fig. 9-27

Fig. 9-26. Knee with findings similar to those in Fig. 9-25, namely, a rolled osteocartilaginous border.
Fig. 9-27. Rolled osteocartilaginous border of patellar facies of lower femur; a suprapatellar approach via arthroscope.

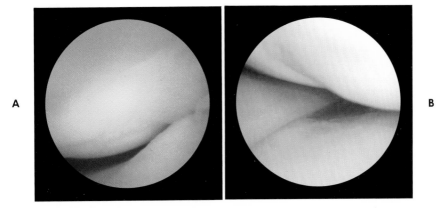

A

B

Fig. 9-28. A, Grade II osteochondritis dissecans with so-called blister formation. **B,** Same lesion as in **A** with methylene blue inserted to reduce highlights and to show marginal fissuring.

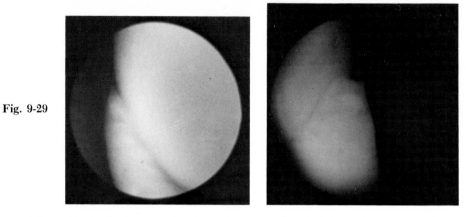

Fig. 9-29

Fig. 9-30

Fig. 9-29. Grade III osteochondritis dissecans of medial femoral condyle with peripheral fracture.

Fig. 9-30. Grade III osteochondritis dissecans with increased separation but no fallout as yet. There is a step-off-like picture to surface of hyaline cartilage.

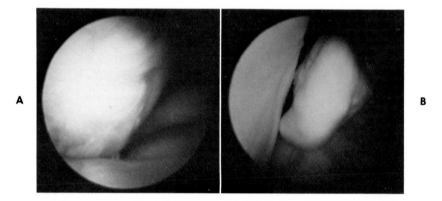

A

B

Fig. 9-31. A, Grade IV osteochondritis dissecans of medial femoral condyle. There exists a complete fallout of the loose body and a lacelike network, covering residual cartilage surface with appearance of a fibrocartilage. **B,** Same knee as in **A** with loose body in medial gutter. Irregularity to area of fallout from substance of medial femoral condyle in same patient. Loose osteochondral body is noted adjacent to femoral condyle.

Grade I. A grade I osteochondral lesion is a smooth surface with no gross evidence of structural change. However, when the area is probed with an instrument such as a spinal needle with stylet a soft sensation is noted after penetration through the outer layer of cartilage. This area of softness is the site of separation of the first few layers of subchondral bone and cartilage from the underlying bone.

Grade II. Grade II is the bulging or blister variety of osteochondral lesion, in which there is a slight elevation of the condylar surface with a marginal fissure. This is usually present along the lateral aspect of the medial femoral condyle. One can barely

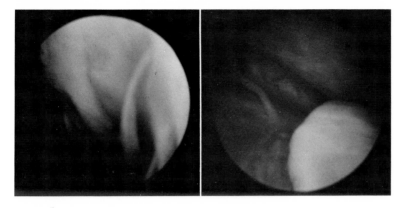

Fig. 9-32. Another patient with same findings as noted in Fig. 9-31.

see the faint bulge, but if this is treated with methylene blue to eliminate the highlights a characteristic demarcation exists (Fig. 9-28).

Grade III. The grade III osteochondral lesion demonstrates a partial dropout of the area of osteochondritis dissecans. There is a step-off, rather sharply demarcated, of the cartilaginous surface (Figs. 9-29 and 9-30).

Grade IV. The grade IV osteochondral lesion exists as a complete separation with fallout of a loose body. The cartilaginous surface at this point is irregular, with a shallow crater; it shows evidence of healing with cartilage that has the gross appearance of a hyalinelike or fibrocartilaginous substance. The loose body is usually found in the vicinity (Figs. 9-31 and 9-32).

SUMMARY

To summarize, lesions of the articular cartilage noted via arthroscopy may be classified in the following way.
  A. By origin
    1. Dechondral: from the surface
    2. Intrachondral: from within
    3. Subchondral: from below
    4. Osteochondral: from both bone and cartilage
  B. By location
    1. Patella
    2. Patellar facies of lower femur
    3. Patellofemoral joint
    4. Condylar: femoral or tibial
  C. By common causes
    1. Congenital
    2. Traumatic
    3. Degenerative
    4. Iatrogenic

Arthroscopic and cadaver knee investigations

S. Ward Casscells

Of all the tissues in or about the knee joint, the articular cartilage is the most important, and, in truth, the fate of the knee joint depends upon the integrity of the articular cartilage. Epiphyseal bone heals promptly and with no particular difficulty, ligaments can be repaired or replaced, torn menisci removed, and diseased synovia excised, but what of articular cartilage? When this cartilage is damaged, will it undergo progressive degradation, or will it at times heal and, if so, under what circumstances? Toward a better understanding of this subject, material will be presented on lesions of the articular cartilage seen arthroscopically; also included are results of an investigation of cadaver knees undertaken some years ago. Material will be presented on the incidence of these lesions, their location in the knee joint, and possible etiology. The discussion will be in two parts, first those lesions involving the patellofemoral joint, and second those involving the weight-bearing area of the tibiofemoral joint.

PATELLOFEMORAL JOINT

Historically chondromalacia has been a term reserved for lesions of the patella, and the older German writers such as Heine[8] and Owre[13] considered it a disease entity and argued about its etiology and its significance. Although the physical appearance of the lesion on the patella is at times different from that seen elsewhere in the knee joint, the patella is peculiar in that it has the thickest cartilage of any joint in the body and is subject to a wider variety of forces than is any other articular surface. However, there is no evidence to suggest that chondromalacia is peculiar to the patella, at least etiologically, and the term will be used to refer to lesions elsewhere in the joint. The word probably should be reserved for mild and early changes in the articular cartilage, which with time may progress to the point where a better term would be "degenerative joint disease" or "osteoarthritis." This is in accord with Sokoloff's use of these terms.

Cadaver knees

In discussing chondromalacia of the patellofemoral area, an understanding of the local anatomy and the forces acting through this joint is important, as they have a direct bearing on the incidence and probably the etiology of these lesions. The figures about to be presented are the result of an investigation I carried out on 369 unselected cadaver knees whose average age was 70 years, with 92% of the specimens 50 years of age or over.[2a]

The width of the lateral femoral condyle anteriorly (Fig. 9-33) is considerably wider than that of the medial condyle, just as the lateral patellar facet is wider than the medial facet; in the femur this lateral-medial ratio is approximately 65:35. Also the average height of the lateral condyle above that of the medial is 4.5 mm with a range of 0 to 10 mm (Fig. 9-33). The intervening groove or sulcus (Fig. 9-34) averaged 5.2 mm in depth, again with a rather wide range of 2 to 10 mm. Some years ago

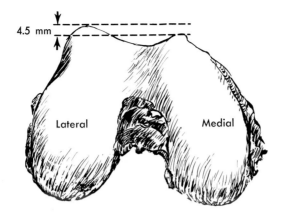

Fig. 9-33. Average increased height of lateral femoral condyle over medial condyle in cadaver knees.

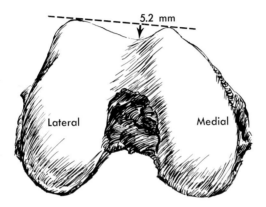

Fig. 9-34. Average depth and configuration of sulcus in cadaver knees.

Brattstrom[2] measured the heights of the condyles by roentgenograms and found the average height of the lateral condyle above the medial condyle to be 4.06 mm. Not too much importance should be attached to these measurements, as considerable variation from the norm is found, both in knees where there were cartilaginous defects and also in those that were perfectly normal. However, gross dysplasia of the anterior femur that predisposes to subluxation and dislocation is an important etiologic factor in patellar chondromalacia.

The clinical significance of forces exerted on the patellofemoral joint is not entirely clear. These forces have been calculated and measured by Haxton,[7] Kettlecamp,[10] and Perry[14]; while not agreeing entirely, they all have found loads much greater than elsewhere in the body, with figures of three or four times the body weight when the weight is borne on the knee flexed at 30° and approximately 7.5 times body weight while squatting. Kettlecamp[10] estimated that the forces were 3.3

times body weight on going up stairs. Thus when one considers that the patel-lofemoral joint is subject to forces such as normal loading of the patella as it moves in a caudad-cephalad direction and is also subject to torsional and shearing stresses, especially in athletes, it is not surprising that this cartilage is most often damaged, and the incidence of chondromalacia of the patella is higher than elsewhere in the body.

Table 1 shows the incidence of these lesions, their location, and severity. A grade I lesion is a small and superficial area of erosion 1 cm or less in diameter (Fig. 9-35). Grade II lesions (Fig. 9-36) are 1 to 2 cm in diameter with some of the deeper layers of the cartilage involved. Grade III lesions (Fig. 9-37) are 2 to 4 cm in diameter with bone exposed. In grade IV lesions (Fig. 9-38) the entire articular cartilage has usually disappeared. As to the location of the lesions, the process does

Table 1. Incidence of patellar lesions by grade and location

Grade	Incidence (percent)	Location	Incidence (percent)
0	37	Medial facet	25
I	25	Ridge	12
II	27	Lateral facet	12
III	6	Generalized	51
IV	5		

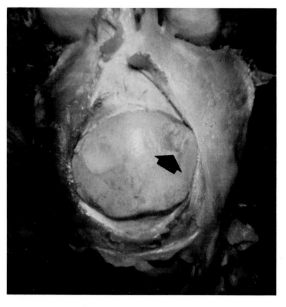

Fig. 9-35. Grade I small superficial lesion, medial facet; base smooth, edges appear to be filling in.

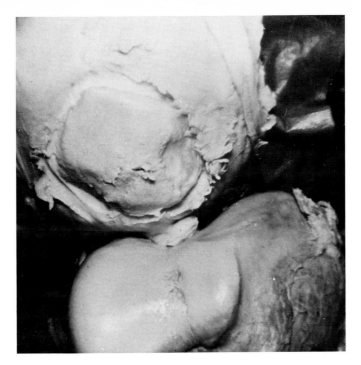

Fig. 9-36. Grade II lesion of femur and patella with deeper layers of cartilage involved.

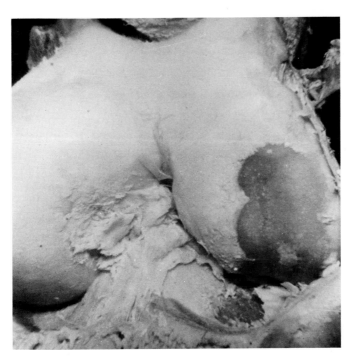

Fig. 9-37. Grade III lesion of lateral femoral condyle and tibia. Edges of lesion are beveled, and there is no spur formation. Gross appearance of a rapidly advancing lesion.

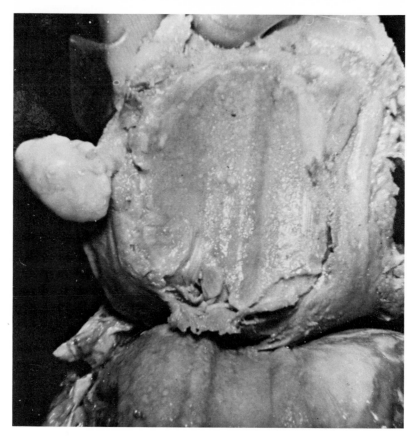

Fig. 9-38. Grade IV lesion with complete loss of articular cartilage in patella and femur with "tram tracks."

Table 2. Incidence of anterior femur lesions by grade and location

Grade	Incidence (percent)	Location	Incidence (percent)
0	52	Medial femoral condyle	19
I	17	Sulcus	34
II	14	Lateral femoral condyle	20
III	8	Generalized	27
IV	9		

not universally start on the medial facet, as has been stated in the past, though isolated lesions do seem to be found medially more often than elsewhere.

Table 2 shows the incidence, severity, and location of the lesions found on the anterior femoral surface; by definition this includes any part of the femur with which the patella articulates, whether in flexion or in extension.

The finding that 37% of the patellae had normal articular surfaces, and only 11%

were graded III or IV may be surprising to those who think that generalized and severe osteoarthritis of the knee is a universal disease of the aged, regardless of their exposure to trauma. Unfortunately no information on the background of these specimens was available, but it is probably true that people born about the turn of the century, as these individuals were, had less opportunity to participate in sports, suffered fewer injuries than the young people of today, and thus suffered less damage to their joints.

Arthroscopic findings

Statistics on the incidence of chondromalacia in clinical practice are not available, and if they were, they would be of doubtful significance, as not being representative of the general population. People who come seeking help from physicians have symptoms and often a history of injury, and the incidence of these lesions would vary with the type of clinical practice of the physician. The great advantage that accrues to the arthroscopist is that he has an abundance of clinical material and can correlate the clinical signs and symptoms with the gross appearance of these lesions, which cannot be done in a cadaver study.

An analysis of a personal series of 1,000 arthroscopic cases of patients from ages 15 to 60 showed that 10.2% of the patients had chondromalacia of the patella as the only pathologic finding in the joint, but it was present in combination with other pathology, such as meniscal tears in 22%.

These lesions of the patella cannot be located and graded as precisely as they can in the cadaver knee, and no attempt was made to do this at arthroscopy. It was noted that not infrequently such lesions were silent, producing no clinical signs or symptoms, and this was especially true of lesions located on the medial half of the medial facet. Even those with the more severe degrees of chondromalacia often had few complaints of pain, although patellar crepitus was usually present.

As was noted in the cadaver knees, lesions of the patella and the anterior femur may exist independently of one another; however, when there was a severe change on one surface, there was at least some minor disturbance of the opposing articular surface in most cases. A representative example of arthroscopic lesions of the patellofemoral joint is given in Fig. 9-39.

The cause of such lesions of the patellofemoral joint is known in some instances but unknown in others. We do know that trauma, such as direct blows over the patella and shearing and torsional forces that drive the patella laterally, can damage the articular surface, as can long-standing chronic subluxation of the patella with a tight lateral capsule that prevents the patella from tracking normally on the femur. In clinical practice, however, I see some lesions grossly similar to those in which there has been known trauma, but the patient recalls no specific injury. In these cases, a traumatic cause is suggested because the appearance is similar to those in which there has been known trauma, but this cannot be proven. The fact that 37% of these cadaver knees, age 70 years, had grossly normal articular cartilage is evidence that the cartilage does not break down and wear out with age. Nor is there much evidence

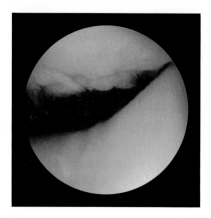

Fig. 9-39. Typical chondromalacia of patella, grade II, with very mild changes of opposing femoral surface.

that climate, diet, or genetic factors have any bearing on the production of these lesions. When one considers the anatomy and mechanical forces at play in the patellofemoral joint, the most likely cause of chondromalacia-type lesions appears to be trauma, either a single episode or repeated minor occurrences or some abnormal mechanical problem such as genu varum or genu valgum.

TIBIOFEMORAL JOINT
Cadaver knees

Lesions in this area of the knee joint occur less frequently than in the patellofemoral joint, where only 23% of the specimens showed lesions of some degree, either in the femur or the opposing tibial surface or both. Almost invariably the pathology was more severe on the femoral side (Figs. 9-37 and 9-45). These lesions were not graded as in the patellofemoral area and were not located as precisely. Although they occur less frequently, lesions in the weight-bearing area of the knee joint are of greater clinical importance, as they may lead to disability such as progressive varus or valgus deformity and are certainly pain producing to a greater extent than are lesions in the patellofemoral joint.

These defects on the articular cartilage vary widely in appearance as well as size (Fig. 9-40). These lesions have a punched-out appearance with sharp edges and the gross appearance of being rather stable. Other lesions (Fig. 9-37) have beveled edges and give the impression of progressing rather rapidly. There are also those lesions (Fig. 9-41) in which the edges are rounding off, and the defect itself seems to be filling in.

Of particular interest to the orthopedic surgeon is the relationship of such lesions to tears or degeneration of the meniscus. Powerful voices have been raised to support the theory that the majority, if not all, of these lesions of the articular surface are the result of torn menisci. Helfet[9] has stated that in the absence of any gross tear of the meniscus, lesions on the articular cartilage of the femur are the result of the so-called

Text continued on p. 131.

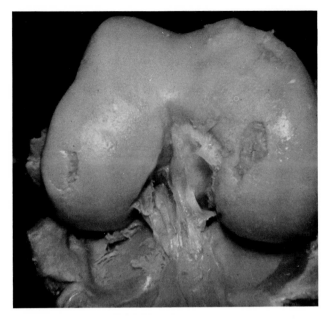

Fig. 9-40. Sharply punched-out lesions of both femoral condyles. Smaller lesion on lateral femoral condyle where meniscus is degenerated. Medial meniscus intact where there is a larger lesion of medial femoral condyle.

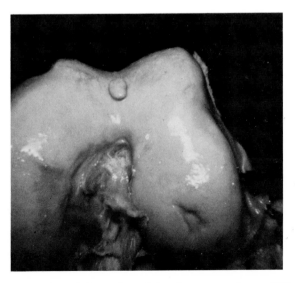

Fig. 9-41. Small defect on lateral femoral condyle, showing evidence of filling in of margins, has appearance of healing lesion with formerly loose body now attached to femur.

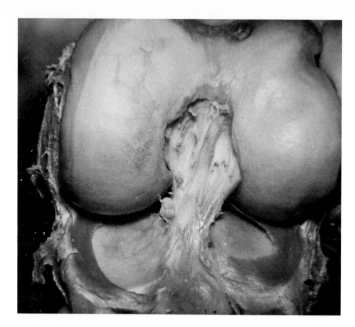

Fig. 9-42. Superficial lesion of medial femoral condyle with very minor changes in opposing tibial condyle; both menisci intact.

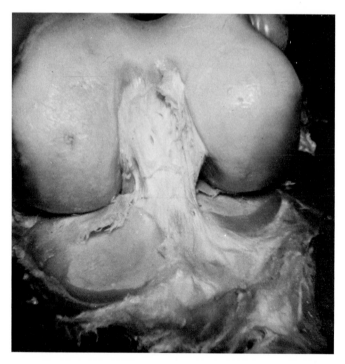

Fig. 9-43. Lateral condyle on right shows normal articular cartilage with tear and degeneration of posterior horn of lateral meniscus. Medial femoral condyle on left shows very small punched out lesion with tear and degeneration of posterior horn of medial meniscus.

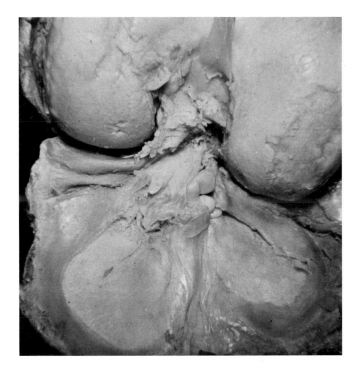

Fig. 9-44. Rather large lesions on both femoral condyles. Medial meniscus on left is intact. Lateral meniscus has small transverse tear of medial third.

"retracted anterior horn of the medial meniscus," which interferes with terminal rotation of the tibia on the femur. Anatomists, however, have always been aware of the fact that the tibial attachment of the anterior horn of the medial meniscus differs from that on the lateral meniscus, in that the anterior horn of the medial meniscus does not attach to the tibia at the base of the cruciate, as it does on the lateral meniscus. Fig. 9-42 shows what Helfet[9] refers to as a "retracted anterior horn," but, in truth, it is perfectly normal anatomy with an area of degeneration of the medial femoral condyle.

Smillie[15] too incriminates the meniscus and has referred to a torn meniscus as a "powerful force with great destructive power." He presents no statistics to support this theory, apparently feeling that the coexistence of a torn meniscus and degeneration of the articular cartilage proves that the latter causes the former.

In my group of 369 cadaver knees, there were 116 knees with some pathologic change in the weight-bearing area of the joint, either in the meniscus or the adjacent articular surface or both. In 52% of the cases, the menisci were essentially normal with varying degrees of degenerative change in the adjacent surfaces of either the tibia, femur, or both (Fig. 9-42). In 7.5% of the cases there was absence or degeneration of the meniscus but normal adjacent joint surfaces (Fig. 9-43). In the remaining 40% changes were present both in the articular cartilage and in the ipsilateral meniscus with no way of proving a cause-and-effect relationship. Fig. 9-44 illustrates

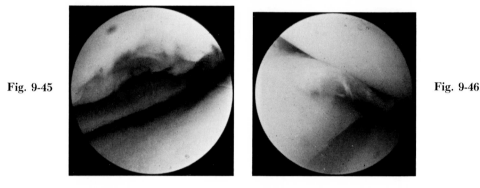

Fig. 9-45. Large punched-out lesion of weight-bearing surface of medial femoral condyle due to injury 1 week previously. Meniscus shows little change.
Fig. 9-46. Flap-type tear of medial meniscus with normal adjacent joint cartilage.

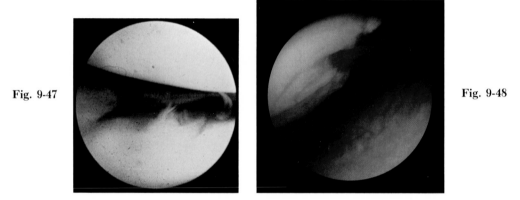

Fig. 9-47. Tear of posterior horn, lateral meniscus, with chondromalacia of lateral tibial condyle.
Fig. 9-48. Chronic degenerative disease of medial femoral condyle with loss of cartilage down to bone. Minor changes in opposing tibial surface.

typical lesions of femoral condyles, in which damage to the articular cartilage was usually more severe than that to the meniscus; it is difficult to think that such minor tears in the meniscus can cause serious damage to the cartilage.

Arthroscopic findings

I felt that it would be of some value to check these findings in the cadaver knees with a comparable but smaller group of patients whose knees were arthroscoped. One hundred and sixty-one consecutive knees that had been examined arthroscopically were reviewed. Of this group there were 100 in which there was some damage either to the meniscus or to the adjacent weight-bearing area of the joint. The average age of this group was 35, just half that of the cadaver knees. In 35% of these cases, there was some pathologic change in the weight-bearing area of the articular

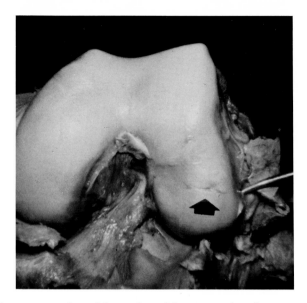

Fig. 9-49. Fine linear scar on lateral femoral condyle, 2 cm in length, opposite pointer. Well-healed lesion.

cartilage, but the adjacent meniscus was normal (Fig. 9-45). In 25% the reverse was true: the meniscus was torn or degenerated, but the joint surfaces were normal (Fig. 9-46). In the remaining 40% just as in the cadaver knees, there were lesions both in the meniscus and in the articular cartilage (Fig. 9-47). Thus just as in the cadaver knees the meniscus could not be incriminated as the cause of damage to the joint surface, and in the remaining 40% its role was undetermined. However, again as in the cadaver knees, the extent of the damage to the articular surface was in almost all the cases much more severe than that in the meniscus (Fig. 9-48).

Evidence in the literature that torn menisci cause any appreciable damage to the articular cartilage is scant. Dandy and Jackson's[4] report in 1975 seems to indicate that the longer a torn meniscus is left in the joint, the more likely the articular cartilage is to be damaged, but damage in their cases was so very minor, one would have to question the clinical significance. Tapper and Hoover[17] in a long-term follow-up of patients who had previously had meniscectomy found that the results were not related to the interval between the injury and the time the meniscus was excised. This was also true of the study done by Appel.[1] A more likely explanation is that the trauma that caused the meniscus to tear also injured the articular cartilage, and one cannot rule out the possibility that a badly damaged articular cartilage can injure the meniscus.

It is interesting and helpful to look critically at the physical appearance of these lesions of the articular cartilage. Those with a punched-out appearance and sharply demarcated edges (Fig. 9-40) are almost surely due to trauma. In the early stages of degenerative arthritis secondary to genu varum one sees a large superficial area of

A

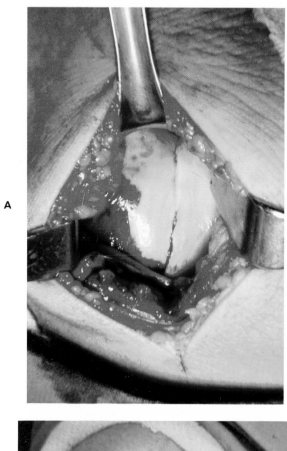

B

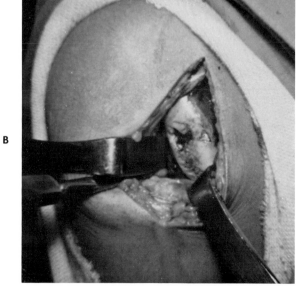

Fig. 9-50. Acute osteochondral fracture 1 week after injury.

cartilage erosion (Fig. 9-42). Occasionally there is definite evidence of repair, as evidenced by the filling in of the defects or even complete healing (Figs. 9-41 and 9-49).

OTHER LESIONS OF ARTICULAR CARTILAGE
Osteochondral fractures

Osteochondral fractures are quite common within the knee joint and may occur anywhere, including the patella, femur, or tibia. They vary widely in appearance, depending upon the direction and magnitude of the forces and may result in a fracture through the condyle (Fig. 9-50, *A*), or there may be much widespread damage to the joint surface (Fig. 9-50, *B*). These lesions can, of course, be seen arthroscopically, if one has the patience to wash the blood out of the knee joint. However, the need for arthroscopy is not as great as in the chondral lesions, as in most cases roentgenograms have already made the diagnosis.

Osteochondritis dissecans

Osteochondritis dissecans is one of the most interesting and perplexing lesions involving the articular cartilage; whether it is the result of trauma or some other factor is still not known. The condition may be unilateral or bilateral and is much more common in young men than in any other group. While the x-ray appearance is fairly characteristic, the gross appearance of the lesion may be quite varied. In the milder cases, there is little more than a softened area on the condyle with slight swelling. In other cases the edges are sharply demarcated, but the lesion is intact (Fig. 9-51). Lastly the lesion may be completely separated and fall into the joint (Fig. 9-52). The advantages of arthroscopy in this condition is obvious. It is of great value not only in planning the proper treatment but also as a follow-up in these cases whether surgery has been performed or not.

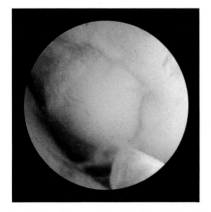
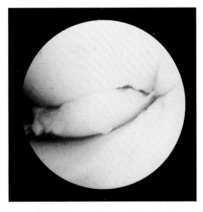

Fig. 9-51

Fig. 9-52

Fig. 9-51. Small area of osteochondritis dissecans, medial femoral condyle, lesion sharply circumscribed but not separated.
Fig. 9-52. Osteochondritis dissecans, medial femoral condyle, with complete separation of lesion.

In the past few years an attempt has been made to promote healing of these lesions by drilling them with a Kirschner wire at the time of arthroscopy, but the effects of this treatment are still unknown. Some lesions heal spontaneously after a period of a year or so, and others may remain unchanged over a period of 6 or 7 years. Removal of the lesion, curettage, and pinning it back with Kirschner wires have been carried out successfully; however, this usually requires a long period in a cast and a further period on crutches, and so the morbidity is rather long.[10a]

Degenerative arthritis

Another type of lesion is degenerative arthritis of the articular surface of the femur or the tibia in the weight-bearing area, which appears to be the result of abnormal mechanics such as genu varum or genu valgum. Such lesions start insidiously, and even when they have reached the stage where they produce some pain, the roentgenogram may show little or no change, although weight-bearing films may indicate some narrowing of one side of the joint. At arthroscopy, damage is more advanced than indicated by the roentgenogram, as it occurs over a wide area of the main weight-bearing portion of the femur and to a lesser extent of the tibia (Fig. 9-48). The meniscus on the ipsilateral side of the joint may show little or no change in the early stages, while later the posterior horn is degenerated to a greater or lesser degree but almost always much less severely than is the articular cartilage. Certainly the meniscal degeneration appears to be the result of the degenerative arthritis rather than the cause.

Rheumatoid arthritis

Other conditions can cause damage to the articular cartilage, such as rheumatoid arthritis, which is primarily a disease of the synovium but which can invade and undermine the cartilage quite rapidly with complete loss of the entire joint cartilage. This is contrasted with osteoarthritis, which tends to involve only one area of the joint.

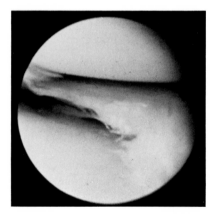

Fig. 9-53. Pseudogout with calcium pyrophosphate crystals in medial meniscus.

Gout and pseudogout

Gout and pseudogout are diseases that involve the articular cartilage, but their potential for doing serious damage to the cartilage is not as great as is that of rheumatoid arthritis. In my experience gout infrequently involves a larger joint such as the knee and is more commonly seen and treated by the rheumatologist rather than by the orthopedic surgeon. Pseudogout is more common than gout in the knee, the process often flaring up, especially after some traumatic episode, and presenting as an acute painful synovitis. In the later stages, roentgenograms show calcification of the meniscus (Fig. 9-53), and these deposits of calcium pyrophosphate are found scattered about in the articular cartilage (Fig. 9-54).

NATURAL HISTORY AND FATE OF ARTICULAR CARTILAGE

Although the older writers of many years ago, mainly the Germans, were uniformly pessimistic about the fate of articular cartilage, recent clinical studies such as this one, as well as laboratory observations by workers such as Meachim,[12] Mankin,[11] and Sokoloff[16] do not bear out this pessimism and strike a more optimistic note. Ekholm[5] in 1951 stated that present experiments demonstrate "that even in unfavorable circumstances, articular surfaces are very resistant to wear and tear, and it is possible under physiological conditions there is so little loss of surface tissue in the healthy adult joint that no multiplication of cartilage cells need occur to sustain cartilage." Sokoloff[16] in referring to the number of chondrocytes in articular cartilage

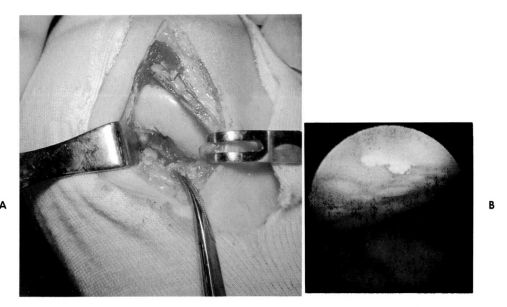

A   B

Fig. 9-54. B, Area of calcium pyrophosphate crystals in medial femoral condyle of a patient who had osteochondritic lesion removed 9 months before. Area shows healing that has taken place in medial femoral condyle since original lesion, **A,** which measured 2.5 cm in diameter.

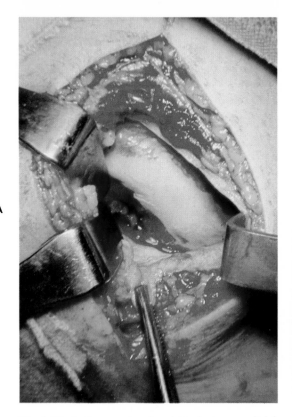

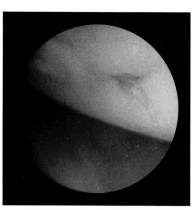

Fig. 9-55. A, Large osteochondritic lesion, medial femoral condyle, measuring 2 × 4 cm was completely separated. **B,** Base was curetted down to bleeding bone. Same lesion as in Fig. 9-24, **A,** 7 months later, showing healing that has taken place, although small defect in articular cartilage remains.

said that "most or all of the decrease per unit volume of histologic area takes place during the years of skeletal growth and not after that." In 1969 Meachim[12] found "surprisingly little evidence of a generalized aging change in properties of human articular cartilage 30 to 40 years of age." He further stated that "in middle and later years of adult life, there is no evidence of a generalized change with age." He regarded such a change, when present, "as a focal process with local factors at least partly responsible for its development." In 1969 Mankin[11] in experiments with rabbits showed that "cartilage is not inert but demonstrates an extremely active anabolic and catabolic system." Although changes in the ratio of the chondroitin sulfate to keratin sulfate appear to be altered in later years, the clinical significance of this is not understood. All these statements, which are for the most part the result of investigations in a laboratory, often using animal models, are certainly supported by the findings in these 369 cadaver knees. When articular cartilage is damaged, the lesions often remain stable for a number of years or progress very slowly. This is supported by the findings of very minor changes in the knees of cadavers in their 60s, 70s, or

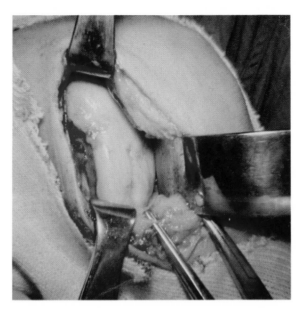

Fig. 9-56. Large healed defect 2 × 5 cm, medial condyle, showing spontaneous healing of an osteochondritic dissecans lesion. Large calcified loose body that originated in this defect was removed 8 years after initial injury in a 25-year-old man.

even 80s. Occasionally the articular cartilage breaks down rather rapidly, and fairly far advanced degenerative changes are seen in the articular cartilage of the knees of persons in their 20s and 30s. What triggers this rapid breakdown is not known, but it may be related to the release of lysosomal enzymes such as cathepsin after injury. Chrisman and Snook[3] have found in experiments with rabbits that salicylates appear to have controlled this response and induce healing. Prostaglandins are also thought to be involved in this process of cartilage breakdown.

As to the ability of cartilage to repair itself, there is no doubt that even some of the larger lesions, those measuring 2 × 4 cm, can fill in these defects when they are deep enough to involve the blood supply of bone, especially when bleeding bone is exposed (Figs. 9-54 and 9-55). This repair tissue does not have the ability to resist wear and tear, as does normal hyaline cartilage; in the experimental animal models, 50% or more of the defects tended to break down 6 to 12 months later. A very limited amount of experience with humans seems to indicate that this repair surface will hold up for a number of years. Fig. 9-56 illustrates a very acceptable surface 8 years after the initial injury. A biopsy of the area showed fibrocartilage (Fig. 9-57). Some 6 years later, when this young man became more athletically active, playing tennis, the joint cartilage, while acceptable, did not look as smooth and healthy as it had previously (Fig. 9-58).

Some years ago fresh defects in the articular cartilage were usually protected by non-weight-bearing and often a cast. However, recent experience, both clinical and experimental, has shown that early motion is desirable if the metaplasia is to proceed

Fig. 9-57. Photomicrograph of margin of lesion, showing fibrocartilage.

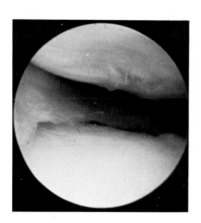

Fig. 9-58. Arthroscopic view of lesion seen in Fig. 9-56 5 years later and 13 years after initial injury. Articular cartilage, while not normal, has survived quite well.

beyond the point of fibrous tissue and become fibrocartilage, and probably, early weight bearing is desirable. The individual shown in Fig. 9-55, *B,* had no treatment in the first 8 years, walking on the joint continuously until the time a large loose body was removed. A photomicrograph of a biopsy taken at the time of surgery is shown in Fig. 9-56.

When the vascular supply to the bone and cartilage has not been violated, the prognosis, of course, is worse, but occasionally the examiner does see small defects fill in (Figs. 9-44 and 9-57). Although the ability of articular cartilage to act in this fashion is doubted by many, it seems to be supported by Green's[6] finding that cartilage can repair itself not only by metaplasia or primitive fibroblast but also by "regeneration, whereby chondrocytes proliferate and produce new matrix."

While much more must be learned about articular cartilage and the way it behaves, the available evidence to date indicates that degenerative arthritis is not a condition brought on simply by aging; it is probably the result of trauma and mechanical factors, which when deep enough to involve the vascular supply to bone have the ability to replace these defects with a fibrocartilaginous surface. If damaged articular cartilage is treated with kindness and consideration, it will provide an acceptable joint surface for an unknown number of years.

References

1. Appel, H.: Late results after meniscectomy of the knee joint, Acta Orthop. Scand. [Suppl.] 133, 1970.
2. Brattstrom, H.: Shape of the intercondylar groove, normally and in recurrent dislocation of the patella, Acta Orthop. Scand. [Suppl.] **68:**1-138, 1964.
2a. Casscells, S. W.: Gross pathological changes in the knee joint of the aged individual, Clin. Orthop. **132:**225-232, 1978.
3. Chrisman, O. D., and Snook, G. A.: Studies on the protective effect of aspirin against degeneration of human articular cartilage. A preliminary report, Clin. Orthop. **56:**77-82, 1968.
4. Dandy, D. J., and Jackson, R. W.: Meniscectomy and chondromalacia of the femoral condyle, J. Bone Joint Surg. [Am.] **57:**1116, 1975.
5. Ekholm, R.: Relationship between articular changes and function, Acta. Orthop. Scand. **21:**81-97, 1951.
6. Green, W. T.: Articular cartilage repair, Clin. Orthop. 124, 1977.
7. Haxton, R.: Function of the patella and effects of its excision, Surg. Gynecol. Obstet. **80:**389, 1945.
8. Heine, J.: Arthritis deformans, Virchows Arch. Pathol. Anat. **260:**521, 1926.
9. Helfet, A. J.: Disorders of the knee, Philadelphia, 1974, J. B. Lippincott Co.
10. Kettlecamp, D.: Personal communication.
10a. Lipscomb, P., Jr., et al.: Osteochondritis dissecans of the knee with loose fragments with treatment by replacement and fixation with readily removed pins, J. Bone Joint Surg. [Am.] **60:**235, 1978.
11. Mankin, H. S., and Lipiello, L.: The turnover of adult rabbit articular cartilage, J. Bone Joint Surg. [Am.] **51:**1591, 1969.
12. Meachim, G.: Age changes in articular cartilage, Clin. Orthop. **64:**33, 1969.
13. Owre, A.: Chondromalacia of the patellae, Acta Chir. Scand. [Suppl.] **77:**41, 1936.
14. Perry, J.: Mechanics of walking, Phys. Ther. **47:**848, 1967.
15. Smillie, I. S.: Injuries of the knee joint, Edinburgh, 1970, Churchill Livingstone.
16. Sokoloff, L.: The biology of degenerative joint disease, Chicago, 1969, University of Chicago Press, pp. 28, 43, and 53.
17. Tapper, E. M., and Hoover, N. W.: Late results after meniscectomy, J. Bone Joint Surg. [Am.] **51:**517-526, 1969.

Arthrography

Harry J. Griffiths

DISEASES OF THE ARTICULAR CARTILAGE

In this section the plain-film and arthrographic changes seen in the various forms of arthritis, including rheumatoid arthritis, osteoarthritis, and pseudogout, will be considered. The earliest arthrographic changes of arthritis will be illustrated, as well as the damage seen in severe degenerative joint disease with complete disorganization and disintegration of the articular cartilage. Baker cysts will be mentioned in association with rheumatoid arthritis, although they are discussed more fully elsewhere. Articular infractions and the formation of loose bodies will be discussed in detail, and the roentgenographic diagnosis of osteochondritis dissecans will also be considered.

Arthritis

The term "arthritis" is derived from the Greek "arthron" or joint and "itis" or inflammation, hence "inflammation of the joint." In the later stages of most forms of arthritis there are obvious plain-film changes that will lead to the correct diagnosis, whether it be one of the commoner types such as osteoarthritis, rheumatoid arthritis, gout, or pseudogout, or one of the rarer forms, such as ochronosis or hemophilia. This is not the place to discuss this plain-film differential diagnosis, and the interested reader is referred to one of the rheumatology texts. However, with the use

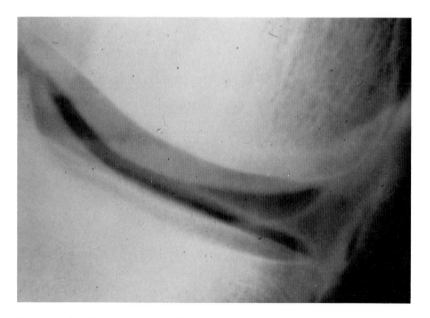

Fig. 9-59. Normal articular cartilage. Note image of articular cartilage running parallel to tibial plateau. Femoral articular cartilage is inclined to thin out at edges of joint.

of arthrography we are able to show changes in the articular cartilage considerably earlier than, for example, the classic appearances of osteophytes and sclerosis in osteoarthritis or the huge destructive erosions seen in rheumatoid arthritis.[1,2,4,6]

The 4 ml of iodinated contrast medium injected into the joint in a double-contrast arthrogram is selectively absorbed by the synovium and the articular cartilage. Hence in a normal arthrogram, the articular cartilage can be easily seen as a somewhat less opaque shadow than the underlying bone, and, of course, it runs roughly parallel to the normal osseous margins of the femur, tibia, and patella (Fig. 9-59). As has been mentioned previously, any disease of the synovium or articular cartilage will cause "imbibition" of contrast, so that the damaged or inflamed area will absorb more contrast more rapidly than do normal areas. Thus damaged cartilage will appear rather denser than do normal parts of the joint and frequently also become somewhat blurred[1,2,4] (Fig. 9-60). These changes in association with a thinning of the cartilage will make the arthrographic diagnosis of arthritis straightforward. As the disease progresses, the cartilage becomes increasingly damaged and ultimately will disintegrate or disappear. This may be associated with large holes in the remaining articular surfaces, which resemble "ulcers" and which may represent one of the places of origin of loose bodies (Fig. 9-61). As a normal person ages, there is progressive narrowing of the articular cartilage. It is important to be able to differentiate this physiologic attrition of cartilage from true early arthritis, but the experienced arthrographer will make the diagnosis of early degenerative joint disease from the blurring of the articular surface and the added imbibition of contrast.[5]

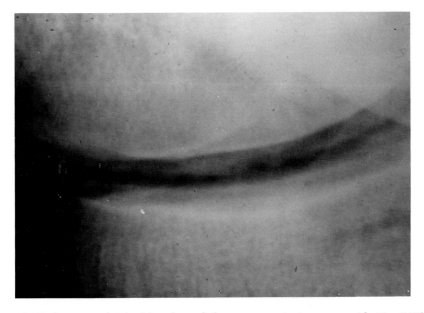

Fig. 9-60. Early osteoarthritis. Note loss of clear-cut margin (compare with Fig. 9-59) and thinning and irregularity of cartilage.

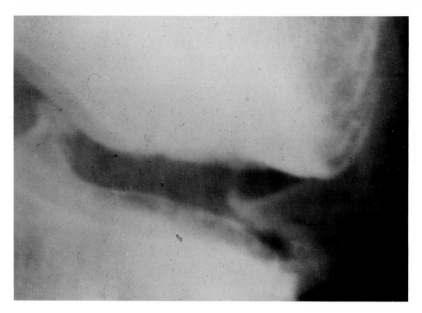

Fig. 9-61. Late osteoarthritis. Note marked loss of articular cartilage both centrally over femoral condyle (where there is also eburnation of bone) and laterally on tibial plateau. This is associated with a degenerated meniscus with increased uptake of contrast (imbibition). (From Griffiths, H. J.: Orthop. Rev. **5**(9):71, 1976.)

The early arthrographic features of most types of arthritis are similar, although the clinical features and presentation may be totally different. But there are often associated roentgenographic signs that will help differentiate the various types of arthritis from each other. In rheumatoid arthritis, there is the synovial overgrowth that has already been discussed, and frequently huge Baker cysts may be seen posteriorly.[6] Routine arthrography in chronic rheumatoid arthritis is rarely indicated unless surgery is contemplated. It is important to confirm the size and ramifications of a Baker cyst and to remember that single-contrast arthrography provides better roentgenograms than do double-contrast techniques; it may be necessary to get the patient to exercise gently and to take delayed films (30 minutes, 1 hour, 2 hours, and even 3 hours) in order to be able to fully define the margins of the cyst (Fig. 9-62).

Patients with chondrocalcinosis and pseudogout often develop secondary degenerative arthritis, but apart from the cartilage calcification seen on plain films, the arthrographic appearance of pseudogout is essentially similar to that of osteoarthritis (Fig. 9-63).

Articular infractions and loose bodies

The diagnosis of a fracture or infraction of the articular cartilage is usually impossible to make on plain films, difficult to make clinically, but easy to demonstrate arthrographically[5] (Fig. 9-64). If articular damage is suspected after trauma, then a double-contrast arthrogram with particular attention to all of the articular cartilage

Text continued on p. 148.

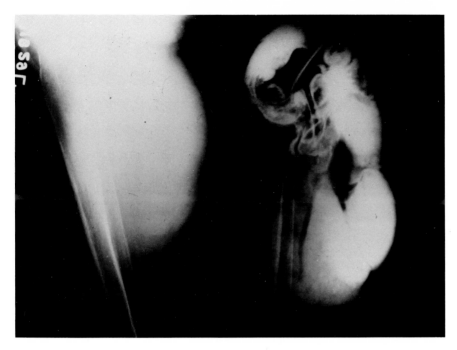

Fig. 9-62. Large Baker cyst in rheumatoid arthritis. Plain film (left) and single-contrast arthrogram demonstrate huge Baker cyst with many ramifications (From Griffith, H. J.: Orthop. Rev. **5**(9):71, 1976.)

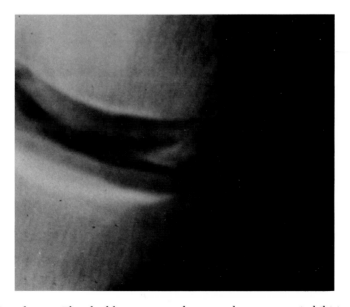

Fig. 9-63. Pseudogout. This double-contrast arthrogram demonstrates imbibition of contrast and chondrocalcinosis in 46-year-old man with pseudogout.

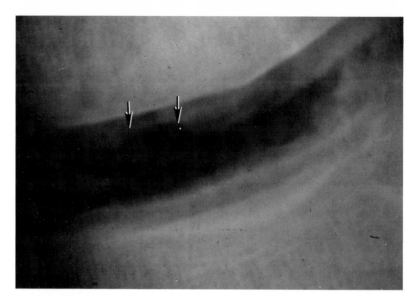

Fig. 9-64. Articular infraction. This 16-year-old girl fell off her horse and complained of pain, swelling, and locking of her knee. A double-contrast arthrogram revealed this defect in femoral articular cartilage.

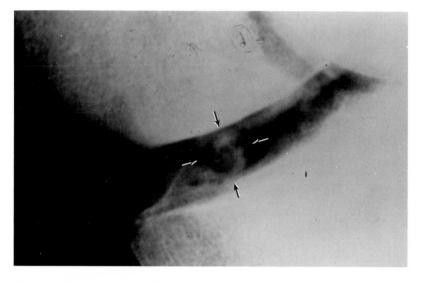

Fig. 9-65. Loose body. This partially calcified loose body is seen in association with a tear of the posterior horn medial meniscus as well as degenerative arthritis and imbibition of contrast in this severely deranged knee (From Griffiths, H. J.: Orthop. Rev. **5**(9):71, 1976.)

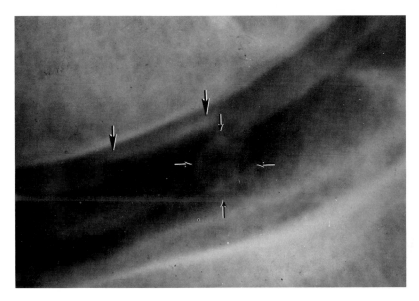

Fig. 9-66. Articular infraction and loose body. This impending loose body is still attached by a pedicle to an area of articular infraction following trauma to knee in this young man.

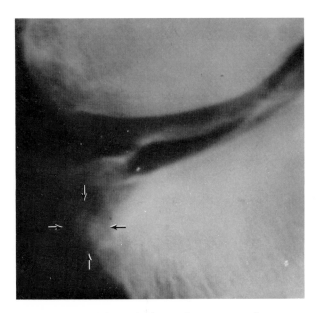

Fig. 9-67. Loose body. A calcified loose body can be seen in inferior recess of this knee in association with tear of middle horn of lateral meniscus.

surfaces will usually show the infraction.[1,4] If the damaged cartilage has actually dropped out into the joint, a loose body should be sought, but it is often difficult to find because of the double-contrast technique (Fig. 9-65). Occasionally one is able to demonstrate the actual formation of a cartilaginous loose body from an area of infraction because the avulsed portion is still attached by a pedicle—not unlike a colonic polyp (Fig. 9-66).

The demonstration of loose bodies is usually best done using single-contrast arthrography as they will show up as radiolucencies against the white contrast medium or as radiodensities against air alone.[2] However, it is usually difficult to anticipate which patients will have loose bodies; thus many loose bodies are found serendipitously with the use of double-contrast techniques (Fig. 9-67). Loose bodies are frequently mobile and may be seen fluoroscopically in different parts of the joint as they move around. They may also get wedged in the intercondylar notch or in one

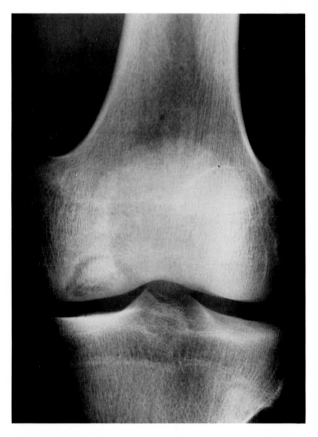

Fig. 9-68. Osteochondritis dissecans. This 14-year-old boy shows typical lucency and irregularity of lateral aspect of medial epicondyle (LAME). Arthrography revealed intact articular cartilage.

of the synovial recesses, in which case they are difficult to see unless they are calcified.[2,5]

Osteochondritis dissecans

Osteochondritis dissecans frequently presents as either pain in the knee joint or with locking of the knee associated with the formation of loose bodies. Osteochondritis dissecans is one of the group of conditions included in the term "osteochondritis" and represents an area of subchondral avascular necrosis. It is of unknown etiology and occurs initially when the patient is in his teens. Many authorities believe that osteochondritis dissecans is preceded by trauma to the rapidly growing epiphysis, although it is obvious that constitutional factors are involved because it may be familial and occur bilaterally. Osteochondritis dissecans may occur adjacent to any articular surface in the body and in the knee is most frequently seen at the lateral aspect of the medial epicondyle (producing the mnemonic LAME). The plain-film changes are characteristic, with a bony defect in this region frequently having a "loose body" contained within it[2,3] (Fig. 9-68). However, the avascular part may either fall out or be knocked out, whereupon it will become a true loose body.

When arthrography is done it is important to define the integrity of the cartilage overlying this bony defect, and so special tangential and oblique views should be obtained under fluoroscopy in order that the examiner can assess the relationship of the articular cartilage to the defect.[2-5] In many patients the articular cartilage remains intact, although there is an obvious bony defect (Fig. 9-69). In some patients the

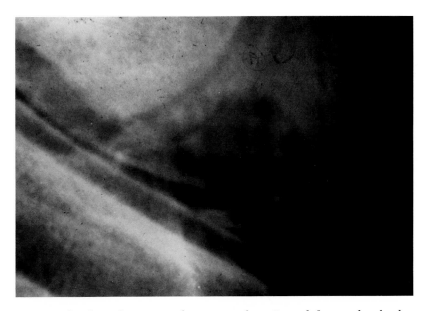

Fig. 9-69. Osteochondritis dissecans with intact cartilage. Bony defect can be clearly seen in this 26-year-old man, but overlying articular cartilage is intact.

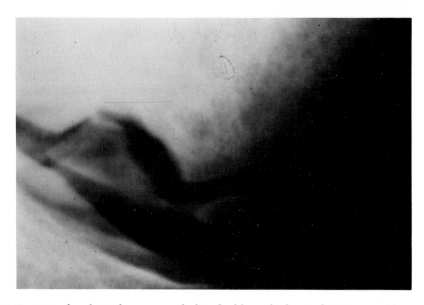

Fig. 9-70. Osteochondritis dissecans with detached loose body. In this 31-year-old man with hemophilia, large bony defect could be seen on plain films of lateral femoral condyle. An arthrogram revealed detached bone and cartilage fragment well outlined by air on this double-contrast arthrogram.

defect will remain in place rather like a plug, but it will in fact be loose and ready to break off at any moment (Fig. 9-70). As has been mentioned, in some patients the avascular part has fallen into the joint and can be seen as a loose body.[2,5]

Summary

Arthrography is particularly useful in defining the degree of articular damage in all forms of arthritis as well as in demonstrating any associated meniscal lesions, loose bodies, and Baker cysts. In patients with osteochondritis dissecans, arthrography is useful in demonstrating either the integrity of the articular cartilage overlying the bony defect or in showing the loose body that has become separated and now lies within the knee joint itself.

DISEASES OF THE PATELLA

Three entities will be considered in this section; the discussion will be brief because the diagnosis is usually best made either clinically or arthroscopically, and arthrography has little to offer in patellar lesions.

Fractures of the patella

The plain-film diagnosis of fractures of the patella is usually simple, although occasionally it is necessary to differentiate a bipartite patella from a minimally displaced fracture of the upper outer pole of the patella. Arthrographically there is little to offer even if there is an associated tendinous rupture.

Rupture of juxtapatella tendons

Rupture of the patella tendon or the quadriceps tendon and insertion is usually diagnosed clinically, although displacement of the patella and avulsion fractures of the tendinous insertions on plain films may help to confirm the diagnosis.[3,7] Arthrography is rarely indicated in such lesions but will demonstrate communication between the knee joint itself and the subcutaneous bursae, of which two are commonly described: the prepatellar bursa and the infrapatellar bursa.[1] There have been a number of case reports in the literature of the arthrographic diagnosis of rupture of the quadriceps tendon,[1,3,7] but in my opinion arthrography is rarely indicated.

Chondromalacia patellae

Unfortunately the diagnosis of chondromalacia patellae is more problematic.[2,5,8] It has proven largely impossible roentgenographically to diagnose this common condition in its early stages. Plain films of the knee are normal, and arthrography has proven disappointing except in the very late stages. Occasionally chondromalacia patellae may be so severe that bony reaction occurs in the patella, and this can be seen on a good lateral view of the knee. However, even with varying the angle of the skyline view from 10° to 70°, it is generally felt that the diagnosis of chondromalacia patellae is difficult to make arthrographically.

The normal patellar cartilage is relatively thicker than the cartilage elsewhere in the knee, and it may be because of the shape of the patellofemoral articulation that we are unable to see the distortion of the cartilage and the associated imbibition of contrast that does occur in chondromalacia patellae.[2] In fact the radiographic diagnosis of chondromalacia patellae has proven so elusive that a number of people are experimenting with intraarticular isotopes to see if they are able to define this condition. Finally some authors[4,6] have advocated the use of lateral tomography of the knee after arthrography in order to demonstrate thinning and irregularity of the patellar articular cartilage.[4,6]

Thus presently neither plain films nor arthrography is capable of demonstrating chondromalacia patellae, and if it is clinically suspected, arthroscopy is the method of choice.

References
Diseases of the articular cartilage

1. Anderson, P. W., and Maslin, P.: Tomography applied to knee arthrography, Radiology 110:271-275, 1974.
2. Horns, J. W.: Single contrast knee arthrography in abnormalities of the articular cartilage, Radiology 105:537-540, 1972.
3. Nicholas, J. A., Freiberger, R. H., and Killoran, P. J.: Double contrast arthrography of the knee. Its value in the management of 225 knee derangements, J. Bone Joint Surg. [Am.] 52:203-220, 1970.

4. Ricklin, P., Rüttiman, A., and Del Buono, M. S.: Meniscus lesions. Practical problems of clinical diagnosis, arthrography and therapy, New York, 1971, Grune & Stratton.
5. Staple, T. W.: Extrameniscal lesions demonstrated by double-contrast arthrography of the knee, Radiology **102**:311-319, 1972.
6. Taylor, A. R.: Arthrography of the knee in rheumatoid arthritis, Br. J. Radiol. **42**:493-497, 1969.

Diseases of the patella

1. Duncan, A. M.: Arthrography in rupture of the suprapatellar bursa with pseudocyst formation, Am. J. Roentgenol. Radium Ther. Nucl. Med. **121**:89-93, 1974.
2. Horns, J. W.: The diagnosis of chondromalacia by double contrast arthrography of the knee, J. Bone Joint Surg. [Am.] **49**:119-120, 1977.
3. Jelaso, D. V., and Morris, G. A.: Rupture of the quadriceps tendon: diagnosis by arthrography, Radiology **116**:621-622, 1975.
4. Lavner. Cited by Ricklin, P., Rüttiman, A., and Del Buono, M. S.: Meniscus lesions, New York, 1971, Grune & Stratton.
5. Outerbridge, R. E., and Dunlop, J. A.: The problem of chondromalacia patellae, Clin. Orthop. **110**:177-196, 1975.
6. Ricklin, P., Rüttimann, A., and Del Buono, M. S.: Meniscus lesions, New York, 1971, Grune & Stratton.
7. Smason, J. B.: Post-traumatic fistula connecting prepatellar bursa with knee joint. Report of a case, J. Bone Joint Surg. [Am.] **54**:1553-1554, 1972.
8. Stougnard, J.: Chondromalacia of the patella. Incidence, macroscopical and radiographical findings at autopsy, Acta Orthop. Scand. **46**:809-822, 1975.

10. Lesions of menisci

Arthroscopy

Robert W. Jackson

HISTORICAL ASPECTS

The first person to recognize rupture of a semilunar cartilage as a clinical entity was William Hey, Professor of Surgery at Leeds University in England. In 1803 Hey described several cases that presented as locked knees. Based on anatomic knowledge only, he suspected that one or the other of the menisci was torn, and the displaced loose fragment was blocking the normal motion of the knee. With the passage of time, the diagnosis and the term "internal derangement of the knee" (or IDK) became popular. Eventually "IDK" became almost synonomous with "I Don't Know," as many knees with obscure diagnoses were labeled "internal derangements." Moreover as surgery became safer and more commonplace the diagnosis of torn meniscus was made more frequently and with less hesitation, leading to an increasing number of torn and normal menisci being removed. The immediate short-term results were quite satisfactory in most instances. Further investigation, however, revealed that the long-term results were often not quite so acceptable, due to the slow and progressive development of degenerative changes.

As the importance of the meniscus in preventing degenerative change was gradually realized, there was an increasing acceptance of the concept that meniscectomy is not an innocuous procedure, and that wherever possible the meniscus should not be removed unnecessarily. There is now no question that the meniscus has several important functions, including lubrication, stability, nourishment of articular cartilage (by providing a surface for intermittent compression), absorption of impact energy, and facilitation of complex movements.

CLINICAL EVALUATION

The importance of taking an adequate history cannot be overemphasized, as it still remains the most informative, noninvasive, quickest, and cheapest method of arriving at a provisional diagnosis of torn meniscus.

The menisci are usually damaged through rotational, angular, or compressive stresses, such as those that occur in strenuous daily activities or in athletics. However, with advancing age, degenerative changes occur that make the meniscus more liable to disruption with less trauma (Table 3).

Table 3. Etiology of meniscal tears (data from 500 consecutive meniscal lesions of all ages)

Cause	Percent	
No injury	41	
Twist	21	62% Minimal trauma
Athletics	16	
Others	22	

Table 4. Site of meniscal pathology

Site	Smillie	Hughston	Nicholas and Freiberger	Lidge	Jackson
Medial	67%	54%	70%	60%	72%
Lateral	31%	27%	26%	30%	23%
Both	2%	19%	3%	10%	5%

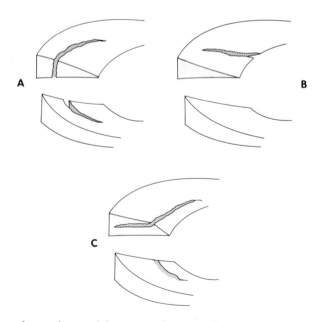

Fig. 10-1. Three basic planes of disruption that can affect a meniscus. **A,** Longitudinal or vertical. **B,** Radial or transverse. **C,** Horizontal or cleavage.

The medial meniscus is damaged two to three times as frequently as is the lateral meniscus. Both menisci may be involved in a lacerating process in anywhere from 5% to 19% of knees seen (Table 4). Bucket-handle tears occur in approximately 24% of cases.

PATHOLOGY
Type of tear

An acute rupture or laceration of the meniscus can occur in one of three basic planes. If the major rupture extends from the posterior to the anterior horn, essentially down the mid portion of the meniscus, it might be considered to be in the *longitudinal* or *vertical* plane (Fig. 10-1, *A*). If the rupture occurs across the sub-

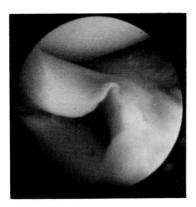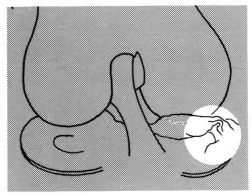

Fig. 10-2. Anterior portion of a longitudinal tear, with displacement of inner border toward intercondylar notch (bucket-handle tear). (From Jackson, R. W., and Dandy, D. J.: Arthroscopy of the knee, New York, 1976, Grune & Stratton.)

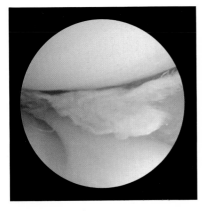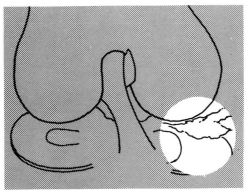

Fig. 10-3. Fresh flap tear of posterior horn, combination of longitudinal and horizontal tearing, with fragment folded forward. (From Jackson, R. W., and Dandy, D. J.: Arthroscopy of the knee, New York, 1976, Grune & Stratton.)

stance of the meniscus, extending from the central area to the periphery, one might consider the tear to be *radial* or *transverse* (Fig. 10-1, *B*). If the tear occurs in the substance of the meniscus, parallel to the upper border of the tibia, it might be considered as a *horizontal* or *cleavage* tear (Fig. 10-1, *C*).

Other types of meniscal lesions, such as bucket-handle (Fig. 10-2), flap (Figs. 10-3 and 10-4), fish-mouth, and parrot-beak tears (Fig. 10-5), are merely variations of this main theme. Radial or transverse tears are more common in the lateral meniscus (Figs. 10-6 and 10-7). Horizontal or cleavage tears are seen in both medial and lateral menisci, usually in the posterior horn region, and more commonly in older persons (Figs. 10-8 and 10-9). Congenital discoid menisci (Fig. 10-10), although not patho-

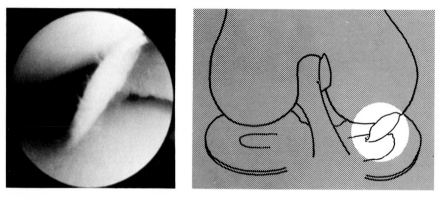

Fig. 10-4. Small flaplike fragment from inner border of meniscus, combination of longitudinal and radial tearing. (From Jackson, R. W., and Dandy, D. J.: Arthroscopy of the knee, New York, 1976, Grune & Stratton.)

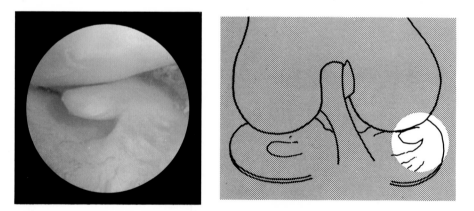

Fig. 10-5. Combination of longitudinal and radial tearing in posterior horn region, allowing inner fragment of meniscus to displace toward center of joint. This is an old tear, as evidenced by increased peripheral vascularity, hyperemia of synovium, and smoothing off of edges of meniscal fragment. (From Jackson, R. W., and Dandy, D. J.: Arthroscopy of the knee, New York, 1976, Grune & Stratton.)

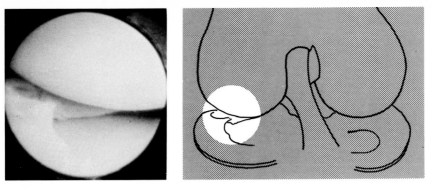

Fig. 10-6. Radial tear with small longitudinal component in lateral meniscus. (From Jackson, R. W., and Dandy, D. J.: Arthroscopy of the knee, New York, 1976, Grune & Stratton.)

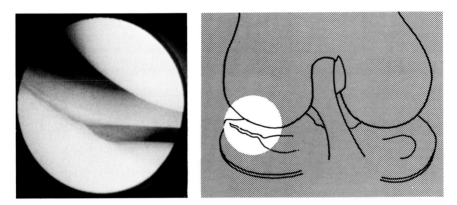

Fig. 10-7. Pure radial or transverse tear in lateral meniscus. (From Jackson, R. W., and Dandy, D. J.: Arthroscopy of the knee, New York, 1976, Grune & Stratton.)

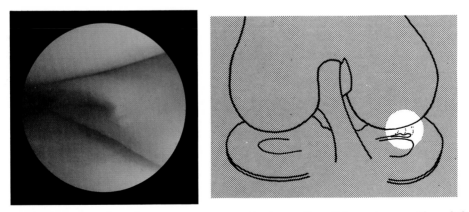

Fig. 10-8. Horizontal or cleavage tear in posterior horn of medial meniscus, with a shift toward center of joint of superior portion of torn meniscus. (From Jackson, R. W., and Dandy, D. J.: Arthroscopy of the knee, New York, 1976, Grune & Stratton.)

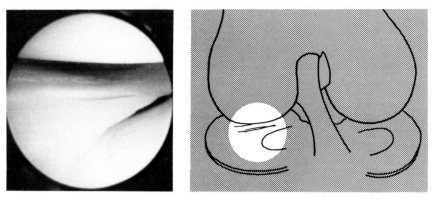

Fig. 10-9. Undisplaced cleavage tear in posterior horn of lateral meniscus. (From Jackson, R. W., and Dandy, D. J.: Arthroscopy of the knee, New York, 1976, Grune & Stratton.)

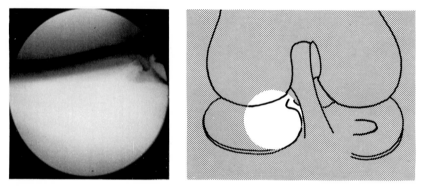

Fig. 10-10. Intact discoid lateral meniscus with inner border of meniscus close to intercondylar notch. (From Jackson, R. W., and Dandy, D. J.: Arthroscopy of the knee, New York, 1976, Grune & Stratton.)

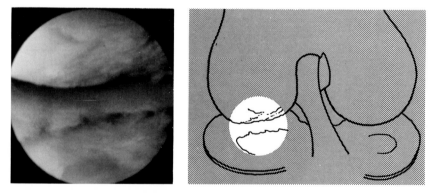

Fig. 10-11. Degenerative posterior horn of lateral meniscus associated with degenerative changes on articular surface of femoral condyle and tibial plateau. (From Jackson, R. W., and Dandy, D. J.: Arthroscopy of the knee, New York, 1976, Grune & Stratton.)

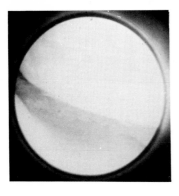 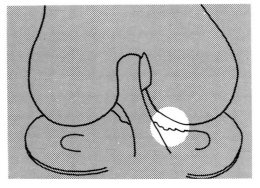

Fig. 10-12. Degenerative posterior horn of medial meniscus. Note loss of definition of inner border. (From Jackson, R. W., and Dandy, D. J.: Arthroscopy of the knee, New York, 1976, Grune & Stratton.)

logic in themselves, are perhaps more prone to laceration, and degenerative menisci presumably develop with the combination of repeated microtraumas and advancing age (Figs. 10-11 and 10-12). Calcification, pseudocysts, and macerations are merely variations of the degenerative process.

Site of tear

The arthroscopist, when describing the type of tear, should specify the location and extent of the lesion. This can be achieved by describing the position within the meniscus itself, such as peripheral, mid portion, or inner border. One also describes the location within the knee, such as anterior, middle, or posterior. For example, a typical bucket-handle lesion could be described as a longitudinal tear from anterior to posterior in mid-portion meniscus (Fig. 10-13), or another lesion might be described as a longitudinal tear in the inner border of the posterior horn (Fig. 10-14).

AIDS TO DIAGNOSIS
Arthrography

The principles of screening, taking multiple views in tangential projections of the menisci, applying varus or valgus strains, and the appearance and interpretation of pathology are discussed later in this chapter.

Arthroscopy

No matter which arthroscope is used, the basic principles of identifying meniscal lesions remain the same. As it is probably easiest to examine the medial compartment from the lateral approach, and as the anterolateral approach permits easy visualization of the posterior horn of the lateral meniscus, the most accepted approach for the identification of meniscal pathology is from the anterolateral aspect.

When the arthroscope enters the medial compartment, its tip is usually on top

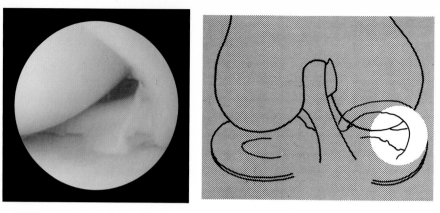

Fig. 10-13. Longitudinal tear from anterior to posterior through midportion of meniscus (bucket-handle tear). Peripheral rim is intact. (From Jackson, R. W., and Dandy, D. J.: Arthroscopy of the knee, New York, 1976, Grune & Stratton.)

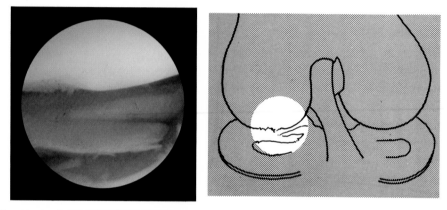

Fig. 10-14. Longitudinal tear, posterior horn, inner border of lateral meniscus, with early degenerative change on lateral femoral condyle. (From Jackson, R. W., and Dandy, D. J.: Arthroscopy of the knee, New York, 1976, Grune & Stratton.)

of the anterior horn of the medial meniscus, and the menisco-synovial junction is easily seen. It is important at this stage to identify the *inner border* of the meniscus. In discoid lesions, this may be very close to the intercondylar spine of the tibia (Fig. 10-10). When the examiner has found the inner border he follows it backward toward the posterior horn region. If there is any disruption in the shape or congruity of the curve of the inner border, he should be immediately suspicious of a tear. A disruption posteromedially will allow the meniscal tissue to in-bulge toward the center of the joint (the so-called "pout sign") (Fig. 10-15). Frequently when a tear is present it is easily seen as a flap of meniscus or as a cleavage tear exiting in a visible area. A displaced bucket-handle tear totally obscures the view of the compartment by virtue of the large mass of meniscal tissue lying in the intercondylar notch (Fig. 10-16).

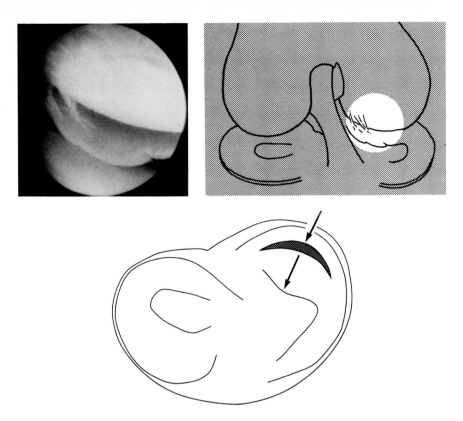

Fig. 10-15. Disruption of posteromedial corner allows meniscal tissue to bulge in toward center of joint. Presence of tear can be confirmed by insertion of palpating tool into joint or by posteromedial insertion of arthroscope and direct visualization of tear. (From Jackson, R. W., and Dandy, D. J.: Arthroscopy of the knee, New York, 1976, Grune & Stratton.)

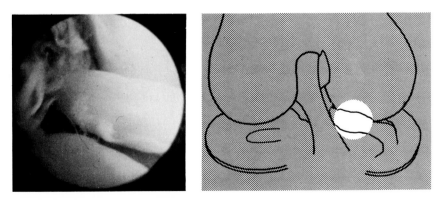

Fig. 10-16. Displaced fragment of meniscus lying in intercondylar notch obscures visualization of medial compartment of joint and is pathognomonic of bucket-handle tear. (From Jackson, R. W., and Dandy, D. J.: Arthroscopy of the knee, New York, 1976, Grune & Stratton.)

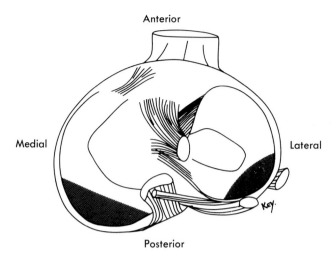

Fig. 10-17. Potential blind spots in posterior corners of joint can be eliminated by application of valgus or varus strain, deeper insertion of arthroscope, or posteromedial or posterolateral insertion of small arthroscope.

Fig. 10-18

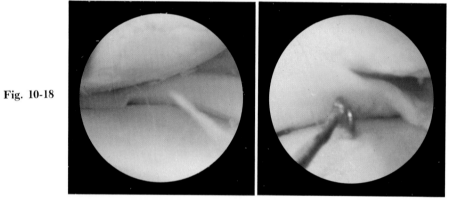

Fig. 10-19

Fig. 10-18. Presence of degenerative changes in articular cartilage of femoral condyles is ancillary or indirect evidence of either meniscal lesion or instability of joint due to ligament or capsular damage.

Fig. 10-19. Instrument has been inserted to lift posterior horn of meniscus to search for cleavage tears exiting in this area. Hypodermic needles, crochet hooks, small Kirschner wires, and other devices can be used to aid visualization of these areas.

Potential blind spots exist in the posterior corners of the joint unless the knee is particularly lax (Fig. 10-17). If there is any difficulty in interpretation, one must make special efforts to visualize the posterior horns clearly. Usually the application of a valgus or varus strain to the knee and deeper penetration with the arthroscope toward the posterior horn region is sufficient. One also looks for the ancillary or

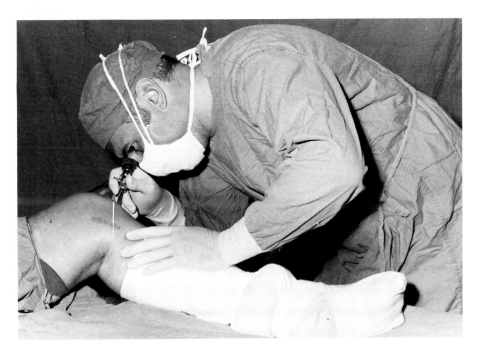

Fig. 10-20. Lateral meniscus is well visualized from lateral approach by placing patient's heel on table and applying varus strain to joint by downward pressure with free hand. (From Jackson, R. W., and Dandy, D. J.: Arthroscopy of the knee, New York, 1976, Grune & Stratton.)

indirect signs of a torn meniscus, such as degenerative changes on the condyle of the femur (Fig. 10-18) or articular cartilage debris in the joint washings. Insertion of an 18-gauge hypodermic needle at the joint line may be useful, as it enables the examiner to probe for a tear and to push or pull the meniscus toward the center of the joint. Crochet hooks and other lifting devices have also been advocated for this same purpose (Fig. 10-19). On occasion a posteromedial insertion of the arthroscope is helpful to directly visualize this area.

The lateral meniscus is seen almost in its entirety from the anterolateral approach, as one looks straight down the length of the compartment. The anterior horn is not seen as it lies beneath the arthroscope. With the knee flexed, the heel on the table, and a varus strain applied to the knee, the posterior horn is easily visualized (Fig. 10-20). Again the inner border of the meniscus must be identified and followed as far as possible to the anterior horn region. Should there be any suspicious but nonconclusive evidence of a lesion in the area, one again uses the ancillary signs of femoral condylar articular cartilage damage, or the additional diagnostic tool of a joint-line needle to probe, palpate, and lift the meniscus to ascertain whether or not it is a solid structure. If the examiner suspects an anterior horn lesion, an anteromedial insertion of the arthroscope enables him to look across at the suspect area.

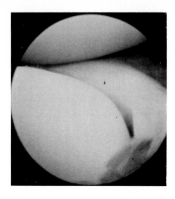 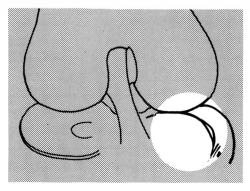

Fig. 10-21. When meniscotibial attachments are torn, anterior horn can extrude from joint, resulting in hypermobile meniscus. (From Jackson, R. W., and Dandy, D. J.: Arthroscopy of the knee, New York, 1976, Grune & Stratton.)

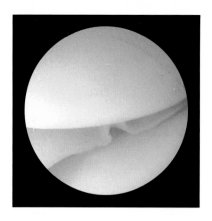

Fig. 10-22. Inner border of meniscus is quite resilient, and on rotation a flounce may be seen. This is normal. However, a change in direction of inner border toward center of joint usually indicates pathology. (From Jackson, R. W., and Dandy, D. J.: Arthroscopy of the knee, New York, 1976, Grune & Stratton.)

Other maneuvers, such as rotation of the tibia on the femur in different degrees of flexion, may reveal an unstable anterior or posterior horn, or an old peripheral tear. A definite clinical entity is the hypermobile meniscus, which results when the coronary ligament is torn, allowing the anterior horn to "dive" over the edge of the tibial plateau (Fig. 10-21). Special attention must be paid to the "flounce," which is not a pathologic condition and which represents the normal resilience of the medial meniscus (Fig. 10-22).

MENISCAL "MIMES"

Numerous conditions can and do present with signs and symptoms similar to those of a torn meniscus and therefore can be considered as meniscal "mimes." It is important to diagnose such meniscal mimes prior to surgery or else there is a risk of excision of a normal meniscus. Some well-recognized meniscal mimes include chondromalacia patellae, isolated rupture of the anterior cruciate ligament, chondral fractures and flaps, osteochondral lesions, synovial impingement, chondrocalcinosis,

Table 5. Results of uncomplicated meniscectomies 2 to 10 years after surgery

	Good to excellent	Fair	Poor
Total meniscectomy (107 cases)	65%	27%	8%
Partial meniscectomy (33 cases)	91%	3%	6%

the fibrosed medial shelf, avulsion of popliteal tendon insertion, and various other rare entities such as synovial hemangiomas or xanthomas.

TREATMENT

If a meniscal lesion is detected, three avenues of treatment remain open. The first is to do nothing except to inform the patient that there is, indeed, some lesion in the meniscus, which might explain his symptoms, and that surgical treatment is not indicated. Consider the situation of a degenerative posterior horn cleavage tear without displacement in an elderly patient with symptoms only on extreme exertion or on full flexion. This patient might be well advised to retain this damaged and imperfect meniscus, on the basis that it is probably doing more good than harm. Such an individual should be advised to modify his way of life in order to cope with this minor imperfection in his body.

In another instance, such as when a small flap tear is noted on the inner border of the meniscus or a single bucket-handle tear is present, a partial meniscectomy or "minisectomy" would appear to be the best method of treatment. By doing a partial meniscectomy, peripheral meniscal tissue is preserved, which provides increased stability and better preservation of articular cartilage with the passage of time. The concept here is to remove only the mobile segment.

The third and classic avenue of treatment is to do a total meniscectomy. If this is determined to be the best possible or, indeed, the only possible method of treatment, the point of excision should be in the avascular zone just inside the meniscosynovial junction. There would appear to be little evidence to support the theory that wide excision (in the vascular area of the synovium) plus early movement promotes regrowth of a functional meniscus. It is probably better to accept the fact that a functioning meniscus of reasonable size rarely if ever regenerates, and to retain a degree of stability by avoiding damage to the meniscal margin and its associated capsule (Table 5).

SUMMARY

With the help of arthroscopy it is possible to make an accurate diagnosis as to the type, location, and extent of meniscal lesions prior to surgery. This knowledge, along with a full appreciation of the total clinical picture (as gained from history and physical examination) enables the surgeon to treat his patient according to a specific plan based on the specific problem. Conditions that mimic a torn meniscus can be identified and treated appropriately. Normal menisci are rarely if ever removed. Partial meniscectomy becomes a rational method of treatment. Overall, the quality of care after meniscal damage is enhanced.

Suggested readings

Huckell, J. R.: Is meniscectomy a benign procedure? A long term follow-up study, Can. J. Surg. **8:**254-260, 1965.

Jackson, R. W., and Dandy, D. J.: Arthroscopy of the knee, New York, 1976, Grune & Stratton.

Smillie, I. S.: Injuries of the knee joint, ed. 4, Edinburgh, 1970, Churchill Livingstone.

Tapper, E. M., and Hoover, N. W.: Late results after meniscectomy, J. Bone Joint Surg. **51:** 517-526, 1969.

Arthrography

Murray K. Dalinka

The precise diagnosis of an internal derangement of the knee is often difficult to make clinically. Arthrography is a relatively innocuous and highly accurate method of diagnosing internal derangements, particularly meniscal abnormalities. Many orthopedic surgeons depend preoperatively on the arthrographic findings, a situation analogous to myelography.[5] In one large series, negative knee explorations fell from 16% to 1% after the introduction of arthrography, and multiple series, many of them weighted with problem cases, demonstrate an accuracy of greater than 90%.[2,4,14] Unsuspected double lesions were found in 6% of Butt and McIntyre's cases.[2]

Meniscal tears have been classified into many subdivisions, but I and others[14] feel that these tears are frequently complex and cannot be accurately described arthrographically. Peripheral tears and occasional bucket-handle tears are exceptions to this rule as they frequently may be classified, and their treatment may differ. The extent of the meniscal lesion is more important than its description, and it is, of course, reported.

MEDIAL MENISCUS

The medial meniscus is a smooth, solid structure made up of dense fibrocartilage that appears triangular in cross section. Any change in its shape or contour is abnormal. Gas or positive-contrast media within the confines of the meniscus indicates a tear (Fig. 10-23).

Fluoroscopic control is extremely helpful in evaluating the menisci, as small tears may only be seen in one projection; slight or questionable abnormalities can be studied with minimal positional changes to clarify these findings (Fig. 10-24).[2,4]

Films must be taken of the entire meniscus from front to back; otherwise, tears, particularly of the anterior horn (Fig. 10-25) or peripheral posterior horn, may be overlooked. Care must be taken to get contrast media beneath the posterior horn of the tibial surface of the medial meniscus; sometimes with oblique tears of the posterior horn this is difficult, and the lesions may be overlooked.[10] Stress, rotation,

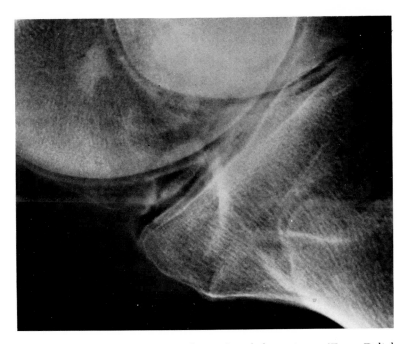

Fig. 10-23. Gas within tear of posterior horn of medial meniscus. (From Dalinka, M. K., Coren, G. S., and Wershba, M.: CRC Crit. Rev. Clin. Radiol. Nucl. Med. 4:1-59, 1973, © 1973 CRC Press, Inc. Used by permission of CRC Press, Inc.)

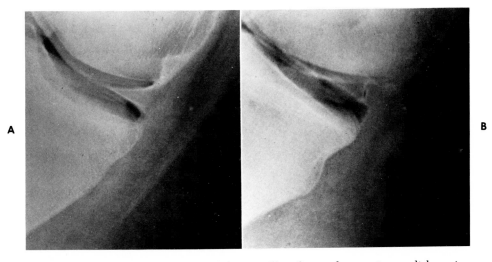

A   **B**

Fig. 10-24. Value on fluoroscopic control. **A,** Spot film of normal-appearing medial meniscus. **B,** Spot film slightly posterior to **A,** showing complete tear of posterior horn of medial meniscus. (From Dalinka, M. K., Coren, G. S., and Wershba, M.: CRC Crit. Rev. Clin. Radiol. Nucl. Med. 4:1-59, 1973, © 1973 CRC Press, Inc. Used by permission of CRC Press, Inc.)

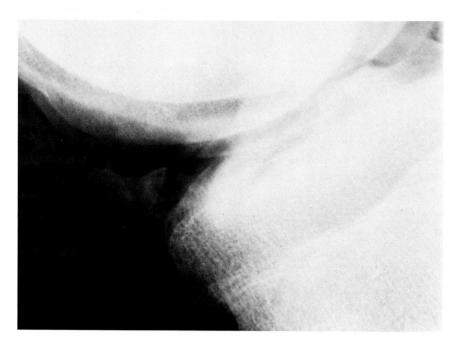

Fig. 10-25. Spot film of very anterior horn of medial meniscus, demonstrating tear in partially detached anterior horn of medial meniscus.

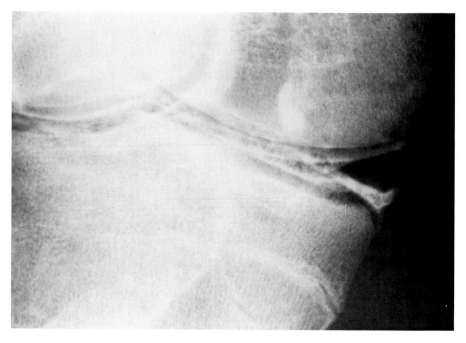

Fig. 10-26. Partial peripheral tear of tibial surface of posterior horn of medial meniscus.

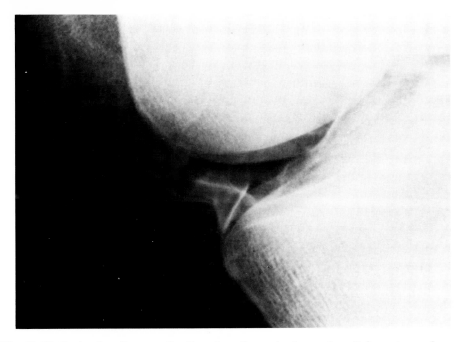

Fig. 10-27. Bucket-handle tear of midportion of anterior horn of medial meniscus, demonstrating two fragments of meniscus with contrast medium coating margins of separated fragment.

and repeat films are extremely helpful. I use a Velcro device to facilitate stress. This has been described elsewhere[3,4] and is now commercially available.*

Peripheral tears may be partial or complete (Fig. 10-26). I and others[6,13] believe that large, posterior, inferior recesses represent healed, partial, peripheral separations. They may be the radiologic counterpart of the hypermobile meniscus. A precise diagnosis of peripheral tears should be made, as these lesions may heal with conservative treatment since the blood supply to the meniscus is through its capsular attachments.

Bucket-handle tears may be recognized when the fragments are adjacent to one another (Fig. 10-27) or when the meniscus has a quadrilateral or blunted inner margin. The abnormal margin indicates separation of the inner meniscal fragment, frequently into the intercondylar notch where it cannot be seen.[2,3] Any variation from the normal triangular shape indicates a torn meniscus. A thorough search should be made for the missing fragment.

Popliteal cysts, recesses, and the anterior fat pad may cause difficulty in the diagnosis of a torn meniscus,[4,6,7] but experience, careful positioning, and attention to detail usually clarify the situation.

---

*Mastrex Medical Systems, Inc., 5 Schoolhouse Drive, Medford, N.J. 08055.

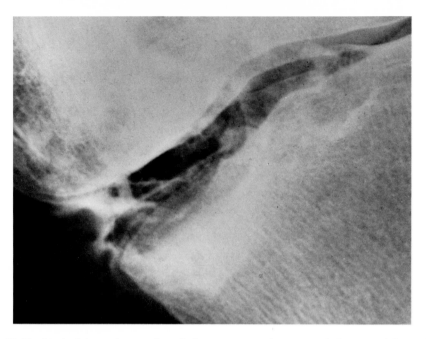

Fig. 10-28. Marked irregularity of medial meniscus with increased density of free edge, indicating contrast trapped within multiple tears. Note almost complete absence of articular cartilage over medial femoral surface. (From Dalinka, M. K., Coren, G. S., and Wershba, M.: CRC Crit. Rev. Clin. Radiol. Nucl. Med. 4:1-59, 1973, © 1973 CRC Press, Inc. Used by permission of CRC Press, Inc.)

Irregularity in the undersurface of the medial meniscus indicates meniscal degeneration,[2] which is often associated with small horizontal tears. Trapping of contrast in these frayed menisci appears as an increased density, usually in the meniscal undersurface. Flattening of the meniscus is a late sign of degeneration and is frequently associated with thinning and irregularity of the articular cartilage (Fig. 10-28). Chand[3] in an autopsy study found abnormal medial menisci in 22 consecutive asymptomatic knees in males over the age of 80: 14 were torn menisci and 8 degenerated. The presence of an abnormal meniscus in the elderly is not in itself sufficient indication for surgery.

Meniscal cysts are uncommon medially, but they are not infrequently palpable clinically. Discoid menisci are very rare medially, but Resnick and associates[16] reported three cases. Norman[15] believes that the large meniscus in Blount disease represents a discoid meniscus.

LATERAL MENISCUS

In the past, authors have commented on the difficulty in diagnosing tears of the lateral meniscus. McIntyre[12] and others[5,8,10] have described the roentgenographic anatomy of the normal posterior horn of the lateral menisci; careful technique and

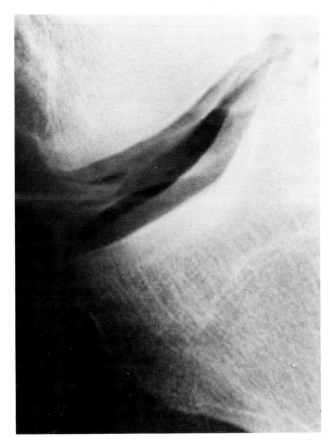

Fig. 10-29. Horizontal tear, demonstrating gas within body of lateral meniscus.

thorough knowledge of this anatomy should lead to a diagnostic accuracy of approximately 90% in lateral meniscal tears. In my experience medial tears were three times as common as lateral tears, and the combination was present in 10% of patients with torn menisci.[5] One third of patients with lateral meniscal tears had associated medial meniscal tears.[5]

Peripheral lateral separations may show a lack of upward mobility of the posterior horn of the lateral meniscus with stress, separation of the meniscus from its capsular attachments, or gas adjacent to the capsule.[12] The meniscal capsular attachments may not be completely visualized, but without these associated findings, peripheral tears cannot be diagnosed.

Tears of all portions of the lateral meniscus may be observed. Bucket-handle tears are somewhat less common laterally, but they do occur. Contrast or gas may be seen within the body of the meniscus (Figs. 10-29 and 10-30), and the tears may be complex.

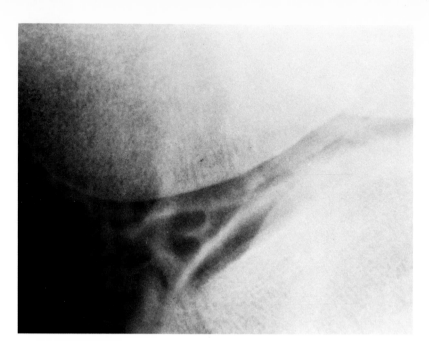

Fig. 10-30. Contrast material within tear of posterior horn of lateral meniscus.

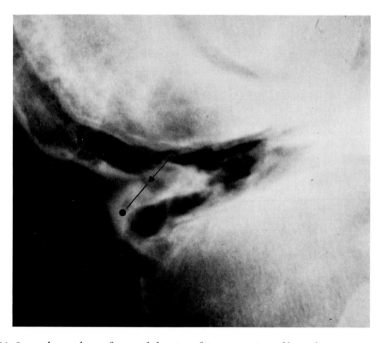

Fig. 10-31. Irregular undersurface and density of inner portion of lateral meniscus, indicating a torn degenerated meniscus. Arrow points to collection of contrast material within meniscal cyst. Note degeneration of overlying articular cartilage. (From Dalinka, M. K., Coren, G. S., and Wershba, M.: CRC Crit. Rev. Clin. Radiol. Nucl. Med. 4:1-59, 1973, © 1973 CRC Press, Inc. Used by permission of CRC Press, Inc.)

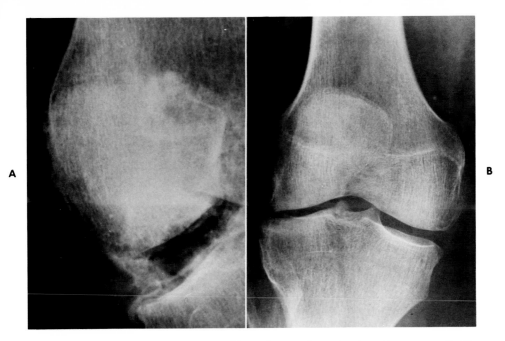

Fig. 10-32. A, Arthrogram demonstrating blunted, irregular, torn, lateral meniscus. **B,** Narrowing of lateral joint compartment. (From Dalinka, M. K., Coren, G. S., and Wershba, M.: CRC Crit. Rev. Clin. Radiol. Nucl. Med. 4:1-59, 1973, © 1973 CRC Press, Inc. Used by permission of CRC Press, Inc.)

Degeneration of the lateral meniscus is less common than degeneration of the medial meniscus but the two have a similar roentgenographic appearance with irregularity, fraying, and increased density of the undersurface.

Cysts of the lateral meniscus are not uncommon pathologically; they occurred in 22% of Smillie's[17] series of lateral meniscectomies. These are not true cysts as they are not synovial lined. They are usually small and peripheral and do not communicate with the synovium. In my experience, they are infrequently demonstrated arthrographically, but fortunately they are frequently palpable or associated with torn or degenerated menisci (Fig. 10-31).

Discoid menisci are thought to be secondary to abnormally strong meniscofemoral ligaments, limiting movement and causing meniscal hypertrophy.[9] These large thick menisci are prone to tear and are probably responsible for the increased percentage of abnormal lateral menisci in pediatric series.[1,13,18] They are discussed in more detail in Chapter 13.

Patients who present with unilateral narrowing of the lateral joint compartment may have unrecognized old lateral meniscal tears rather than degenerative arthritis (Figs. 10-27 and 10-32). Arthrography in these patients may change the treatment from an osteotomy to a meniscectomy with gratifying results.

References

1. Bramson, R. T., and Staple, T. W.: Double contrast knee arthrography in children, Am. J. Roentgenol. Radium Ther. Nucl. Med. **123:**838-844, 1975.
2. Butt, W. P. and McIntyre, J. L.: Double-contrast arthrography of the knee, Radiology **92:**487-499, 1969.
3. Chand, K.: Horizontal (cleavage) tears of the knee joint menisci in the elderly, J. Am. Geriatr. Soc. **20:**430-433, 1972.
4. Dalinka, M. K., Coren, G. S., and Wershba, M.: Knee arthrography, CRC Crit. Rev. Clin. Radiol. Nucl. Med. **4:**1-59, 1973.
5. Dalinka, M. K., Lally, J. F., and Gohel, V. K.: Arthrography of the lateral meniscus, Am. J. Roentgenol. Radium Ther. Nucl. **121:**79-85, 1974.
6. Dalinka, M. K., and Brennan, R. E.: The technique, evaluation and significance of knee arthrography, Rad. Sci. Update Series 3, 1976.
7. Hall, F. M.: Pitfalls in knee arthrography, Radiology **118:**55-62, 1976.
8. Jelaso, D. V.: The fascicles of the lateral meniscus: an anatomic-arthrographic correlation, Radiology **114:**335-339, 1975.
9. Kaplan, E. B.: Discoid lateral meniscus of the knee joint—nature, mechanism and operative treatment, J. Bone Joint Surg. [Am.] **39:**77-87, 1957.
10. Kaye, J. J.: Personal communication.
11. Lindblom, K.: Arthrography of knee: roentgenographic and anatomic study, Acta Radiol. [Suppl.] (Stockh.) **74:**1-112, 1948.
12. McIntyre, J. L.: Arthrography of the lateral meniscus, Radiology **105:**531-536, 1972.
13. Moes, C. A. F., and Munn, J. D.: The value of knee arthrography to children, J. Canad. Ass. Radiol. **16:**226-233, 1965.
14. Nicholas, J. A., Freiberger, R. H., and Killoran, P. J.: Double-contrast arthrography of the knee, J. Bone Joint Surg. [Am.] **52:**203-220, 1970.
15. Norman, A.: Personal communication.
16. Resnick, D., Goergen, T. G., Kaye, J. J., Ghelman, B., and Woody, P. R.: Discoid medial meniscus, Radiology **121:**575-576, 1976.
17. Smillie, I. S.: Injuries of the knee joint, ed. 4, Edinburgh, 1970, Churchill Livingstone, p. 102.
18. Stenstrom, R.: Arthrography of the knee joint in children. Roentgenologic anatomy, diagnosis and the use of multiple discriminant analysis, Acta Radiol. [Suppl.] (Stockh.) **281:**5-86, 1968.

11. Lesions of the ligaments

Arthroscopy
Robert W. Jackson

CLINICAL ASPECTS

When a patient presents with a painful swollen knee after trauma, a complete and detailed history must be obtained. The type of trauma, the mechanism and magnitude of the injury, the degree of initial stability or instability, and the length of time prior to presentation for treatment should be considered. The ideal time to assess a ligament injury is in the early stages before there is pain due to swelling and reactive inflammation, which can severely compromise the physical examination. Often if some time has passed prior to presentation, more useful information can be obtained from the history than from the physical examination. It should be remembered that noticeable swelling within an hour of the time of the injury must be due to bleeding from a vascularized structure. The commonest causes of hemarthrosis therefore are rupture of the anterior cruciate ligament, osteochondral fracture, and a peripheral separation of a meniscus. Damage to an avascular structure will not produce swelling until several hours after the injury and often not until the next day. This is due to a reactive effusion, and the commonest cause is a torn meniscus.

The responsible physician should also be aware of the paradox that while pain is very common in minor and moderate degrees of ligament injury, it may be relatively minimal in the grossly disrupted knee. In the latter case, leakage of blood and inflammatory effusion occurs through holes in the torn capsule. As a result the hemarthrosis does not accumulate and distend the joint, and pain is minimal. Moreover the blood and inflammatory effusions that leak out of the joint may track downward, producing a swollen calf that can be mistakenly diagnosed as thrombophlebitis. Again the time elapsed from injury is an important consideration when the examiner is assessing the severity of the problem.

As a general rule, the examiner should be quite aggressive in making an accurate diagnosis in acute knee injuries, as a delay in appreciation of the severity of the injury may lead to further damage or may compromise treatment. Recent studies on consecutive cases of traumatic hemarthrosis showed a 67% incidence of anterior cruciate injury and a 20% incidence of meniscal injury in 70 cases reported by De Haven, and Ericksson reported anterior cruciate injuries in 70% of a series of 50 cases, with a 36%

incidence of meniscal injury. It would appear therefore that two thirds of knees presenting with a traumatic hemarthrosis have an anterior cruciate lesion, and approximately one in four have an associated meniscal injury. The medial collateral ligament is significantly damaged in approximately one fourth of the cases of hemarthrosis. Other problems such as posterior cruciate tears and osteochondral fractures are noted less frequently.

AIDS TO DIAGNOSIS

If from the initial clinical appraisal one suspects a ligament injury of some magnitude, it is wise to conduct a definitive examination under general anesthesia. Such an examination would not only include the clinical assessment of ligament stability (and possibly stress roentgenograms) but also an arthroscopic examination of the interior of the knee. In an adolescent patient stress views should always be carried out, because an epiphyseal separation may well be mistaken for ligament instability.

Ideally an examination with anesthesia and arthroscopy should be done within 1 week of the time of injury in order not to miss the optimal time for correcting the problems that can be repaired surgically. Although an examination of the acutely injured knee with the patient under local anesthesia is technically feasible, it is usually difficult to completely assess ligament stability without undue discomfort for the patient. A relaxing anesthetic, general, spinal, or epidural, is therefore preferred.

Irrigation of the joint at the time of arthroscopy is also beneficial, in that blood and inflammatory debris are washed from the joint. Even in instances where surgery is not indicated, the joint irrigation itself appears to lessen the period of morbidity to a considerable degree, as the body is not obliged to absorb the hemarthrosis.

During the arthroscopic examination, failure of the joint to contain the irrigating

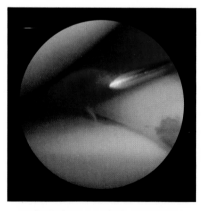

Fig. 11-1. Blood clot being washed from medial compartment of joint through 18-gauge needle inserted at joint line. Copious irrigation is necessary to clear joint of hemarthrosis.

fluid and therefore distend may indicate a major tear of the capsule. The examiner should be careful that the additional fluid that is being infused into the joint does not increase tension in the calf to such an extent as to compromise the vascular supply to the lower limb.

The usual anterior approaches to the knee are utilized for this acute examination, and copious irrigation of the joint is always necessary to wash out blood clots. Perhaps the ideal time to perform arthroscopy is within the first 10 to 12 hours after injury, as at this point the hemarthrosis has not clotted. A tourniquet may be necessary to prevent bleeding during the examination. Should the patient not be seen until the second or third day after injury, it is sometimes advantageous to wait another 4 or 5 days before performing arthroscopy on the joint. This allows early resolution of the clot to occur and enables a better joint irrigation to be carried out. Pressure pumps or syringes can be used to flush the irrigating fluid in and out of the joint through large-bore needles (Fig. 11-1) or water-sleeves from the arthroscope. It may take some time, but a complete joint washout and good visualization are possible.

ACUTE DISORDERS
Anterior cruciate ligament

The anterior cruciate ligament (Fig. 11-2) is ruptured in two thirds of traumatized knees presenting with a hemarthrosis. Consequently this ligament should be studied carefully (arthroscopically) for the type and location of the tear, as this might well influence further management. Complete rupture may occur at its proximal attachment (Fig. 11-3), its distal attachment (Fig. 11-4), or in its mid structure. Surgical repair is feasible and definitely advisable if the tear has occurred at either end of the ligament. If it is a mid-substance tear, there is still controversy as to whether or not surgical reapposition of the tattered ends is of much value.

It should be noted that a partial tear of the anterior cruciate is a common occurrence, although statistics are lacking as to incidence. This occurs when the ligament is stretched to its maximum, and there is partial giving way of some of the fibers without total loss of continuity of the structure. As the ligament is normally covered by synovium, a partial tear is identified by the presence of subsynovial hemorrhages (Fig. 11-5). Occasionally a break in the synovium is visible, and portions of the torn ligament are seen to extrude from the synovial sheath (Fig. 11-6). The insertion of a second instrument, a palpating or pulling probe, such as a blunt nerve hook, can be of value in assessing the integrity of the anterior cruciate ligament. Moreover if a drawer sign is attempted while the arthroscope is in position, undue laxity may be visualized.

Should the anterior cruciate ligament be the only significant structure to show signs of traumatic disruption within the joint, it may well be considered as an "isolated" anterior cruciate ligament tear. One should realize, however, that this is almost always associated with some degree, however minor, of sprain or strain of the medial collateral ligament or posterior capsule. The treatment of the true "isolated" anterior cruciate lesion should be conservative.

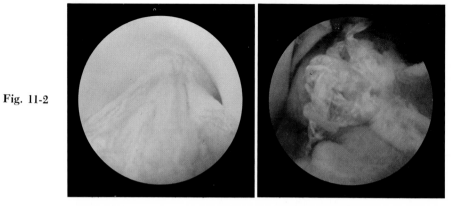

Fig. 11-2   **Fig. 11-3**

Fig. 11-2. Normal anterior cruciate ligament, showing origin in intercondylar notch and insertion on tibial spine (magnified by its closeness to lens of arthroscope).

Fig. 11-3. Rupture of anterior cruciate ligament close to proximal attachment. Frayed ends of ligament are clearly visible.

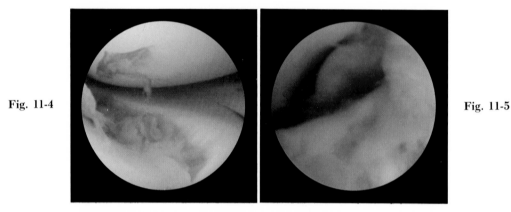

Fig. 11-4   **Fig. 11-5**

Fig. 11-4. Osteochondral fracture due to avulsion of distal insertion of anterior cruciate ligament. Note normal meniscus in background.

Fig. 11-5. Partial tear of anterior cruciate ligament, identified by presence of subsynovial hemorrhages.

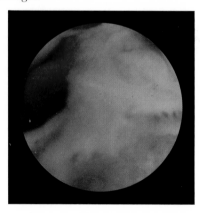

Fig. 11-6. Partial tear of anterior cruciate ligament with break in synovial sheath, allowing some frayed ends of ligament to extrude.

Posterior cruciate ligament

If there is suspicion that the posterior cruciate may be injured (from the mechanism of injury or from physical examination) special efforts should be made to confirm or deny the diagnosis, as an unrecognized posterior cruciate rupture may be a source of continued disability in the future. Clinically a posterior drawer sign or excessive laxity in full extension, on varus or valgus strain, is the diagnostic point. Roentgenograms may reveal the avulsion of a small fragment of bone above the posterior edge of the tibia. Should the posterior cruciate be torn from its upper end, it can sometimes be recognized from the routine anterior approach. Should it be ruptured in the middle or near its insertion on the tibia without a bony fragment, it may be seen from one of two alternative arthroscopic approaches. A posteromedial approach enables one to visualize the posterior cruciate along with the posterior horn insertion of the medial meniscus. An anterior patellar tendon–splitting approach with a small arthroscope or a 70° forward-oblique arthroscope enables the examiner to see between the anterior cruciate and the medial femoral condyle and to visualize the posterior cruciate behind the anterior cruciate. Increasing awareness of this lesion, plus improved arthroscopic techniques, is allowing this diagnosis to be made more frequently.

Medial collateral ligament

The medial collateral ligament may be injured by itself or concomitantly with the anterior cruciate ligament. Testing by valgus strain must be done in both extension and 30° of flexion. Often this ligament is torn either proximal or distal to the joint line. Therefore the tear may be extraarticular and only diagnosed by clinical examination. The arthroscopic clue to a medial collateral ligament rupture is laxity of the medial compartment when a valgus strain is applied to the joint. In such an instance the medial meniscus can usually be seen in its entirety because the compartment

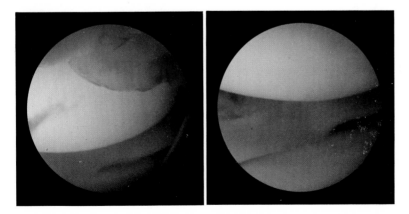

Fig. 11-7. With rupture of medial collateral ligament, medial compartment opens widely on valgus strain, allowing excellent visualization of medial meniscus.

opens widely (Fig. 11-7). Should the ligament rupture be at the level of the joint line, the examiner may see a capsular or synovial disruption in the region of the tear. Should the rupture be fairly significant, and again at the joint line level, he may also see infolding of the soft tissues either above or below the meniscus.

It is also important to assess whether or not the meniscus rises with the femur on valgus strain or remains with the tibia. This gives the examiner some indication as to whether the capsular and ligamentous rupture is on the tibial side of the meniscus (the coronary ligament) or on the femoral side.

Lateral collateral ligament

This ligament is also an extraarticular structure, and assessment of its integrity is basically a clinical diagnosis. If the ligament is torn, the lateral meniscus becomes more easily visualized at arthroscopy because of increased opening of the lateral compartment on varus strain. However, one must remember that the popliteal tendon is an intraarticular structure and passes through the joint in close proximity to the lateral collateral ligament. The popliteal hiatus should not be confused with a peripheral tear or separation of the lateral meniscus (Fig. 11-8).

Popliteal tendon avulsion

Several cases have been identified in which the popliteal tendon insertion has been avulsed from the lateral femoral condyle. When this happens a small bony fragment is pulled into an intraarticular site (Fig. 11-9). On x-ray examination it is seen in the slightly oblique view. This avulsion fragment from the femoral condyle should not be confused with the fabella. Treatment of choice, if the fragment is recognized, is to reinsert it back into its normal extraarticular situation.

Fig. 11-8

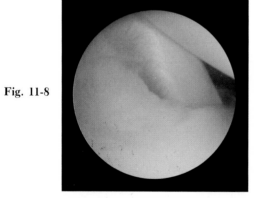 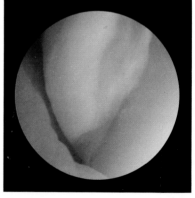

Fig. 11-9

Fig. 11-8. Normal popliteal tendon passing through popliteal hiatus. This hiatus should not be confused with peripheral tear of lateral meniscus.

Fig. 11-9. Bony fragment avulsed from insertion of popliteal tendon has been pulled into joint. This relatively rare condition, if recognized, is best treated by replacement of fragment in its anatomic site.

Capsular tears

The coronary ligament stabilizing the anterior horn of the meniscus may well be ruptured by a mechanism similar to that which would produce a meniscal tear. This lesion is recognized arthroscopically by the presence of blood in the joint (not seen in a pure meniscal lesion) and extrusion of the anterior horn of the meniscus from the joint, as the knee is brought into full extension. Treatment should consist of reattachment of the coronary ligament if the problem is recognized in the acute stage.

CHRONIC DISORDERS
Anterior cruciate ligament

The long-standing anterior cruciate ligament tear characteristically demonstrates a positive anterior drawer sign, which may or may not be associated with the "pivot shift" sign (indicating anterolateral rotatory instability) or the Slocum sign (antero-medial instability). Clinical evaluation is most important in assessing this problem.

Arthroscopy should be done with the patient under general anesthesia to permit adequate examination of ligament stability. In chronic anterior cruciate problems, the examiner may encounter an absent space where the anterior cruciate normally would traverse the intercondylar notch. Occasionally there is a stub of anterior cruciate remaining at its distal insertion. This fragment of cruciate ligament is usually rounded off by attrition (Fig. 11-10). Occasionally it enters the medial compartment of the joint, causing clicking and a sensation of giving way similar to that of a torn meniscus. Also, because of associated instability the synovium in the area is often profusely hypertrophied and obscures visualization of the intercondylar region. In cases of anterior cruciate instability with a positive pivot shift sign, the lateral meniscus is ruptured in approximately 50% of cases. If the anterior cruciate is torn the posterior cruciate may be seen from the anterior approach (Fig. 11-11).

Fig. 11-10
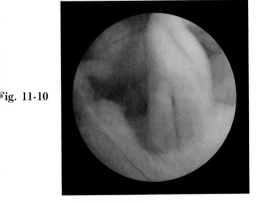
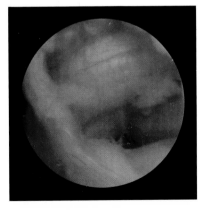
Fig. 11-11

Fig. 11-10. Distal stub of torn anterior cruciate, rounded off by attrition.
Fig. 11-11. Intact posterior cruciate ligament seen from anterior approach only when anterior cruciate is absent.

Posterior cruciate ligament

This ligament can be visualized arthroscopically through a central patellar tendon approach or through a posteromedial approach, if a chronic tear is suspected. If there has been a significant degree of instability for a period of time, there may well be degenerative changes on the articular surface of the femur or the tibia or both.

SUMMARY

Arthroscopic examination soon after a serious injury to the knee that has produced a hemarthrosis can be invaluable in the total understanding of the existing lesions and consequently can lead to appropriate therapy. Anterior cruciate lesions can be identified with accuracy, and with increasing experience, ruptures of the posterior cruciate will undoubtedly be diagnosed with greater frequency.

Damage to the collateral ligaments and associated capsular structures may be identified by direct visualization of a tear, or through the ancillary finding of increased joint laxity. Washout of blood and inflammatory debris during the irrigation process appears to have a beneficial effect in cases where surgery is not indicated, and conservative management is carried out. As stated, however, the greatest value of arthroscopy lies in the fact that the surgeon can quickly determine the complete extent of the lesions within the traumatized knee and consequently deal with it appropriately.

Arthrography
Harry J. Griffiths

Although it is true that the diagnosis of many ligament injuries to the knee joint is primarily a clinical one, the radiologist, using arthrography, may be able to help with the definition of the amount of damage present, as well as with the demonstration of concomitant meniscal injuries. In this section the plain-film diagnosis of ligament tears as well as the arthrographic appearance of cruciate ligament tears and capsular rupture will be considered. Moreover many ligament injuries are associated with effusions, and this is an appropriate place to discuss the plain-film diagnosis of a knee effusion.

PLAIN-FILM DIAGNOSIS OF LIGAMENT INJURIES

Many tears of the collateral ligaments are produced by indirect trauma with forced rotation and slight flexion as well as with forced abduction or adduction of the leg. These injuries often result in a strain with no roentgenographic features. Tears of the lateral collateral ligament are less common than those of the medial ligament, which is more firmly attached both to its osseous origins and to the joint capsule. But if there is a true tear of a collateral ligament, the joint can be opened on a stress film. This is performed by abducting or adducting the knee joint as is appropriate and taking a plain film at rest and under stress. This will often cause the patient some pain, and if the pain is too severe an injection of local anesthetic into the most painful place will allow the roentgenogram to be taken.

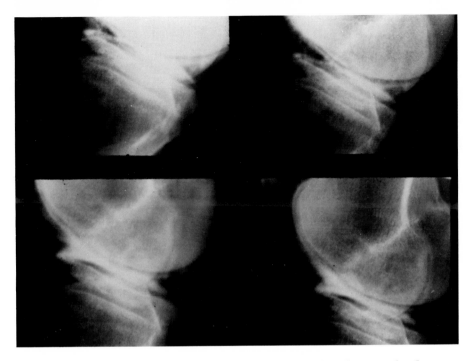

Fig. 11-12. Instability. By rocking tibia backward and forward on femur under fluoroscopy or with cine roentgenography, some idea of degree of instability can be seen on these four selected films.

Occasionally in an acute tear, a small avulsion fracture from the epicondyle of the femur or the head of the fibula can be seen at the point of origin of the ligament. In chronic or long-standing tears, it is frequently possible to visualize a linear calcification adjacent and often parallel to the femoral condyle. This represents calcification in the site of origin of the ligament and is known as Pellegrini-Stieda syndrome. When it is present, this syndrome is indicative of a previous collateral ligament tear.

There are also few if any plain-film roentgenographic features of cruciate ligament tears, unless the tear is an old one, and the ligament calcifies, or there is an associated fracture of a tibial spine. However, with the use of either cine roentgenography or of 105 mm spot-filming, instability in a joint may be demonstrated when a sequence of pictures is taken while stressing the joint backward and forward and relating the relative position of the femur (intercondylar notch) to the tibial spines (Fig. 11-12). Many cruciate ligament injuries are associated with capsular tears as well as meniscal injuries, and an arthrogram is indicated to define the overall problem with respect to the internal derangement of the knee joint.[9-11]

PLAIN-FILM DIAGNOSIS OF AN EFFUSION
IN THE KNEE JOINT

Most of us were trained to diagnose knee effusions by looking at the region of the popliteal fossa posteriorly and observing the bulge made by the joint capsule, which

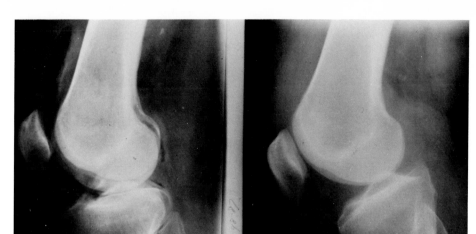

Fig. 11-13. Effusion. On right is knee of a 39-year-old woman with rheumatoid arthritis and a knee effusion. Arthrogram performed 1 month later shows position of suprapatellar bursa where effusion can be identified on earlier film.

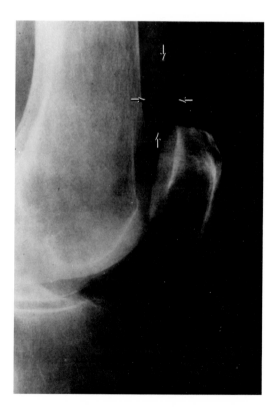

Fig. 11-14. Rheumatoid effusion. In this slightly flexed view of knee, this 15 ml effusion can be identified lying between suprapatellar fat pad and fat anterior to femur *(arrows)*.

will displace the normal soft tissues. However, in older patients it is often difficult to differentiate tortuosity of the popliteal artery or a popliteal artery aneurysm from an effusion. Recently it became obvious that it is possible to diagnose a knee effusion by looking in the region of the suprapatellar bursa, where a very small amount of fluid will displace the normal fat pads that are present: one above the patella itself and the other anterior to the femur (Fig. 11-13).[5] On either a straight lateral view of the knee or with the joint flexed about 20°, Weissman and Sosman[15] showed in autopsy studies that an effusion of only 3 ml can be seen. In vivo an effusion of perhaps 10 or 15 ml is easily visible, for example, as is frequently seen in rheumatoid arthritis (Fig. 11-14), and larger effusions are extremely easy to diagnose using this method.[2,5,6,8,15]

ARTHROGRAPHIC DIAGNOSIS OF LIGAMENT TEARS

Collateral ligament tears are often associated with capsular tears, and these will appear as either irregularities or as increases in capsular size, particularly laterally or inferiorly. However, the main use of the arthrogram in patients with collateral ligament tears is to exclude an associated meniscal lesion. A capsular tear is diagnosed arthrographically when contrast leaks outside the normal confines of the joint (Fig. 11-15).[7,13,14]

On the other hand the cruciate ligaments have invaginations of synovium that

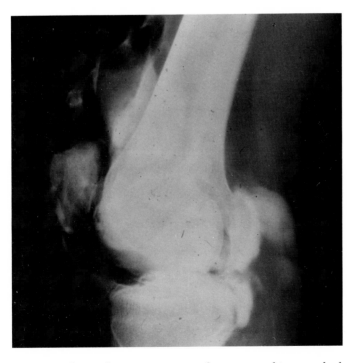

Fig. 11-15. Ligament and capsular tears. During arthrogram on this severely deranged knee, contrast and air ran into soft tissues anteriorly and posteriorly. Tears of lateral collateral and quadriceps ligaments were present.

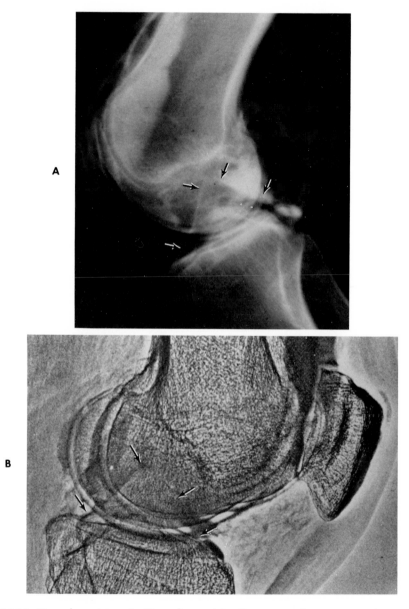

Fig. 11-16. Normal cruciates. **A,** Normal synovial reflection overlying cruciate ligaments can be seen as a synovial "tent" in center of most knee joints at arthrography *(arrows).* **B,** Xero-radiograph.

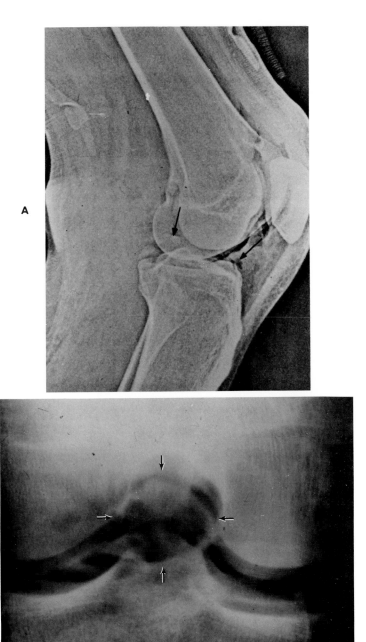

Fig. 11-17. Tears of cruciates. Although deflections of synovium over posterior cruciate are diagnostic of tear *(posterior arrow)*, **A,** often tears of anterior cruciate are seen only as large "loose body" within intercondylar notch *(arrows),* **B.** (**A** from Griffiths, H. J.: Orthop. Rev. **5**(9):71, 1976.)

outline their course arthrographically. In the normal knee the two cruciates form a "tent" in the intercondylar notch (Fig. 11-16). This can be seen on a true lateral roentgenogram but is best shown with a 5° rotated view off true lateral. The normal cruciates have very clear margins, and these are easy to see using either single- or double-contrast arthrography.[12] A tear of either of the cruciate ligaments will produce irregularity and narrowing of the normal contours (most often true of tears of the anterior cruciate) or will produce marked displacement of the normal synovial reflections (best seen with posterior cruciate tears) (Fig. 11-17).[7,9,13,14]

A final arthrographic appearance of note is that a cruciate tear will often be associated with rupture of the capsule; on a tunnel view of the knee done at arthrography the torn cruciate may appear as a rounded opacity (loose body) within the intercondylar notch.

Lateral tomography has been advocated by a number of authors in order to better delineate this synovial "tent."[1-4] However, tomography is rarely indicated because the diagnosis of cruciate ligament tears is usually a clinical one, and tomography increases the time taken for arthrography as well as the radiation exposure to the patient. Similarly xeroradiography has been used to enhance the soft tissue detail of the joint capsule and surrounding ligament structures, but it also entails a higher radiation dose and usually involves moving the patient from one x-ray room to another, lengthening the procedure unnecessarily.

SUMMARY

The roentgenographic features of both collateral and cruciate ligament injuries may be of help to the orthopedist in the demonstration of joint space widening on stress views, instability of the joint, and the irregularities in contour of the synovial "tent" seen in cruciate injuries at arthrography. However, the principle use of arthrography in patients with suspected ligament injuries is to exclude associated meniscal damage.

References

1. Anderson, P. W., and Maslin, P.: Tomography applied to knee arthrography, Radiology **110:**271-275, 1974.
2. Bachman, A. L.: Roentgen diagnosis of knee-joint effusion, Radiology **46:**462-469, 1946.
3. Dalinka, M. K., Gohel, V. K., and Rancier, L.: Tomography in the evaluation of the anterior cruciate ligament, Radiology **108:**31-33, 1973.
4. Fagerberg, S.: Tomographic studies on the normal and injured knee, Acta Radiol. [Suppl.] (Stockh.) 138, 1956.
5. Hall, F. M.: Radiographic diagnosis and accuracy in knee joint effusions, Radiology **115:**39-54, 1975.
6. Harris, R. D., and Hecht, H. L.: Suprapatellar effusions: a new diagnostic sign, Radiology **97:**1-4, 1970.
7. Horns, J. W.: Single contrast knee arthrography in abnormalities of the articular cartilage, Radiology **105:**537-540, 1972.
8. Lewis, R. W.: Roentgenographic study tissue pathology in and about the knee joint, Am. J. Roentgenol. Radium Ther. Nucl. Med. **65:**200-220, 1951.

9. Liljedahl, S. O., Lindvall, N., and Wetterfors, F.: Roentgen diagnosis of rupture of anterior cruciate ligament, Acta Radiol. [Diagn.] (Stock.) **4:**225-239, 1966.
10. Lindblom, K.: Arthrography of the knee: a roentgenographic and anatomical study, Acta Radiol. [Suppl.] (Stock.) 74, 1948.
11. Ricklin, P., Rüttiman, A., and Del Buono, M. S.: Meniscus lesions, New York, 1971, Grune & Stratton.
12. Roebuck, E. J.: Double contrast knee arthrography. Some new points of technique including the use of Dimer X, Clin. Radiol. **28:**247-257, 1977.
13. Staple, T. W.: Extrameniscal lesions demonstrated by double-contrast arthrography of the knee, Radiology **102:**311-319, 1972.
14. Wang, J. B., Rubin, R. M., and Marshall, J. L.: A mechanism of isolated anterior cruciate ligament rupture, J. Bone Joint Surg. [Am.] **57:**411-413, 1975.
15. Weissman, B. N. W., and Sosman, J. L.: The radiology of rheumatoid arthritis, Orthop. Clin. North Am. **6:**653-674, 1975.

12. The previously operated knee

Arthroscopy

John J. Joyce III
Houshang Farahver

The importance of performing prompt and adequate surgery on the knee joint has been repeatedly emphasized by many authors. In order to achieve this goal various surgical exposures have been proposed. Several observers[1,6] in the past have suggested that total meniscectomy had undesirable long-range sequelae, and more recent reports have tended to confirm the earlier data. The parapatellar incision[2] has been indicted as a factor in at least some of the unsatisfactory long-term results. Few of these studies have noted the condition of the joint at the time of the original operation.

This report presents the arthroscopic findings observed in 88 knees examined between 1971 and 1975. All patients had undergone prior operations about the knee joint for various reasons. All patients had complaints relating to the previously operated knee joint (Table 6). There were 59 males and 29 females. The ages varied from 13 years to 70 years with an average age of 34. The right knee was involved in 42 instances, the left knee in 44, and in two patients both previously operated joints were symptomatic.

During the early period of our arthroscopic investigations, the examination was performed using general anesthesia. For this reason, 42 patients were admitted to the hospital for arthroscopy. As it became evident that many of these individuals could be examined with the patient under local anesthesia, 46 patients were done on an outpatient basis. Arthroscopy was performed with the patient under general anesthesia on 41 knees and under local anesthesia on 47 knees.

Among the previously performed surgical procedures, medial meniscectomy alone had been done on 47 patients. Lateral meniscectomy alone was the prior operation on eight patients, and both medial and lateral menisci had been excised in six patients. Four individuals had undergone medial meniscectomy plus a ligament repair. A variety of operations had been performed on the knees of the remaining patients.

As one would anticipate, degenerative change was found to be the chief problem in 47 of the 88 knees examined (Table 7). It was of interest to note that lesions of the remaining meniscus were found in 12 of the patients who had undergone prior arthrotomy. Nine patients had a tear of the remaining meniscus, while a discoid

Table 6. Prior procedures

Operation	No.
Meniscectomy	
Medial	49
Lateral	8
Medial and lateral	6
Meniscectomy and ligamentous repair	4
Loose bodies	4
Patelloplasty	4
Excision scar	1
Meniscectomy on both knees	1
Synovectomy	1
Exploration	1
Patellectomy	1
Hauser and loose body	1
Hauser alone	2
Osgood-Schlatter operation	1
Condyle repaired	1
Fractured patella repaired	1
Bullet removed	1
Baker cyst	2
Prosthesis	1

Table 7. Arthroscopic findings

Finding	No.
Degenerative change	
Mild	9
Moderate	31
Severe	9
Retained posterior horn	6
Tear of other meniscus	9
Discoid lateral meniscus	3
Cruciate tear	2
Condyle defect	5
Synovitis and scar	7
Research only	4
Adhesions	2
Patellar fissure	1
Pigmented villonodular synovitis	1
Loose prosthesis	1

lateral meniscus was present in the other three. All of the discoid lateral menisci were found to be torn, and symptoms had appeared shortly after the original operations. A retained posterior medial meniscal horn of significant size was found in six knees, while only two showed a definite tear of the anterior cruciate ligament. Femoral condylar defects were observed in five patients, while a significant synovial scar was noted in seven. Adhesions were seen in two instances. In one patient lysis of these scars resulted in a rather dramatic improvement in symptoms and motion so that the patient was able to return to a part-time job. Fissuring of the patella, recurring pigmented villonodular synovitis, and a loose femoral component of a unicompartmental knee prosthesis comprised the remaining causes for patients' difficulties.

The loosened knee prosthesis was of particular interest. The device had been inserted several months previously to correct a severely damaged tibial plateau. Although x-ray studies had shown the device to be apparently well fixed in satisfactory position, the knee could not be extended beyond 15° or flexed beyond 40°. Arthroscopic examination revealed loosening of the femoral component. Motion of the joint caused the unicompartmental device to change position, thus limiting motion to the above range. Revision of the prosthesis resulted in marked improvement of the patient's problem.

Accuracy of clinical diagnosis made prior to arthroscopic evaluation revealed 34 diagnoses to be correct and 22 diagnoses to be partly correct. Evaluation of the patient's problem was indefinite in 13 cases and incorrect in 17. Second arthroscopic examinations were done on two asymptomatic knees 1 year after meniscectomy so that their conditions could be assessed.

Complications were few in number and, for the most part, to be expected. Four patients experienced a significant effusion that lasted for more than a week. Two patients in whose knees cortisone had been instilled immediately after arthroscopy developed leakage of synovial fluid from the stab wound through which the arthroscope had been inserted. Fortunately both wounds closed uneventfully without any infection, and this practice has been discontinued. Severe pain was experienced by an alcoholic individual who had undergone medial meniscectomy 38 years earlier and whose severe degenerative changes led eventually to a total-knee replacement. Severe disabling joint pain had been the reason for arthroscopic evaluation. Discomfort in the joint that lasted up to a month was present in seven knees, and one person developed a transitory phlebitis of an arm vein in which intravenous sedation had been administered. The remaining 72 patients had either minimal effusion or nondisabling discomfort that lasted up to a week after examination.

DISCUSSION

Arthroscopy has come to assume an important role in the evaluation of knee problems. The patients included in this presentation had all been examined and treated by well-qualified orthopedists and were referred because of difficulty in the identification of the patient's problems by conventional means. Several investi-

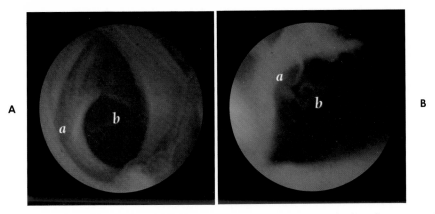

Fig. 12-1. A, Six months prior to arthroscopy this 26-year old woman had undergone medial meniscectomy and repair of medial capsule and collateral ligament in left knee. Persistent pain and decreased motion ensued. Dense and extensive synovial scarring was noted in suprapatellar pouch area of scar, *a*. Suprapatellar pouch, *b*. **B,** Appearance of suprapatellar pouch immediately after division of adhesions with arthroscope. Six months after arthroscopy patient was able to return to a part-time job that required standing for long periods. Residual synovial scar, *a*. Suprapatellar pouch, *b*.

Fig. 12-2

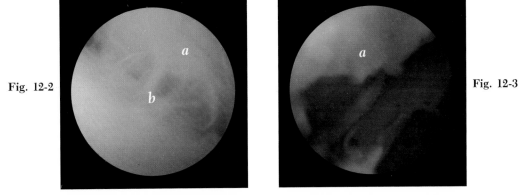

Fig. 12-3

Fig. 12-2. Severe degenerative changes seen in medial side of left knee joint of 55-year-old woman who had had medial meniscectomy 40 years prior to arthroscopy. Marked improvement after partial joint replacement. Medial femoral condyle, *a*. Tibial plateau, *b*.
Fig. 12-3. Fifteen years prior to arthroscopy this 60-year-old man had his torn medial meniscus excised by a well-known orthopedist. Gradually increasing pain on weight-bearing activities led him to seek aid. Note severe degenerative change in femoral condyle, *a*.

gators previously demonstrated that total removal of a meniscus is sometimes followed by later changes that can cause disability.[1,5-7]

The role of synovial scar tissue in producing occasional postoperative difficulties is again suggested by several cases in this series. These patients, in whom a retained posterior meniscal tag was noted, as well as those patients in whom other knee ab-

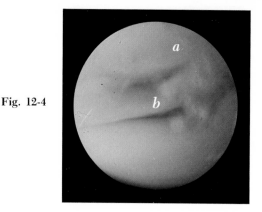
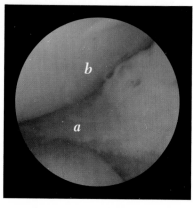

Fig. 12-4

Fig. 12-

Fig. 12-4. Left knee. Three years previously this 24-year-old man had his torn medial meniscus excised elsewhere through a minimal incision. Continued symptoms of pain, locking,
and swelling caused him to seek further aid. Arthroscopy showed a torn discoid lateral meniscus, excision of which relieved his symptoms. Femoral condyle, *a*. Flap of lateral meniscus
in notch, *b*.

Fig. 12-5. After two medial meniscectomies this 44-year-old man again developed right knee
pain. In addition to rather extensive scarring of synovium and meniscus area, *a*, moderate
degenerative changes were observed in medial femoral condyle, *b*, and there was considerable
chondromalacia of patellofemoral joint.

normalities were observed at the time of arthroscopy reemphasize the limitations
imposed by conventional surgical exposures.

Improvement in the patient in whom adhesions in the pouch were visualized
arthroscopically illustrates the potential value of the arthroscope as a therapeutic
device. Other investigators have demonstrated that such procedures as removal of
loose bodies, synovial biopsies, and partial meniscectomies can be performed arthroscopically with apparent minimal time of disability.[10,14] It is important to realize
that the procedure is a new one, and further evaluation of it must be undertaken
before final conclusions can be drawn (Figs. 12-1 to 12-5).

CONCLUSIONS

1. Arthroscopic findings in 88 previously operated knees are presented.
2. The arthroscope is helpful in the evaluation of the previously operated knee
   and in planning further therapy.
3. The arthroscope is useful in the treatment of certain specific knee problems.

References

1. Böhler, L.: The treatment of fractures, New York, 1958, Grune & Stratton, vol. 3, p.
   1608.
2. Charnley, J.: Horizontal approach to the medial semilunar cartilage, J. Bone Joint Surg.
   [Br.] **30**:659, 1948.
3. Dandy, D. J., and Jackson, R. W.: The diagnosis of problems after meniscectomy, J. Bone
   Joint Surg. [Br.] **57**(3):349-52, 1975.

4. Fairbank, T. J.: Knee joint changes after meniscectomy, J. Bone Joint Surg. [Br.] **30**:664, 1948.
5. Huckell, J. R.: Is meniscectomy a benign procedure? A long-term follow-up study, Can. J. Surg. **8**:254-260, 1965.
6. Jackson, R. W.: Arthroscopy of the knee. In Ahstrom, J. P., Jr., editor: Current practice in orthopaedic surgery, vol. 5, St. Louis, 1973, The C. V. Mosby Co., pp. 93-117.
7. Watanabe, M. In Helfet, A. J., editor: Disorders of the knee, New York, 1974, J. B. Lippincott Co., pp. 139-149.

Suggested readings

Casscells, S. W.: Arthroscopy of the knee joint. A review of 150 cases, J. Bone Joint Surg. [Am.] **53**:287-298, 1971.
Dandy, D. J., and Jackson, R. W.: Meniscectomy and chondromalacia of the femoral condyles, J. Bone Joint Surg. [Am.] 57(8):116-119, 1975.
Jackson, R. W., and Dandy, D. J.: Arthroscopy of the knee, New York, 1976, Grune & Stratton.
Jackson, R. W.: Arthroscopy of the knee. In Ahstrom, J. P., Jr., editor: Current practice in orthopaedic surgery, vol. 5, St. Louis, 1973, The C. V. Mosby Co., pp. 93-117.
Jackson, R. W., and deHaven, K.: Arthroscopy of the knee, Clin. Orthop. **107**:87, 1975.
Smillie, I. S.: Injuries of the knee joint, ed. 2, Edinburgh, 1951, E. & S. Livingstone.
Watanabe, M., Takeda, S., and Skeuchi, H.: Atlas of arthroscopy, ed. 2, Tokyo, 1969, Igaku Shoin Ltd.

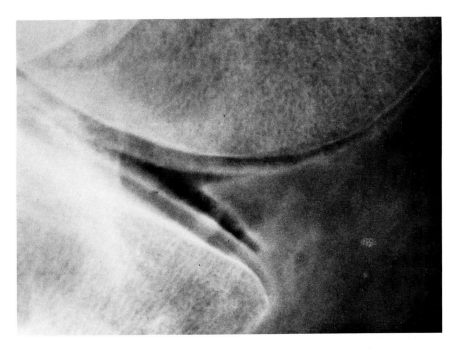

Fig. 12-6. Regenerated posterior horn of medial meniscus. Note triangular appearance and lack of normal recesses.

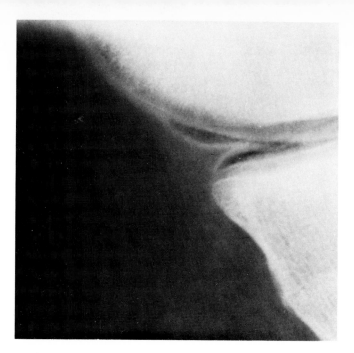

Fig. 12-7. Regenerated midportion of medial meniscus, showing small meniscus with equilateral triangular appearance. (From Dalinka, M. K., Coren, G. S., and Wershba, M.: CRC Crit. Rev. Clin. Radiol. Nucl. Med. **4**:1-59, 1973, © 1973 CRC Press, Inc. Used by permission of CRC Press, Inc.)

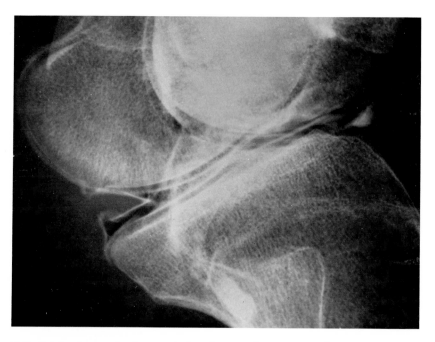

Fig. 12-8. Retained posterior horn, which is large and retains its inferior recess. (From Dalinka, M. K., Coren, G. S., and Wershba, M.: CRC Crit. Rev. Clin. Radiol. Nucl. Med. **4**:1-59, 1973, © 1973 CRC Press, Inc. Used by permission of CRC Press, Inc.)

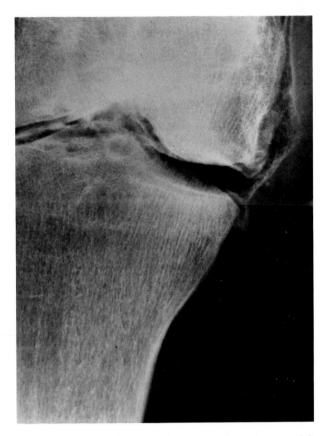

Fig. 12-9. Postmeniscectomy knee, showing almost complete absence of femoral and tibial articular cartilage. Note spur on femoral surface and flat edge of capsule along cleavage plane. (From Dalinka, M. K., Coren, G. S., and Wershba, M.: CRC Crit. Rev. Clin. Radiol. Nucl. Med. 4:1-59, 1973, © 1973 CRC Press, Inc. Used by permission of CRC Press, Inc.)

Arthrography

Murray K. Dalinka

The presence of knee symptoms after meniscectomy is significant. In one large series[7] only 38% of patients were symptom free after surgery.

Smillie[6] emphasizes the importance of total meniscectomy, and some surgeons make two incisions to accomplish this. Cargill and Jackson[1] feel that more conservative surgery should be performed in bucket-handle tears. Cox and associates[2] have shown that partial meniscectomy leads to less severe degenerative changes than does total meniscectomy. His experiments in dogs showed that the degree of degenerative change is directly related to the amount of meniscus removed. In partial meniscectomies, the cartilage surface covered by the regenerated meniscus was protected from degenerative change.

After complete meniscectomy, fibrous regeneration of the meniscus occurs and is usually complete within 3 months.[5] The regenerated meniscus is thinner than normal and is shaped like an equilateral rather than an isoceles triangle (Figs. 12-6 and 12-7). It has a dense broad capsular attachment, and there is no cleavage plane between the meniscus and the joint capsule. The recesses are lost.[4] Grossly the regenerated meniscus has a glistening surface that resembles hyaline cartilage. The surface area of the regenerated meniscus is 50% to 60% of the normal meniscal size.[5] The regenerated fragment has decreased mobility and hence is rarely torn.

The retained posterior horn appears normal in size (Fig. 12-8) but changes abruptly from posterior to anterior. Occasionally when a portion of the posterior horn is not completely removed, the tear may be left in situ.

The partially resected bucket-handle tear shows a blunted periphery, simulating

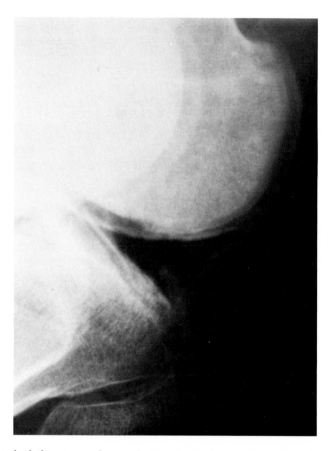

Fig. 12-10. Marked thinning and irregularity of articular cartilage about lateral joint compartment after meniscectomy. (From Dalinka, M. K., Coren, G. S., and Wershba, M.: CRC Crit. Rev. Clin. Radiol. Nucl. Med. 4:1-59, 1973, © 1973 CRC Press, Inc. Used by permission of CRC Press, Inc.)

a fresh tear. The lack of a free fragment and a meniscectomy scar differentiate the two.

The commonest abnormality in our patients has been degeneration of the femoral articular cartilage (Figs. 12-9 and 12-10). Dandy and Jackson[3] have seen this in 55% of their postmeniscectomy arthroscopies. In 40% of their cases, it was thought to be the major or only cause of symptomatology.

In Debnam and Staple's[4] arthrographic series, multiple lesions were seen in 25% of their cases. Abnormalities of the anterior cruciate ligament, tears of the opposite meniscus, and torn remnants were not infrequent. We have seen occasional tears of the opposite meniscus and absent or attenuated cruciate ligaments, but these abnormalities only accounted for a small percentage of cases. The retained posterior horn is common in our experience, but we are loath to attach significance to it unless it is torn.

We have seen small contracted joints in a number of patients, probably secondary to chronic synovitis. In one postmeniscectomy patient, the symptoms were dramatically relieved by arthrography. We felt that joint distension probably lysed small adhesions that were responsible for the symptomatology.

We feel that arthrography is a simple, safe, and accurate method of evaluating the postmeniscectomy knee. The source of symptoms is most frequently chondromalacia of the femoral articular cartilage, which usually can be recognized at arthrography. The torn opposite meniscus, abnormal anterior cruciate ligament, and retained fragment are considerably less common but can easily be identified.

References

1. Cargill, A. O., and Jackson, J. P.: Bucket-handle tear of the medial meniscus. A case for conservative surgery, J. Bone Joint Surg. [Am.] **58:**248-251, 1976.
2. Cox, J. S., Nye, C. E., Shaefer, W. W., and Woodstein, I. J.: Comparison of partial and total resection of the medial meniscus in dogs' knees, Jefferson Ortho. J. **3:**57-63, 1974.
3. Dandy, D. J., and Jackson, R. W.: The diagnosis of problems after meniscectomy, J. Bone Joint Surg. [Br.] **57:**349-352, 1975.
4. Debnam, J. W., and Staple, T. W.: Arthrography of the knee after meniscectomy, Radiology **113:**67-71, 1974.
5. Doyle, J. R., Eisenberg, J. H., and Orth, M. W.: Regeneration of knee menisci: a preliminary report, J. Trauma **6:**50-55, 1966.
6. Smillie, I. S.: Injuries of the knee joint, ed. 4, Edinburgh, 1970, Churchill Livingstone, p. 102.
7. Tapper, E. M., and Hoover, N. W.: Late results after meniscectomy, J. Bone Joint Surg. [Am.] **51:**517-526, 1969.

13. Arthroscopy and arthrography in children and adolescents

Arthroscopy

Robert E. Eilert

As arthroscopy has gained wide acceptance, its place in the diagnosis and treatment of knee disorders in children has become better established. It is a medical dictum that the efficacy of treatment improves with greater accuracy of diagnosis. As the etiology and natural history of disease is understood, treatment becomes more rational and direct. Arthroscopy assists in diagnosis, treatment, and definition of the natural history of disease.

This section of this chapter is based on experience gained from arthroscopic examination of the knees in 129 patients under 19 years of age. Eighteen of these patients were 12 years or younger when examined, and the remainder were teenagers from 13 to 18 years of age. The new fiber optic arthroscopes with improved lens systems have permitted arthroscopy to be done with excellent clarity and minimal trauma. I have found an arthroscope of 3 mm diameter to be the most useful size for examinations in children. The procedure is done as though it were an arthrotomy with sterile preparation and draping in the operating room. Local anesthesia has been used routinely for purely diagnostic procedures in teenagers, although general anesthesia is the rule for the smaller child. The uses and benefits of arthroscopy in children will be discussed according to the diagnoses of the patients examined.

CONGENITAL ANOMALIES

As can be seen from Table 8 a variety of congenital anomalies were explored mostly in patients under 12 years of age. Discoid lateral meniscus may not be a problem other than that it involves a snapping sensation in the knee. Other patients have pain and swelling, prompting surgical excision. In such cases it was beneficial to observe the mechanism by which the discoid meniscus snapped. By watching the meniscus while the knee was passively flexed and extended I observed that the central thin portion of the meniscus tended to buckle up and snap beneath the condyle. This finding is consistent with the tears that are usually seen in the central abnormal portion of the meniscus. The peripheral moorings of the meniscus were normal. Based on these findings it is reasonable to trim out the abnormal central portion and leave the semilunar peripheral portion of the meniscus.

200

Table 8. Arthroscopy of the knee in children 12 years and under

Diagnosis	Age (years)
Congenitally absent anterior cruciate ligament and fibula	1
Postinjection quadriceps fibrosis, internal joint normal	2
Hemangioma	2
Congenital flexion contracture, capsular hypoplasia	3
Discoid lateral meniscus	6
Foreign body (sewing needle) in upper tibia	7
Infectious synovitis	8
Juvenile rheumatoid arthritis	8
Foreign body (sewing needle fragment) in joint	8
Synovial plica	9
Nonspecific synovitis	9
Discoid lateral meniscus	10
Minimal traumatic chondromalacia of femur	10
Osteochondritis dissecans	11
Discoid lateral meniscus	11
Juvenile rheumatoid arthritis	11
Puncture wound (pitchfork)	12
Traumatic chondromalacia of tibia, flexion contracture	12

Congenital flexion contracture of the knee may be associated with other congenital anomalies of the limb, such as absence of the fibula. The abnormality noted in these joints consisted of diminution of capsular volume and usually absence of the anterior cruciate ligament. In two adolescents, one with nail-patella syndrome and another with spondyloepiphyseal dysplasia, it was possible to define the contracted joint space as well. In the patient with nail-patella syndrome there was a shallow patellar groove and obvious easy dislocation of the patella, which could be seen during passive manipulation of the joint. The patient with dysplasia had an acute exacerbation of her chronic knee pain, and an irregular condyle was seen on x-ray examination. It was not possible to define whether or not there was a loose fragment within the joint. Arthroscopy helped by ruling out the loose body and defining the expected arthritic changes of the articular cartilage.

DISEASES OF THE SYNOVIUM

One of the great advantages of arthroscopy as a diagnostic tool is the fact that the synovium and cartilaginous surfaces of the knee joint can be directly examined. This type of view can only be obtained at arthrotomy by a wide anatomic dissection. Several diseases of the synovium have been defined and studied by synovial biopsy in children with persistent swelling and discomfort. The most significant diagnosis is juvenile rheumatoid arthritis. When the disease involves only a single joint the diagnosis is difficult based on clinical and laboratory examination alone. The synovium shows proliferative changes with early pannus formation and fibrinous "floaters" in the joint (Figs. 13-1 and 13-2). Under direct visual examination biopsies of typical pathologic areas can be performed for histologic confirmation. With a more

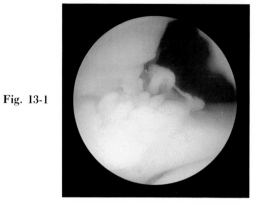
Fig. 13-1
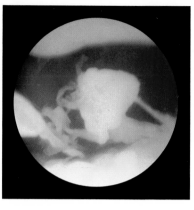
Fig. 13-

Fig. 13-1. Juvenile rheumatoid arthritis with pannus overgrowing meniscus.
Fig. 13-2. Juvenile rheumatoid arthritis with "floater" in suprapatellar pouch.

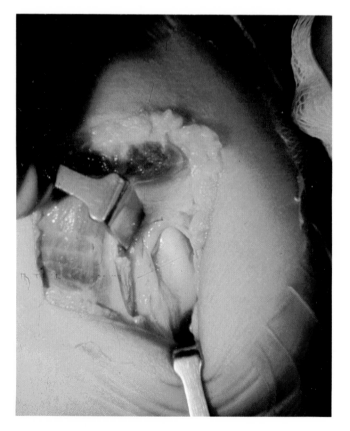

Fig. 13-3. Synovial plica. At arthrotomy, plica is seen crossing femoral condyle between retractors.

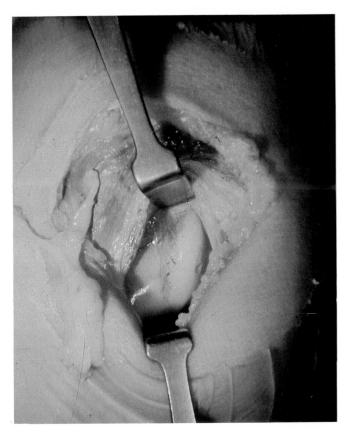

Fig. 13-4. Synovial plica. After partial synovectomy, plica is placed on skin adjacent to incision. It is thick and fibrotic. Hemorrhagic impression on femoral condyle is seen between two retractors.

accurate diagnosis, aggressive medical therapy can be reasonably instituted. It is important in these patients to examine the eyes under slit lamp for evidence of chorioretinitis as this complication of the disease is more common in the monarticular than in the polyarticular form of rheumatoid arthritis.

The anatomy of the synovium with its folds and pleats is generally not appreciated at arthrotomy, but when the knee joint is distended for better visualization during arthroscopy these structures become important in that they obstruct the movement of the arthroscope at times and may be a source of pain for some patients. There is a fold of synovium that is a normal structure in many individuals; this fold extends from above the patella on the medial side downward and laterally crosses the medial femoral condyle, ending in the synovial fat pad (Fig. 13-3). When it is traumatized this synovial fold swells, and fibrous reaction follows, producing a thickened, tight, fibrous band that cuts into the margin of the medial femoral condyle during knee motion between 60° and 90° of flexion (Fig. 13-4). If this condition is suspected, often the band may be palpated through the skin. The synovial fold can be seen with the arthroscope and divided by the use of biopsy forceps or scissors passed through a second puncture. The simple division of the band allows it to separate much as a bowstring that is under tension. Thus the patient's symptoms can be relieved by a procedure done through two small wounds.

Hoffa disease or thickening and fibrosis of the infrapatellar fat pad may follow a direct injury to the knee, during which time the synovium is swollen and pinched between the femur and the tibia. In this series there was one child in whom the fibrotic edge of the fat pad masqueraded as a tear of the anterior portion of the lateral meniscus. Correct localization, however, led to partial synovectomy and pain relief.

Synovitis about the patella likewise may be proliferative, and the thickened synovial fronds may be pinched between the patella and the femur (Fig. 13-5). This type of peripatellar synovitis is common in adolescence. Because of the tenderness under and about the patella, the diagnosis of chondromalacia may be made mistakenly. Delineation of a patellar pain problem as peripatellar synovitis suggests rational treatment by exercise, splinting, and aspirin.

Synovitis is caused by various irritative agents. Traumatic synovitis may follow fracture or operation and may produce fibrinous or fibrous adhesions. These adhesions can be broken by the use of the blunt obturator and the arthroscope sheath, relieving troublesome pain without the necessity for arthrotomy. Foreign bodies such as fragments of sewing needles may produce synovitis. It is possible for the examiner to remove such fragments using the arthroscope and to resolve the synovitis. Infectious synovitis will be covered later in this chapter. At times there is no obvious inciting cause such as a foreign body, trauma, or infection. In these instances of nonspecific synovitis, the examiner can pursue conservative treatment, knowing that there is no internal derangement of the knee that requires operation.

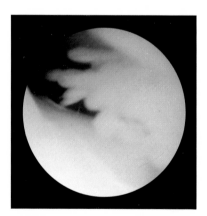

Fig. 13-5. Peripatellar synovitis. Fronds of swollen synovium are seen between patella in upper right and intercondylar notch running from 10 o'clock to 6 o'clock.

DISEASES OF CARTILAGE

The cartilaginous joint surfaces over the femur, tibia, and patella can be thoroughly explored by arthroscopy. The term "chondromalacia" is reserved for those lesions of cartilage that are manifested by softening and irregularity associated with fissuring and frond formation. In advanced stages there may be loss of articular cartilage with the exposure of eburnated cancellous bone. In the population studied these degenerative changes of cartilage were not seen as isolated diseases except in instances in which there had been direct trauma or in which the changes were secondary to subluxation or to dislocation of the patella. Degenerative changes of the articular cartilage were likewise seen after infection, rheumatoid arthritis, or secondary to separation of a loose body generated by osteochondritis dissecans.

Osteochondritis dissecans

Osteochondritis dissecans is the disease for which arthroscopy has provided a new dimension in diagnosis and treatment. It is well known that these lesions will heal spontaneously in children. To follow the natural history of this disease, x-ray films of 43 patients who had been treated for osteochondritis dissecans at the Alfred I. duPont Institute were reviewed. The lesions healed in some of the children; this healing was within 4 or 5 months and showed progressive bony bridging on x-ray examinations during that time. Healing occurred most consistently in the group with an open growth plate. Among individuals for whom growth was ceasing there was a certain percentage of patients whose lesions did not heal and went on to fragmentation with loose body formation and early degenerative changes over the next few years. X-ray examination showed only the bony part of the disease, so arthroscopy was begun to study the cartilage changes associated with the disease. In those instances where patients were not responding to joint rest and had persistent pain or swelling associated with a lack of healing response as shown on x-ray examination,

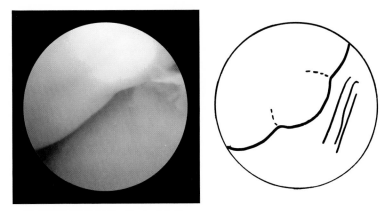

Fig. 13-6. Osteochondritis dissecans. Stage I: bubble.

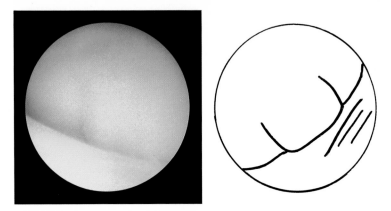

Fig. 13-7. Osteochondritis dissecans. Stage II: crack.

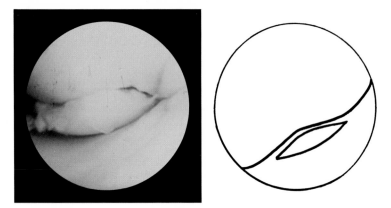

Fig. 13-8. Osteochondritis dissecans. Stage III: separation. (Courtesy Dr. S. W. Casscells.)

arthroscopy was performed. By these examinations the cartilaginous progression of the disease could be staged.

Figs. 13-6 to 13-8 illustrate the stages of osteochondritis dissecans. In stage I of the disease there is softening of a circular area of the articular cartilage associated with a dulling of the surface reflection; a color change toward yellow and softening are noted when the area is probed with the end of a Kirschner wire (Fig. 13-6). In stage II a fissure forms in the cartilage, outlining the margin of the lesion (Fig. 13-7). In stage III there is a frank separation of the osteochondritic fragment from its bed, with formation of a flap or a loose body attached only by a thin synovial pedicle (Fig. 13-8). Serial examination in a few cases showed these stages to be progressive in those lesions that did not heal spontaneously. For stage I and II lesions it was possible to drill percutaneously through the lesion, stimulating the ingrowth of blood vessels and fibrous tissue, or to insert pins to stabilize late lesions in the stage II group.

INTERNAL DERANGEMENTS OF THE KNEE

In the adolescent group of patients internal derangement was the most common difficulty, which connotes problems of a mechanical nature, producing pain, locking, swelling, or instability of the knee joint. The topic will be divided into those problems arising either from a disorder of the meniscus, the patella, or the ligaments. The usefulness of arthroscopy for acute hemarthrosis in children and adolescents will be discussed.

The menisci are valuable biomechanical units, converting the upper surface of the tibia from a flat plane to a cup-shaped structure that helps to stabilize the spheroid femoral condyles. The menisci are also important for nutrition as well as for protection of the articular cartilage that they cover. For all these reasons it is important to conserve the menisci in the young if this is feasible. An accurate diagnosis of torn meniscus, either medial or lateral, can be made with the arthroscope. In several instances the pain and clinical examination pointed toward the wrong side of the knee, particularly with medial pain secondary to a torn lateral meniscus. It is possible to make an accurate assessment of the extent of damage to the meniscus and to adjacent articular cartilage. In those instances in which the meniscus was causing more disservice than service to the knee, a complete meniscectomy was performed. On the other hand, when a bucket-handle tear was the cause for locking and pain, it was possible to examine the remaining rim of the meniscus, and if this tissue was in satisfactory condition, the bucket-handle tear alone was removed. This conservation of tissue appears to be worthwhile and concurs with the studies of others who had done partial meniscectomy.

Peripheral tear of the medial meniscus usually heals in a child because of the vascularity present at the menisco-synovial junction. Some of these lesions do not heal, however, and produce an unstable meniscus that causes pain and locking sensation in the knee joint. Because of the success experienced with the surgical repair of such peripheral detachments in instances where there were associated major collateral ligament ruptures, I elected to attempt direct repair of these tears rather than to sacrifice valuable tissue. In four instances the detachment was repaired with plication of the capsule. These patients have not required excision of their meniscus and have been able to return to vigorous athletic activities without pain or swelling. In these cases the arthroscope helped to define the healthy character of the meniscus and articular cartilage so that preservation of the meniscus was reasonable.

The classic problem plaguing many orthopedic surgeons is the adolescent girl with pain about the patella. Most of these problems are associated with ligament laxity, poor muscle control, or tightness of the hamstring muscles, which will respond to exercise, splinting, and aspirin. On the other hand there are some individuals who have persistent pain with or without swelling for whom this conservative program is not effective over a period of several months. Arthroscopy is valuable for these individuals to determine whether or not they have synovitis or some internal derangement. Gross degrees of subluxation and dislocation of the patella can easily be determined by clinical examination. Arthroscopy is an ancillary test when lateral release of the retinaculum is considered for rebalancing forces on the patella. In these circumstances the patella is observed throughout flexion and extension of the knee. This examination can be done during active motion with the patient under local anesthesia.

The anterior and posterior cruciate ligaments can be viewed directly. The anterior cruciate ligament is easily picked up at its upper attachment in the lateral portion of the intercondylar notch. When no tourniquet is used the blood vessels over the surface of the anterior cruciate ligament differentiate it from the synovial reflections. When the ligament is not seen as a definitive structure it is because it has been torn and partially resorbed. Laxity of the anterior cruciate ligament can be demonstrated by watching while anterior and posterior drawer signs are used to displace the tibia anteriorly and posteriorly on the femur. The posterior cruciate ligament can be viewed from the front with an oblique arthroscope passed into the intercondylar notch, but this technique is difficult to perform unless the anterior cruciate ligament is missing. It is simpler to visualize the posterior cruciate ligament by introducing the arthroscope through a second puncture wound posteriorly behind the medial capsular ligament and visualizing it across the medial compartment as it arises from the tibia and goes almost directly superiorly to insert into the femur.

Acute hemarthrosis of the knee has been lightly treated in the past, especially in those instances where no instability of the joint could be demonstrated. With a more aggressive approach to diagnosis there are many surprises. The joint is aspirated in those patients who have a history of rapid swelling after injury. If blood is found, an arthroscopic examination is scheduled in the operating suite. The joint is copiously irrigated, and a tourniquet is used. A large-bore arthroscope sheath, 6 mm in diameter, is useful for clearing the joint with 1,000 to 2,000 ml of saline used to wash out all the clots. The bleeding may be caused by a tear of the anterior cruciate ligament, by osteochondral fractures off the patella (Fig. 13-9) or femur, or by a marginal detachment of the meniscus, all of which have been seen in adolescents. It is easy to wash small loose bodies out of the joint or to extract them with forceps, thus allowing rapid healing of the joint (Fig. 13-10). In other instances if a peripheral tear of the meniscus does not heal with splinting of the joint, an earlier decision can be made to repair it. There is controversy regarding repair of the anterior cruciate ligament, but certainly if this structure is to be repaired, the success rate is much higher in the first few days after injury. In any instance an accurate diagnosis obtained by a small intrusion leads to an intelligent therapeutic decision. On the one hand, early diagnosis of acute hemarthrosis avoids unnecessary surgery, and on the other hand, an accurate diagnosis avoids unnecessary delay.

INFECTION

Arthroscopy has been useful in the treatment of certain types of joint infections. Particularly in cases where treatment has been inadequate or partially done, the arthroscope may be helpful to the examiner in making decisions regarding future management. An example of this situation is the puncture wound seen several days

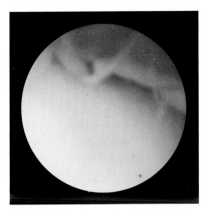

Fig. 13-9. Osteochondral fracture of patella. Hemorrhagic site of fracture is seen in upper left; femoral condyle below.

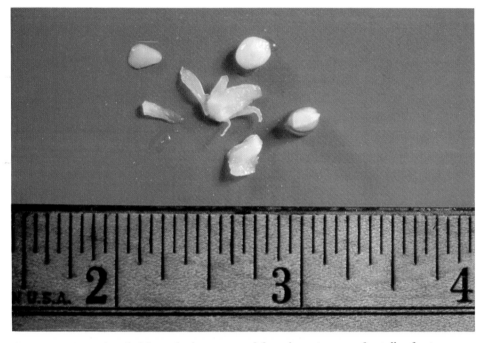

Fig. 13-10. Osteochondral loose bodies removed from knee in case of patellar fracture seen in Fig. 13-9.

late, in which there is some swelling of the joint but no severe skin reaction or general inflammatory reaction, such as fever or increased white blood cell count. The joint can be examined through a small wound and copiously irrigated. Acute pyarthrosis has been treated by use of the arthroscope to drain the knee joint, but I did not use it in this series. For cases of partially treated pyarthrosis not responding to treatment, there exists a condition that can be termed "infectious synovitis." There is no gross pus within the joint, but there is a marked synovial reaction with many inflammatory cells on synovial biopsy. After the joint has been copiously irrigated it is splinted, and antibiotics are given, without the need for a large arthrotomy.

Another type of infectious synovitis is that due to gonorrhea. In cases treated early with penicillin, there is a rapid cure. In late cases that have been inadequately treated the appearance of the synovium is almost diagnostic. The synovium is beefy red, thickened, and swollen. In one instance the synovitis was so typical for gonorrhea that the history was retaken. A positive vaginal culture had been obtained elsewhere 2 weeks previously, but a full course of penicillin had not been given. The diagnosis of infectious synovitis secondary to gonorrhea was made in retrospect.

FRACTURES

Intraarticular fractures of the knee joint may involve any one of the three bones forming the joint and may be associated with damage to the meniscus or the cruciate ligament. An osteochondral fracture is often difficult to define by routine x-ray examination but presents as an acute hemarthrosis. Often these fractures are the result of acute traumatic dislocation of the patella with spontaneous reduction. For fractures either off the patella or off the lateral condyle of the femur, the fragments may be extracted through the arthroscope without the necessity for further therapy. In one instance a girl had a fracture of the tibial spine associated with a femoral shaft fracture. The tibial spine fracture was not recognized and healed with a malunion. With the arthroscope it was possible to see that this fragment blocked full extension of the knee by striking the intercondylar notch. Once the fragment was removed, full extension was gained. The arthroscope was useful in this instance in defining the dynamic status of the joint.

TUMOR

In this series there were three patients with tumor problems. One boy had hemangioma that was partially intrasynovial and partially extrasynovial and was the cause for repeated hemarthrosis. The second patient was a girl who had had a hemangioma excised previously and had some recurrent pain that proved to be secondary to a synovial plica and not recurrence of the tumor. The third patient had an osteochondroma excised from the knee joint and had some secondary degenerative changes of the patellofemoral joint. Acute hemarthrosis is so uncommon in children under 12 years of age, it is worthwhile to think about a hemangioma, glomus tumor, or bleeding disorder.

SOCIAL INDICATIONS

At times social circumstance has been the primary indication for arthroscopy in children. One example is that of the hysterical patient who has loss of function or claims discomfort in the knee joint with absolutely no clinical abnormality. Several times it has been valuable to perform an arthroscopic examination in order to reassure the family and other treating physicians that the joint itself is normal, and treatment can then be directed toward the underlying psychiatric condition. Occasionally a child is involved in litigation, such as one patient with mild knee pain 2 years after being knocked off his bicycle. The arthroscope provided the diagnostic basis to make a settlement. Another child was constantly complaining about his knee and missing school. Because of persistent complaints and failure to respond, an arthroscopic examination was done to rule out any serious disease of the knee joint. Once the normal examination was established, more aggressive work with the school counselor and social worker helped this boy to get rid of his remaining complaints.

PROGNOSTIC EXAMINATIONS

One of the great advantages of the arthroscope is that it can be used for follow-up examination with the patient under local anesthesia. In this instance the patient, with only a bandage on his knee, is able to leave the operating room at the same time as the surgeon. Regeneration of cartilage has been documented in osteochondritis dissecans and osteochondral fractures when the base of the lesion has been cleaned

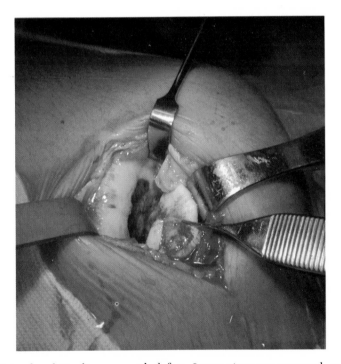

Fig. 13-11. Osteochondritis dissecans with defect. Loose piece was removed, and crater was cleaned of fibrous tissue.

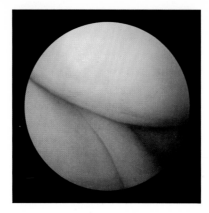

Fig. 13-12. Osteochondritis dissecans in patient shown in Fig. 13-11. Arthroscopic view of articular cartilage 2 years after operation, showing fill-in by cartilage.

down to bleeding bone (Figs. 13-11 and 13-12). Healing of meniscal repairs has also been documented as well as follow-up of ligament repairs, rheumatoid arthritis, and drilling of osteochondritis dissecans, stages I and II. Prognostic information can be gained in regards to the quality of cartilage regeneration, which was remarkably good in young individuals.

CONTRAINDICATIONS

An obvious contraindication to arthroscopy is the presence of infection of the overlying skin. The risk is that infection may be carried into the joint itself. Lack of full joint motion is a relative contraindication in that complete examination of the joint is difficult, although valuable information may be gained from a partial examination. With any new procedure there is a tendency to overenthusiasm once its value is demonstrated. It is a well-known fact that hip joint pathology may be referred to the area of the knee. One patient with a slipped capital femoral epiphysis had a normal arthroscopic examination of his knee 1 year previously. Obviously the hip joint cannot be visualized with an arthroscope placed in the knee. A complete history and physical examination should be done, especially regarding the hip joint, before arthroscopy. In instances of complete rupture of the collateral ligaments of the knee, the integrity of the joint capsule is lost, and the irrigating fluid tends to accumulate in the subcutaneous tissue, compressing the joint. This compression along with the blood makes visualization difficult. Since wide anatomic dissection is necessary, arthroscopy adds little in these cases.

SUMMARY

Arthroscopy of the knee is a useful procedure for diagnosis and treatment of disorders of the knee joint in children and adolescents. Indications for its use in the child under 12 years of age are uncommon, but it is especially helpful in the adolescent age group for direct viewing of the synovium and cartilage in order to define the extent and type of internal derangement. Also arthroscopy of the knee can be helpful for treatment of certain infections and fractures.

Arthrography
Murray K. Dalinka

Arthrography of the knee in children and adolescents is of considerable value. In addition to its use in suspected internal derangements[1,2,11,12] it has been used in osteochondritis dissecans,[15] Blount disease,[5] popliteal cysts, and miscellaneous abnormalities, including unexplained knee pain. I use fluoroscopic control with spot-filming, stress, and a 0.6 mm focal spot for all studies. Arthrography of the uncooperative infant may be done with the patient under general anesthesia or heavy sedation, but anesthesia is not necessary in the cooperative child or adolescent. The technique is similar to that in the adult except that less contrast, 1 to 3 ml of meglumine diatrizoate (Renografin 60%) as opposed to 4 ml in the adult, and gas are used because of the smaller joint capacity.[3]

MENISCAL ABNORMALITIES

We agree with Bramson and Staple,[1] who state that children with internal derangements can be divided into two groups, those above and those below the age of 12. Children 12 years of age or older have abnormalities almost identical to those of

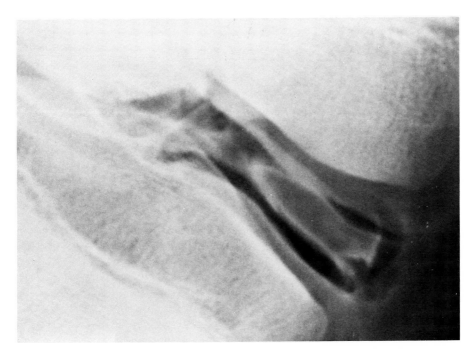

Fig. 13-13. Discoid lateral meniscus. Note large size and parallel shape.

adults, while in the younger child, lateral tears are more common than are medial tears.[1,10-12] This distribution is thought to be secondary to the discoid lateral meniscus, which frequently presents in childhood and almost always occurs laterally. The discoid meniscus may be bilateral[10] or familial.[6] It is thought to be secondary to strong meniscofemoral ligaments, causing limitation of movement during extension with dislocation of the meniscus into the intercondylar notch.[9] On flexion the meniscus is pulled laterally by the coronary ligament and the popliteal tendon. The medial-to-lateral mobility is thought to be responsible for the characteristic click and the meniscal thickening, causing the irregular discoid form.[9]

These abnormally thick menisci are prone to tear. The arthrographic diagnosis can be made as the meniscus extends to the intercondylar notch, with the body of the meniscus having a parallel rather than a triangular shape (Fig. 13-13).[7,10,11] These large menisci with strong posterior attachments are difficult to remove with a standard anterior incision. They are frequently accompanied by large geniculate vessels that may be predisposed to postoperative hemorrhage.[9]

OSTEOCHONDRITIS DISSECANS

Arthrography has been used in osteochondritis dissecans to determine the status of the overlying articular cartilage, which may be bulging, normal (Fig. 13-14), or

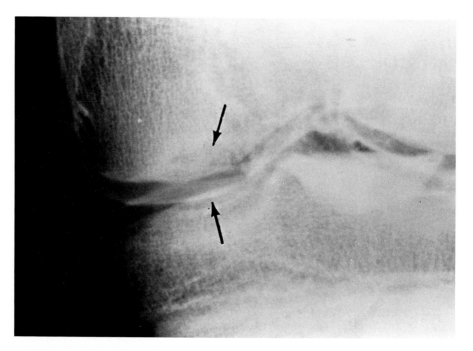

Fig. 13-14. Osteochondritis dissecans. Note bony defect *(upper arrow)* and normal-appearing articular cartilage *(lower arrow).*

retracted and irregular (Fig. 13-15).[15] Loose bodies in these patients are better evaluated on plain films, but associated meniscal tears are not infrequent.

BLOUNT DISEASE

Arthrography has been performed to evaluate the unossified cartilage of the medial tibial plateau.[5] Early in this deformity the epiphyseal cartilage is hypertrophied (Fig. 13-16), and the medial meniscus is large to compensate for the abnormal bony development. There is a disparity between the abnormal plain films and the relatively normal arthrogram. As the deformity progresses there is a depression of the bony epiphysis and metaphysis, but the epiphyseal cartilage maintains a relatively normal appearance. Later the cartilage becomes depressed posteromedially and is no longer parallel to the depressed medial metaphysis. When the epiphyseal cartilage is depressed more than is the metaphysis, the ligaments are lax, and an osteotomy is usually insufficient treatment. In these cases a relative laxity of the

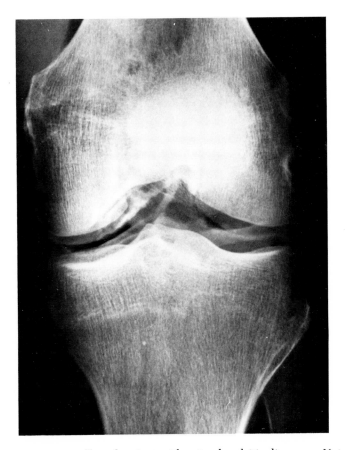

Fig. 13-15. Posteroanterior film of patient with osteochondritis dissecans. Note irregularity of articular cartilage, which is also slightly thinned.

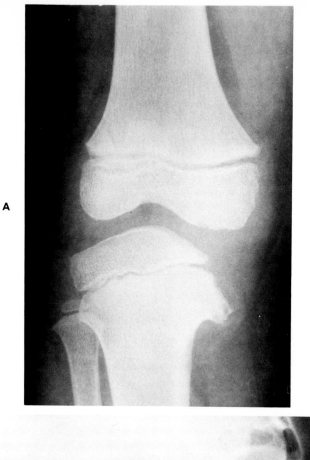

A

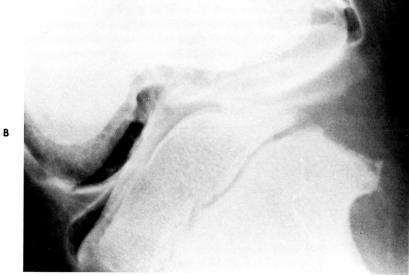

B

Fig. 13-16. Blount disease. **A,** Note depression and beaking of medial tibial metaphysis and lack of ossification of medial aspect of tibial epiphysis. There is thickening of medial tibial cortex. **B,** Arthrographic spot-film of same patient, showing large calcified portion of tibial epiphysis, which is fairly anatomic despite metaphyseal depression.

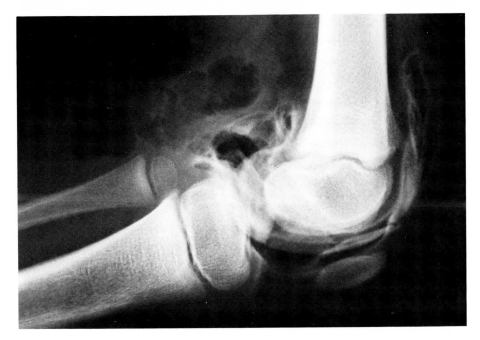

Fig. 13-17. Lateral film, demonstrating popliteal cyst in a 5-year-old girl.

medial collateral ligament is frequent, and ligament stabilization procedures are often necessary to prevent recurrent deformity.

POPLITEAL CYSTS

The presence of a popliteal cyst is an indication for arthrography in adults because of the association of these cysts with meniscal tears. I feel that any cause of increased intraarticular pressure may lead to communication between the posterior portion of the knee joint and the semimembranosogastrocnemial bursa and hence a popliteal cyst. Bryan and associates[2] have stated that popliteal cysts in children rarely have associated internal derangements of the knee. In my experience with two cases of popliteal cysts in children (Fig. 13-17), no internal derangement was present. Arthrography was of value in excluding a solid mass.

•　　•　　•

Arthrography has demonstrated synovial tumors in the pediatric age group.[16] Although I have had no personal experience with these lesions in children, I have seen pigmented villonodular synovitis and intrasynovial hemangiomas in adolescents.[4]

Opaque loose bodies are best demonstrated on plain films. Nonopaque loose bodies are difficult to see on double-contrast arthrography, particularly if they are in the suprapatellar pouch. Gas arthrography is the procedure of choice when looking for nonopaque loose bodies.

Although Horns[8] and Thijn[13] have reported success in the arthrographic diagnosis of chondromalacia patella, I do not feel confident in making this diagnosis. I feel that the arthrogram can be used in these cases to rule out associated meniscal abnormalities.

SUMMARY

Knee arthrography is a useful procedure in the evaluation of knee injuries in children and adolescents. Its accuracy in the diagnosis of meniscal abnormalities is greater than 90%.

Arthrography is of considerable help in the evaluation and treatment planning of patients with osteochondritis dissecans. When the osteochondritic fragment is intact with normal or bulging cartilage, a conservative or extraarticular approach can be used, and revascularization can be attempted without disruption of the overlying articular cartilage.[3]

In Blount disease the angulation necessary for osteotomy can be determined as can the need for ligament stabilization procedures.[3,5] Arthrography can also confirm the presence of synovial tumors and can aid in the diagnosis of internal derangements associated with osteochondritis dissecans, popliteal cysts, or chondromalacia patella.[9]

References

1. Bramson, R. T., and Staple, T. W.: Double contrast knee arthrography in children, Am. J. Roentgenol. Radium Ther. Nucl. Med. 123:838-844, 1975.
2. Bryan, R. S., DiMichele, J. D., and Ford, G. L.: Popliteal cyst. Arthrography as an aid to diagnosis and treatment, Clin. Orthop. 50:203, 1967.
3. Dalinka, M. K., Brennan, R. E., and Canino, C.: Double contrast knee arthrography in children, Clin. Orthop. 125:88-193, 1977.
4. Dalinka, M. K., Coren, G. S., and Wershba, M.: Knee arthrography, CRC Crit. Rev. Rad. Sci. 4:1-59, 1973.
5. Dalinka, M. K., Coren, G., Hensinger, R., and Irani, R. N.: Arthrography in Blount's disease, Radiology 113:161-164, 1974.
6. Dashefsky, J. H.: Discoid lateral meniscus in three members of a family, J. Bone Joint Surg. [Am.] 53:1208, 1971.
7. Haveson, S. B., and Burton, I. R.: Lateral discoid meniscus of the knee: arthrographic diagnosis, Am. J. Roentgenol. Radium Ther. Nucl. Med. 109:581-586, 1970.
8. Horns, J. W.: The diagnosis of chondromalacia by double contrast arthrography of the knee, J. Bone Joint Surg. [Am.] 59:119-120, 1977.
9. Kaplan, E. B.: Discoid lateral meniscus of the knee joint—nature, mechanism and operative treatment, J. Bone Joint Surg. [Am.] 39:77-87, 1957.
10. Moes, C. A. F., and Munn, J. D.: The value of knee arthrography in children, J. Can. Assoc. Radiol. 16:226-233, 1965.
11. Stenstrom, R.: Arthrography of the knee joint in children. Roentgenologic anatomy, diagnosis and the use of multiple discriminant analysis, Acta Radiol. [Suppl.] (Stockh.) 281:5-86, 1968.

12. Stenstrom, R.: Diagnostic arthrography of traumatic lesions of the knee joint in children, Ann. Radiol. (Paris) **18:**391-394, 1975.
13. Thijn, C. J. P.: Double-contrast arthrography in meniscal lesions and patellar chondropathy, Radiol. Clin. Basel **45:**345-362, 1966.
14. Thomas, M. L., and Andress, M. R.: Angioma of the knee demonstrated by angiography and arthrography, Acta Radiol. [Diagn.] (Stockh.) **12:**217-220, 1972.
15. Wershba, M., Dalinka, M. K., Coren, G. S., and Cotler, J.: Double contrast knee arthrography in the evaluation of osteochondritis dissecans, Clin. Orthop. **107:**81-86, 1975.

14. Acute injury to the knee

Arthroscopy
Kenneth E. DeHaven

Acute injury to the knee is common in athletics, vehicular and pedestrian accidents, and certain occupational accidents. Successful return to preinjury functional capacity is largely dependent upon accurate diagnosis and appropriate treatment. Many of these injuries warrant surgical management, and often early primary surgical intervention provides more favorable results than does late secondary treatment. Obviously recognition of those injuries that do warrant surgical treatment and in particular those that are best treated with prompt primary surgical intervention is of critical importance. This section of this chapter will review these categories of injuries, outline the clinical and diagnostic approaches for identification of surgical candidates, and emphasize the important role of arthroscopy in dealing with these problems.

TECHNICAL ASPECTS

Hemarthrosis was formerly listed as a contraindication or at least a relative contraindication to arthroscopy because of poor visualization.[1,4,5] However, experience has shown that a satisfactory arthroscopic examination can be obtained with a slightly modified technique, using a large-bore (13-gauge) suprapatellar outflow needle and florid irrigation through the arthroscope sleeve (Fig. 14-1); sometimes 2 to 4 liters of irrigation fluid is required to sufficiently clear the hemarthrosis to permit arthroscopic visualization. In addition, inflation of the tourniquet may be required in certain cases. This technique has been successful in allowing satisfactory arthroscopic examination in 70 of the last 72 cases of acute injuries with hemarthrosis.

ACUTE KNEE INJURIES OF SURGICAL SIGNIFICANCE

The diagnostic categories of acute knee injuries that warrant surgical intervention are listed below.
1. Ligament tears
   a. Collateral
   b. Cruciate
2. Extensor mechanism ruptures
   a. Quadriceps tendon
   b. Patellar tendon

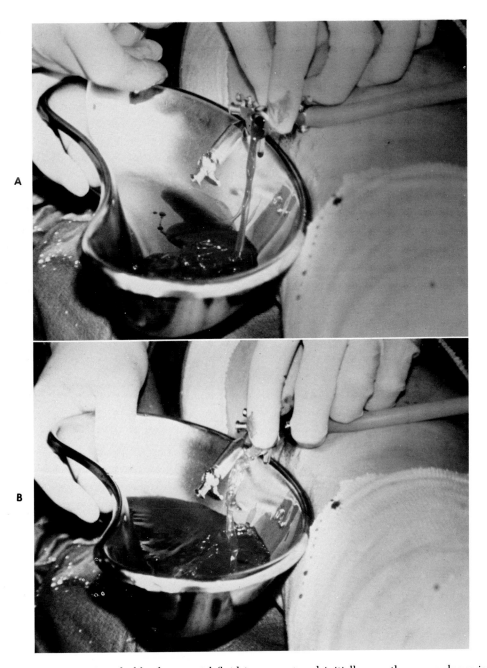

Fig. 14-1. A, Grossly bloody synovial fluid is encountered initially as arthroscope sleeve is inserted into acutely injured knee. **B,** Copious irrigation is continued until fluid becomes sufficiently clear of blood to provide adequate arthroscopic visualization.

3. Meniscus tears
4. Intraarticular fractures
   a. Tibial plateau
   b. Tibial intercondylar eminence
   c. Femoral condyle
   d. Patella
   e. Osteochondral fractures with loose body formation
   f. Popliteal tendon avulsion fracture

The clinical approach to these problems continues to rely on the time-honored principles of a careful history, thorough physical examination, and standard roentgenograms. In addition the currently available diagnostic adjuncts of arthrography and arthroscopy can provide valuable assistance.

Injuries amenable to definitive clinical evaluation

The decision regarding the need for surgical treatment can definitively be made on the basis of the clinical examination or standard roentgenograms in several of these types of knee injuries. Medial or lateral collateral ligament tears are usually associated with diagnostic medial or lateral laxity. Diagnostic adjuncts are usually not necessary to delineate the need for surgery, but in questionable cases stress x-ray films and limited arthrograms with single contrast can be helpful in documenting lesions.[7] Arthroscopic examination is of limited benefit in defining the need for surgery but can be useful in demonstrating whether the lesion is in the meniscofemoral or meniscotibial portion of the ligament and certainly can be instrumental in demonstrating associated meniscus pathology, particularly in the compartment opposite the collateral ligament injury.

Posterior cruciate ligament tears can also be diagnosed clinically by demonstrating a positive posterior drawer sign or, when in combination with collateral ligament injury, by demonstrating significant straight medial or lateral laxity with the knee in full extension, as described by Hughston and associates.[3] The role of arthroscopy in cases involving the posterior cruciate lesion is primarily confirmatory rather than diagnostic, but arthroscopy can be extremely helpful in demonstrating unsuspected associated meniscus pathology. The posterior cruciate ligament can be acutely torn in an "isolated" fashion, however, with no associated posterior or rotational instability. In these cases arthroscopic examination can be the key to diagnosis. When the ligament is torn from the femoral attachment, it is easily visualized through an anterior approach, but when the tear is at or near the tibial attachment, it may be visualized only through a posteromedial approach (Fig. 14-2).

The diagnosis of extensor mechanism ruptures rests with a high index of suspicion and clinical testing to indicate lack of functional integrity. These disabling injuries are deceptive and are frequently missed initially because of unremarkable x-ray films and the absence of instability; also frequently the patient is not asked to actively extend the knee, or the ability to partially extend the knee to 45° misleads the examiner.

Several types of intraarticular fractures frequently occur with acute trauma and

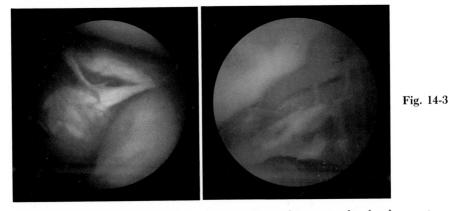

Fig. 14-2

Fig. 14-3

Fig. 14-2. "Isolated" tear of posterior cruciate ligament from tibia as visualized arthroscopically from posteromedial approach. Corner of posterior femoral condyle is seen in upper portion of photograph, and periphery of posterior horn of medial meniscus is seen below.
Fig. 14-3. Typical arthroscopic appearance of acute tear of anterior cruciate ligament. Hemorrhagic edematous ligament is found lying horizontally in intercondylar notch rather than in its normal anatomic position.

are associated with pain, disability, and hemarthrosis. Definitive diagnosis can usually be made roentgenographically in tibial plateau fractures, tibial intercondylar imminence fractures, fracture of the femoral condyle, and fractures of the patella. Demonstration of significant depression or displacement will define the need for surgical intervention, and arthrography and arthroscopy would play little if any role in those injuries. However, if there is any question as to the presence of significant displacement or depression or of associated internal derangement, arthroscopic examination will help define the need for surgical treatment. Also, more subtle osteochondral fractures with loose body formation, and avulsion fractures of the popliteal tendon may be associated with such a small amount of bone that roentgenograms are normal, but these lesions can be visualized arthroscopically.

Injuries with no instability and normal x-ray films

There remains a sizable group of patients with the history of significant trauma, immediate disability, and the early onset of hemarthrosis, who have no demonstrable ligament laxity and who also have normal x-ray films. These patients are normally not considered to be surgical candidates, but in fact they frequently harbor diagnoses of surgical significance, including anterior cruciate ligament tears, meniscus tears, and osteochondral fractures.

It has been my preference to proceed with the arthroscopic examination of these acute knee injuries with hemarthrosis, with the patient under anesthesia. In the last 70 consecutive cases lesions have been identified that warrant definitive surgical intervention in 62 cases.[2]

The most frequent (67%) lesion encountered in these knees has been anterior cruciate ligament tears (Fig. 14-3).[2] Most have been acute lesions, but a few have been acute episodes of chronic problems related to old anterior cruciate ligament injuries (Fig. 14-4). In acute cases the tear is usually proximal, near the femoral origin (Fig. 14-5), but mid-third (Fig. 14-6) and distal tears also occur. It is recognized that repair of acute anterior cruciate ligament tears is controversial, but it is my preference to proceed with repair whenever possible, and 60% of these acute lesions have been favorable for repair, the remainder being either nonrepairable (23%) or partial

Fig. 14-4 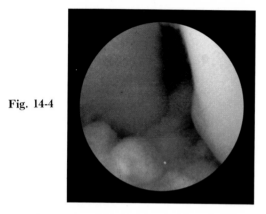 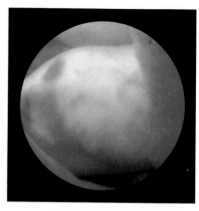 Fig. 14-

Fig. 14-4. Remote anterior cruciate ligament tears are recognized arthroscopically by degenerated nubbin of anterior cruciate ligament tissue at tibial insertion of ligament and by empty space in lateral aspect of intercondylar notch where ligament normally courses toward its femoral attachment.

Fig. 14-5. Acute anterior cruciate ligament tear from femur, which was amenable to repair. Hemorrhagic edematous ligament is seen lying horizontally in intercondylar notch.

Fig. 14-6 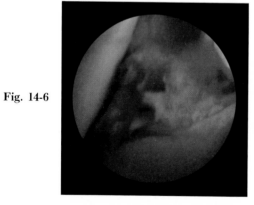 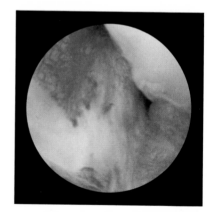 Fig. 14-

Fig. 14-6. Acute midsubstance tear of anterior cruciate ligament, which was not amenable to repair.

Fig. 14-7. Acute partial anterior cruciate ligament tears are recognized arthroscopically by appearance of hemorrhage within synovial sheath around anterior cruciate ligament, which remains in continuity and in its normal anatomic position.

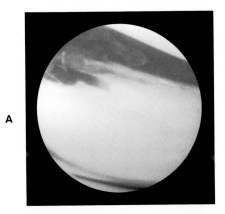

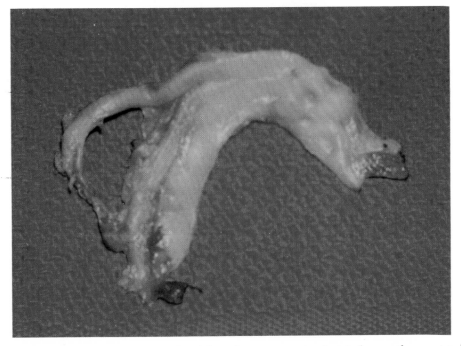

Fig. 14-8. Type of posterior peripheral lateral meniscus tear that is frequently associated with anterior cruciate ligament injury. **A,** Close-up arthroscopic appearance of posterior horn of lateral meniscus, which occupies majority of field, with a small corner of femoral condyle seen above and a small portion of tibial plateau seen below. Hemorrhagic split tears are seen on both superior and inferior surfaces of meniscus out near periphery. **B,** Resected lateral meniscus shown arthroscopically in **A,** demonstrating extensive posterior horn tears.

(17%) lesions (Fig. 14-7). Initially it was believed that the extent and type of anterior cruciate ligament tears could be determined from the arthroscopic appearance, but because of numerous misinterpretations, we no longer attempt to decide whether a particular case is a complete or incomplete tear, repairable or nonrepairable from the arthroscopic appearance alone, but rather we perform an arthrotomy to make this determination.

Two thirds of all cases with anterior cruciate ligament lesions have been found to also have associated meniscus tears, which have been visualized arthroscopically. There is a surprisingly high incidence (66%) of lateral meniscus lesions in association with the anterior cruciate ligament tears,[2] and frequently these are peripheral tears through the posterior horn (Fig. 14-8), which are difficult if not impossible to visualize at arthrotomy, even knowing that they are present.

Arthrography for meniscus lesions in acute injuries has been disappointing, with numerous false-negative results (especially for the lateral meniscus), which are possibly related to the presence of blood in the joint and resultant "coating" of the menisci to obscure pathologic lesions.

Meniscus lesions with no associated anterior cruciate ligament tears are also encountered in acute knee injuries with hemarthrosis (21%).[2] The vast majority are displaced bucket-handle tears (Fig. 14-9) or peripheral tears of other types, which result in synovial injury and hemarthrosis.

Another category of lesion encountered in acute knee injuries with hemarthrosis is osteochondral fracture with loose body formation, which we have found in approximately 10% of these cases.[2] Usually these result from patellar dislocation (Fig. 14-10), with the loose body located in the lateral sulcus between the lateral femoral condyle and the lateral capsule (Fig. 14-11). These lesions also can occur in either femoral condyle, however, (Fig. 14-12) and there may be associated meniscus tears. When the loose body is the only lesion of surgical significance, it can frequently be removed under arthroscopic control and open arthrotomy thereby avoided (Fig. 14-13).

The final category of acute injury with hemarthrosis is that injury in which no discernible internal derangement has occurred, which in our experience has been infrequent (3%).[2] These cases have all been grade II sprains of the medial collateral ligament with synovial bleeding but no internal derangement.

In patients with hemarthrosis but no demonstrable laxity, definitive surgical treatment has been carried out following arthroscopic visualization of significant pathology in 88% of the cases. It is recognized that repair of anterior cruciate ligament tears is controversial, and in deference to the "anterior cruciate nonbelievers"[6] the cases in which repair of the anterior cruciate ligament was the only surgical procedure performed could be eliminated from the definitive surgery group. This still leaves 73% of the cases who underwent definitive surgery. The role of arthroscopy in this group of patients is extremely significant, not only in clarifying the need for surgical treatment by documenting the presence of a surgically significant lesion but in demonstrating the frequent posterior peripheral tears of the lateral meniscus, which may be difficult if not impossible to visualize in any other way.

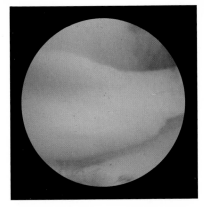

Fig. 14-9

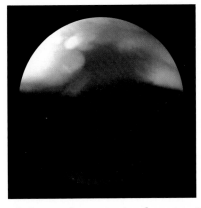

Fig. 14-10

Fig. 14-9. Representative example of meniscus pathology without associated cruciate injury encountered in acute knee trauma with hemarthrosis. Large, displaced bucket-handle tear of medial meniscus is pictured, with displaced portion occupying medial portion of intercondylar notch, blocking arthroscopic visualization of medial compartment.

Fig. 14-10. Arthroscopic photograph of articular surface of patella after an acute dislocation, which caused an osteochondral fracture. Crater left by osteochondral fracture is visualized.

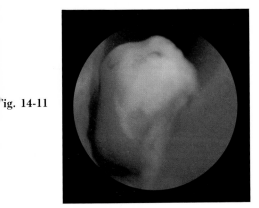

Fig. 14-11

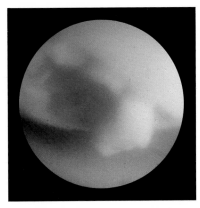

Fig. 14-12

Fig. 14-11. Loose bodies arising from patellar dislocation with osteochondral fracture are usually found lying in lateral sulcus between lateral femoral condyle and lateral capsule, as shown in this arthroscopic view.

Fig. 14-12. Arthroscopic appearance of acute osteochondral fracture involving main weight-bearing portion of medial femoral condyle.

Fig. 14-13. When a loose body is the only lesion of surgical significance, it can frequently be removed under arthroscopic control without a formal arthrotomy. In this arthroscopic photograph, forceps can be seen grasping a loose body in posterior portion of lateral compartment.

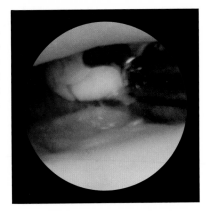

SUMMARY

Acute knee injuries are frequently associated with major disruption of critical structures, and prompt definitive diagnosis and treatment are essential to provide the best opportunity for optimal functional recovery. The important role of arthroscopy in these patients is to help clarify the need for surgical treatment by direct visualization of the pathology and to demonstrate unsuspected associated lesions that may be very difficult to visualize by any other means, including arthrotomy. The arthroscopic examination adds no significant morbidity to that of the injury itself and affords the opportunity to "go in or stay out" with a high degree of confidence. Rather than being a contraindication to arthroscopy, the acute knee injury with hemarthrosis is, in fact, one of the very best indications for this procedure.

References

1. Casscells, S. W.: Arthroscopy of the knee joint. A review of 150 cases. J. Bone Joint Surg. [Am.] **53:**287-298, 1971.
2. DeHaven, K. E.: Diagnosis of acute knee injuries with hemarthrosis. The role of arthroscopy. In manuscript.
3. Hughston, J. C., Andrews, J. R., Cross, M. J., and Moschi, A.: Classification of knee ligament instabilities, J. Bone Joint Surg. [Am.] **58:**159-179, 1976.
4. Jackson, R. W., and Abe, I.: The role of arthroscopy in the management of disorders of the knee. An analysis of 200 consecutive examinations, J. Bone Joint Surg. [Br.] **54:**310-322, 1972.
5. Jackson, R. W., and DeHaven, K. E.: Arthroscopy of the knee, Clin. Orthop. **107:**87-92, 1975.
6. Kennedy, J. C.: The enigma of the anterior cruciate ligament, Paper presented at AAOS Postgraduate Course on The Knee in Sports Medicine, Houston, 1976.
7. Marshall, J. L.: A diagnostic aid in the treatment of ligamentous injuries of the knee, Paper presented at AAOS Postgraduate Course on Skiing Injuries, Snowmass, Colo., 1974.

Arthrography

Jeremy J. Kaye

Arthrography of the knee in the acutely injured patient presents no more problems than does physical examination. If the patient can be examined in the very acute state, as in the case of the professional athlete examined by the orthopedic surgeon on the field, then physical examination may be extremely reliable. Most patients, however, are seen after the onset of muscle spasm and protection, and physical examination without an anesthesic can be less reliable.

In this situation it is no more difficult to perform arthrography than to perform a physical examination. Additional information that may be valuable in patient management may be forthcoming.

The restraints in terms of knee arthrography on the acutely injured patient are primarily technical. The *truly* locked knee presents particular problems to the arthrographer in terms of his vertical x-ray beam. If the meniscus cannot be brought parallel to the x-ray beam, a technically adequate examination cannot be expected. Many patients with "locked" knees are suffering from muscle spasm or are in a semiacute situation with mild flexure contractures. Most of these can be corrected during arthrography and an adequate examination obtained.

A second technical factor pertains to the total evacuation of any effusion. This may be difficult and time consuming when a large effusion is present. Particularly when a hemarthrosis is present, it is my opinion that the coating of the meniscus may not be optimal. The presence of a significant hemarthrosis should suggest to the arthrographer that there may be a significant ligament injury in addition to the possibility of a meniscus injury.

The arthrographic features of meniscus and extrameniscus injuries seen in acute trauma are identical to those listed in the foregoing sections. When it is desirable to examine the medial collateral ligament by means of arthrography, this examination should be performed within the first 42 to 78 hours after injury. This is important since the medial collateral ligament may become watertight (although not structurally intact) within this period, due to the accumulation of fibrin and clot.

In my opinion arthrography can provide valuable information in the management of acutely injured patients.

15. Arthroscopic surgery of the knee

Richard L. O'Connor

Any orthopedic surgeon working with diagnostic arthroscopy must on occasion look at an abnormality within the knee and sense frustration at being unable to reach and remove that which he can visualize so clearly. The initial response is a desire to put in a probe or nerve hook and palpate the lesion. Unfortunately this maneuver requires a well-developed stereotactic sense, which comes only with practice. Once this sense has developed, however, it is not long before the probe can be replaced with a grasping and then a cutting instrument.

ADVANTAGES AND DISADVANTAGES

The value of diagnostic arthroscopy is now accepted by most surgeons. However, few realize that not only can a better understanding of the patient's knee pathology be achieved with arthroscopy, but often an arthrotomy can be avoided by removing the source of the patient's symptoms through incisions only large enough to admit the arthroscope. The advantages of arthroscopic surgery are as follows. (1) There is a very short recovery period, one that is measured in hours and days rather than in weeks or months, as compared to the recovery period after arthrotomy used to achieve the same end. (2) The small incision required for arthroscopy does not cause the quadriceps inhibition seen after arthrotomy. Also the inflammatory response of arthroscopy is not as intense as that of arthrotomy. (3) The complication rate after arthroscopic surgery is not greater than that following diagnostic arthroscopy. In over 1,900 cases of diagnostic arthroscopy, including perhaps 600 involving arthroscopic surgery, there have been no cases of joint sepsis and two cases of deep-vein thrombosis without embolization. Anesthetic complications have been minimal, despite the almost exclusive use of general anesthesia. (4) Secondary effects of arthrotomy, such as neuroma formation, a painful scar over the femoral condyle, or patellofemoral imbalance are avoided with arthroscopy. (5) The laxities, especially posterior medial capsular laxity, that may occur after total meniscectomy are not seen after partial meniscectomy performed with the arthroscope.

The disadvantages of arthroscopic surgery, however, are numerous. (1) Particularly in the early stages, arthroscopic procedures are time-consuming. (2) There is a normal aversion to making several additional small incisions; hence attempting to work through a single incision with poor mechanical advantage is an early tendency. As the examiner gains experience, however, the visual and operative limitations of each portal of entry become familiar, and if one portal is difficult, another can be quickly made. (3) The extensive specialized equipment (including telescopes of different sizes) necessary at the onset may also inhibit the interest of the beginning arthroscopist. (4) Not all orthopedists have personalities capable of dealing with the frustrations of working in the depths of a small hole, with a limited field of vision, using equipment with working parts the size of those on instruments used in hand surgery. Quite often the working area is covered by the condyle, and the field is obscured by flagellating fibrillated articular cartilage, articular debris, or blood. These conditions can tax the patience of the most long-suffering surgeon.

EQUIPMENT

Necessary equipment for arthroscopy includes the standard diagnostic arthroscope. The arthroscope itself should have a large diameter with sufficient clearance between the telescope and the water-sleeve to provide an unremitting flow of fluid to remove blood and debris (Fig. 15-1). A straight-ahead lens is preferable at least initially in order to minimize frustration by removing the variable of instrument rotation. Occasionally a small, (2.5 mm diameter) telescope is useful for getting into small, relatively inaccessible areas (Fig. 15-2). The operating arthroscope is often necessary for partial meniscectomy (Fig. 15-3). Quite often the meniscus that is to be excised must be placed under tension with a retractor through an ancillary portal. The operating arthroscope with a lens system parallel to the operating chamber permits observation in the same plane as the dissection. Operating instruments of 3 and 5 mm diameter are essential. The 3 mm instruments are inserted through the operating channel of the operating arthroscope, while the 5 mm instruments are used through an ancillary portal. Meniscus scissors have a hooked end, allowing them to retract tissue forward (Fig. 15-4). Basket biopsy forceps are used to trim the peripheral meniscus rim and synovial biopsy (Fig. 15-5). A small amount of tissue may be stored in the center of the instrument so that the basket forceps do not need to be removed after every cut. A 3 mm meniscus knife, used through the operating channel, is frequently necessary for excising the posterior tibial attachment of the displaced bucket-handle tear (Figs. 15-6 to 15-9). Nonarthroscopic equipment that I have found useful includes a set of Zimmer 3 mm pituitary ronguers (downward, straight ahead, and upward blunting) (Fig. 15-10). The downward ronguer is especially useful in working around the posterior tibial attachment of the medial meniscus. A small Kocher clamp is used as a retractor for the displaced fragment, and a small osteotome is handy for excision of an occasional osteophyte.

TECHNIQUES

1. *Single-puncture technique:* Work is done through one portal, using an operating arthroscope; a retractor is not required. This method is limited to an occasional

Text continued on p. 237.

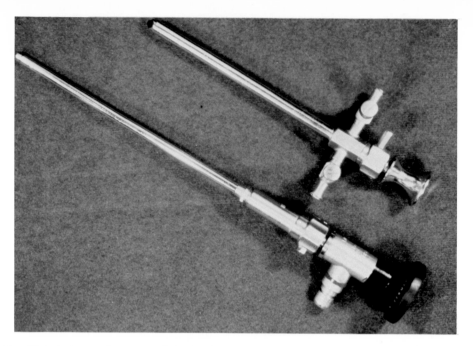

Fig. 15-1. A 5 mm telescope with bridge fits into water-sleeve above. Large-diameter arthroscope is invaluable in operative work since fibrillated cartilage, synovial villi, and debris often obscure vision when a small-diameter instrument is used.

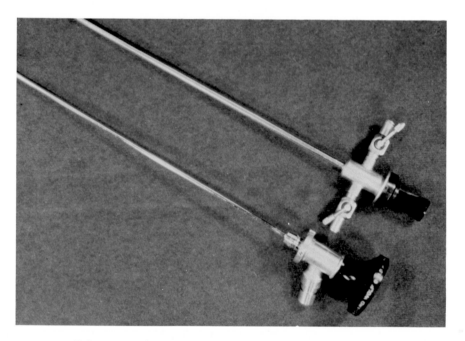

Fig. 15-2. Small-diameter arthroscope may be of use in special situations. This telescope is 2.5 mm in diameter.

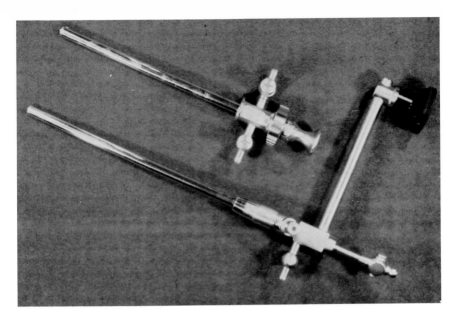

Fig. 15-3. Operating arthroscope also is inserted into knee through water-sleeve, shown above. By removing operating unit and adding an adapter the 5 mm diagnostic telescope can be used through this water-sleeve without removing instrument from joint. Offset eyepiece allows operator to view straight ahead while working. Operating accessories are introduced down shaft of arthroscope.

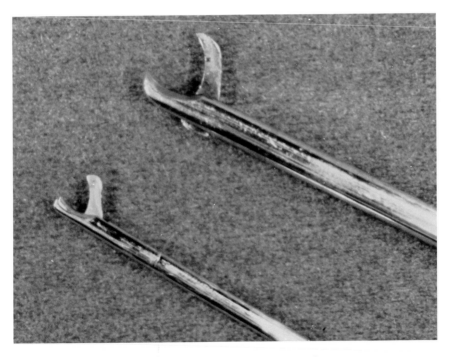

Fig. 15-4. Hooked meniscus scissors, 3 and 5 mm.

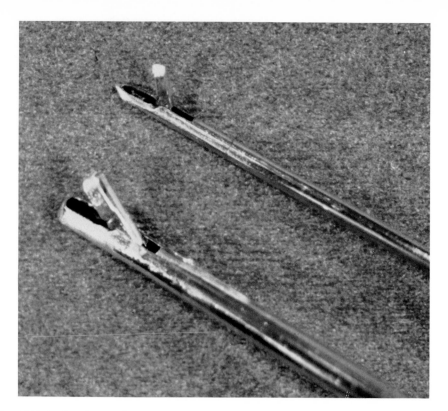

Fig. 15-5. Basket biopsy forceps, 3 and 5 mm, are used to trim peripheral meniscus rim. Serrated upper jaws fit into lower; stationary lower jaw stores fragment so that forceps need not be removed after every cut.

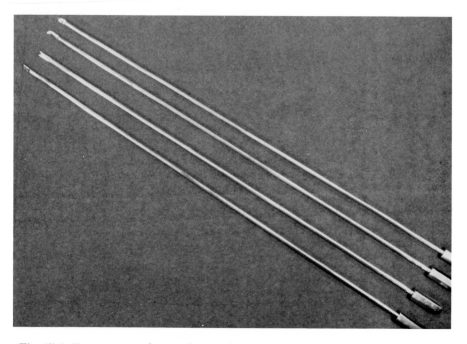

Fig. 15-6. Four meniscus knives that can be inserted through operating arthroscope.

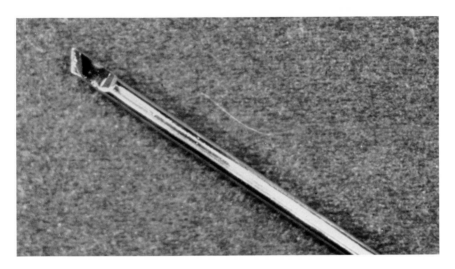

Fig. 15-7. Retrograde meniscus knife.

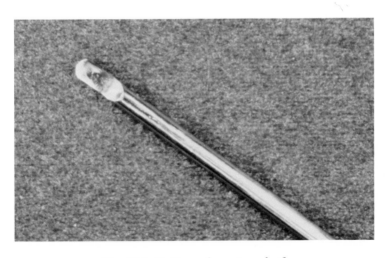

Fig. 15-8. Half-round meniscus knife.

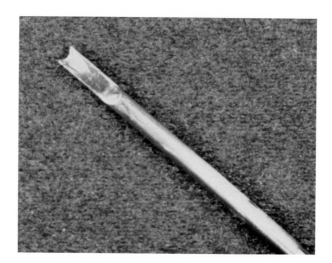

Fig. 15-9. The 3 mm Smillie knife.

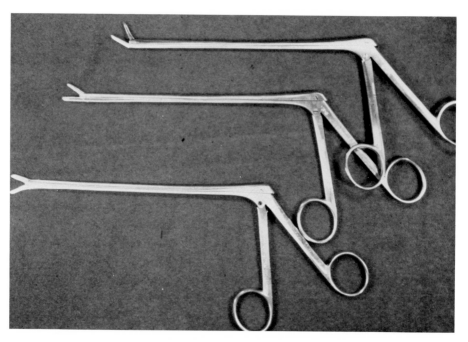

Fig. 15-10. Three 3 mm pituitary rongeurs. These may be used either as retractors or to excise a flap of tissue.

excision of the shelf, suction irrigation removal of multiple cartilaginous loose bodies, and the very occasional removal of a small, localized meniscus tear.

2. *Double-puncture technique:* This method requires the use of two or more portals of entry to allow viewing and dissection through one portal and retraction through a second portal. The shelf is *best* excised using this technique, and large osteochondral loose bodies can be removed as well as torn mobile meniscus fragments. Common double portals include the superolateral and inferolateral for the shelf, anteromedial and anterolateral for meniscus tears, and anteromedial and posteromedial for meniscus tears and osteocartilaginous loose bodies.

USES FOR ARTHROSCOPIC SURGERY
Soft tissue

Since in any pathologic process not all areas are involved to the same degree at the same time, synovial biopsy is most effective when performed arthroscopically. In a blind synovial biopsy, a normal area of meniscus tissue may accidently be selected that will result in either noncontributive or misleading information. Direct visualization of the pathologic synovium will allow separate aliquots of different stages of synovial involvement.

Soft tissue fronds may occasionally cause joint-line pain by getting trapped between the femoral condyle and tibia during flexion, extension, or rotation. These fronds may be excised arthroscopically.

Localized pigmented villonodular synovitis is an infrequent cause of knee discomfort. Upon three occasions, I have found this lesion attached by a stalk to the floor of the quadriceps bursa, interfering with patellar excursion. In one instance, the lesion was found beneath the middle third of the lateral meniscus, protruding beneath the meniscus during tibial rotation. These lesions were excised arthroscopically.

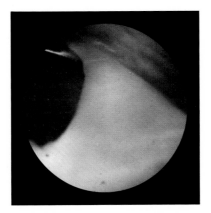

Fig. 15-11. Shelf in a right knee. This shelf is quite fibrotic, without vessels on its surface. This structure is also referred to as Iino's band, medial intraarticular band, or medial patellar plica.

The shelf (Fig. 15-11), also known as the medial patellar plica or Iino's band, is a frequent but infrequently recognized cause of knee discomfort. Present in a high percentage of patients, it is a structure of variable length and width. It traverses the medial side of the quadriceps bursa and often reaches its proximal limit at the superior pole of the patella when the knee is extended, running distally to the fat pad. It runs beneath the patella and over the medial femoral condyle, occasionally leaving an indentation on the cartilaginous surface of the medial femoral condyle. The pressure exerted by this band against the condyle increases with flexion.

Not to be confused with the shelf is the plica synovialis or suprapatellar plica, (Fig. 15-12), which runs in a plane at right angles to the shelf, with the knee in

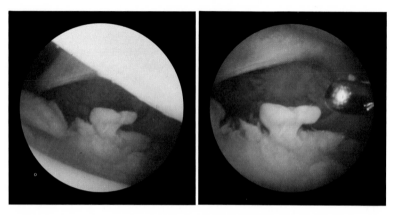

Fig. 15-12. Plica synovialis seen from lateral inferior patellar portal. On right, medial pillar of plica is partially covered by a blunt probe. On left, lateral pillar of plica inserts into suprapatellar recess. Lateral aspect of patellofemoral joint is seen in foreground.

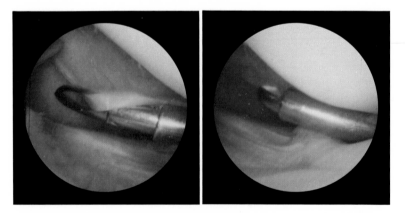

Fig. 15-13. Shelf has been split from medial sidewall as result of a twisting injury and is being manipulated with a forceps introduced through inferior lateral portal. Telescope has been inserted lateral and superior to patella.

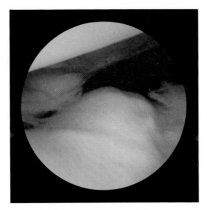

Fig. 15-14. Patellofemoral joint of left knee is studied from superior lateral patellar approach. Distal insertion of shelf into fat pad can be seen.

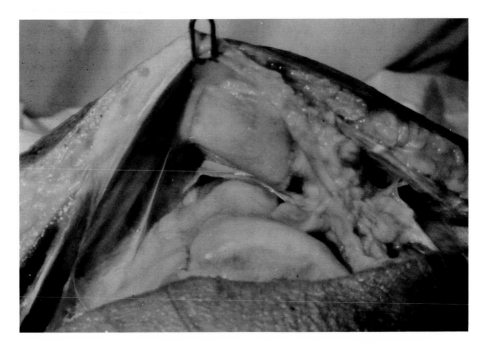

Fig. 15-15. Patella has been reflected laterally in this left cadaver knee. Shelf can be seen crossing medial femoral condyle, and just superior to patella, medial pillar of plica synovialis can be seen to lie in a plane at right angles to shelf. As knee goes into flexion both plica and shelf rub against medial femoral condyle.

extension. The suprapatellar plica rises from the medial sidewall, runs superiorly 1 mm from the most proximal portion of the patella, and inserts laterally into the suprapatellar bursa by a fibrotic pillar. The opening beneath the plica has been named the porta. The plica is variable in size and appears to be a fibrous septum, separating the joint proper from the quadriceps bursa. In flexion the plica slides centrally to the shelf via a groove just adjacent to the cartilage of the medial femoral condyle. In only one case that I have treated was the plica synovialis thought to be pathologic. Resection alleviated the patient's pain.

The shelf is often injured either by a direct blow to the anteromedial aspect of the knee in 90° of flexion when the band is taut over the medial femoral condyle, or as a result of a twisting injury. The latter may actually avulse the band from the medial capsule, allowing it to intermittently trap in the patellofemoral joint (Fig. 15-13). Injury by a direct blow is apt to cause edema, followed by replacement with fibrosis, resulting in a localized loss of elasticity of the involved synovium. Symptoms include tenderness over the shelf (one finger's breadth above the inferior pole of the patella), a snapping sensation on flexion and extension, nocturnal aching over the medial joint line, aching on acute flexion of the knee, and occasional pseudolocking. This damage to the shelf is often confused with a torn medial meniscus, chondromalacia of the patella, or patellar malalignment or subluxation. Treatment consists of removal of a wedge of the shelf, or excision, best performed arthroscopically (Figs. 15-14 and 15-15).

Cartilaginous and osteocartilaginous loose bodies

Frequently, cartilaginous loose bodies are encountered during arthroscopy. These cartilaginous fragments are not perceptible preoperatively, due to their radiolucency. The lateral joint line and to a lesser degree the medial joint line are the areas most often sought by these highly mobile fragments. Most often, cartilaginous fragments, unless unusually large, can be removed by using alternating positive and negative pressure through the water-sleeve connected to an irrigating syringe.

Because of their incompressibility and round configuration, osteocartilaginous loose bodies are most often found in the quadriceps bursa, intercondylar notch, lateral gutter, or posterior compartment (Fig. 15-16). Even loose bodies in the posterior compartment can be removed with arthroscopic equipment. Large fragments in the intercondylar notch are best brought into the lateral gutter and then into the quadriceps bursa. Because of the elasticity of the soft tissues, the incision through the lateral capsule and the quadriceps bursa in line with the fibers of the capsule can be enlarged to remove even the largest loose body.

Partial meniscectomy for meniscus tears

In no area of the knee is there a greater potential for avoiding arthrotomy and relieving symptoms than in the joint lines. Quite often in patients seen relatively soon after a meniscus tear, the rupture (as it appears at arthroscopy) is relatively localized, sparing the peripheral attachments of the meniscus. In these cases it is

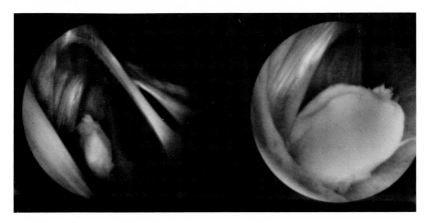

Fig. 15-16. An osteochondral loose body enmeshed in adhesions in quadriceps bursa. Lysis of these adhesions and removal of this loose body arthroscopically resulted in marked clinical improvement.

quite tempting to resect the localized area of torn meniscus, using arthroscopic equipment. Over an 8-month period this was attempted in carefully selected patients with what appeared to be amenable tears. As I gained experience and the results of these patients were compared to those of patients who had undergone arthrotomy, it became obvious that the concept of partial meniscectomy was valid. An effort was made to improve the arthroscopic equipment and technique so that more complex tears might be dealt with in this manner.

Clinical correlation of the patient's symptoms, physical findings, and the arthroscopic appearance of many meniscus ruptures shows that meniscus pain results from the trapping of the mobile "fragment" of meniscus between the femoral condyle and tibial plateau (especially on the medial side where the congruence between the medial femoral condyle and medial tibial spine is greater than on the lateral). A trapped fragment still attached to the periphery of the meniscus will, upon rotation, produce pain (Fig. 15-17). Thus the longitudinal tear is only minimally associated with pain, while the horizontal cleavage tear with flaps is very painful. If this reasoning is correct, it follows that by resecting the mobile fragments, traction and thus pain are eliminated. The results of partial meniscectomy seem to support this contention.

That a meniscus tear will cause degeneration of the overlying articular cartilage is accepted by most orthopedic surgeons as fact. However, evidence obtained from diagnostic arthroscopy does not completely support this premise. In several instances, longitudinal tears, with a patient's history of intermittent locking and unlocking, have been present for as long as 35 years without alteration of the contiguous articular cartilage. Conversely degeneration of the posterior, inner, medial, femoral condyle is often seen in the absence of a demonstrable tear. Certain specific tears, however, are almost always associated with condylar degeneration. These are trans-

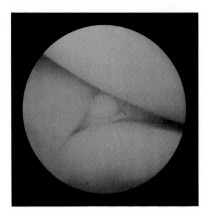 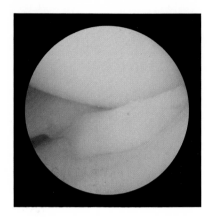

Fig. 15-17. Flap tear of medial meniscus can be seen sequestered beneath medial meniscus with tibia in internal rotation. On right, tibia has been externally rotated, and flap swings centrally into intercondylar notch.

verse tears of the lateral meniscus (Fig. 15-18) and flap tears of the medial meniscus, which flip from the posterior and rotate on their bases to rest between the inner medial condyle and medial meniscus (Fig. 15-19). At arthroscopy this latter tear resists movement as if it were being pressed on its superior surface. Both tears exert localized pressure over their respective condyles. Tears other than these do not seem to have the same propensity for causing hyaline cartilage degeneration since they may not localize stress. One objection to partial meniscectomy is that the peripheral rim may cause localized pressure, leading to hyaline cartilage degeneration. However, in the limited number of patients on whom we have been able to do another arthroscopic examination after partial meniscectomy, the articular cartilage has been unchanged and the thickened peripheral rim triangulated.

Another (less valid) objection to partial meniscectomy is that resecting only the bucket will fail to disclose additional tears that may be present in the periphery of the meniscus. However, arthroscopic study after partial resection can establish the presence of additional tears, and these may also be treatable by arthroscopic excision.

There have been a wealth of reports written in the 1960s and 1970s which indicate that total or subtotal meniscectomy may be associated with marked degenerative changes in the compartment operated upon, with less than optimal 10-year results in 50% of the patients treated (Jackson, Gear, Huckell, Tapper and Hoover, Cargill). Tapper and Hoover in a small series of partial meniscectomies associated with arthrotomy and excision of only the displaced longitudinal tear noted a high percentage of good results, and Cargill found short-term improvement from excision of only the displaced bucket to be equal to that derived from total meniscectomy.

The advantage of partial meniscectomy performed with arthroscopic equipment is that only the mobile fragments are excised, and the peripheral rim can be studied

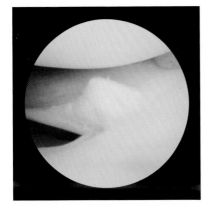

Fig. 15-18. Transverse tear at junction of posterior and middle thirds of lateral meniscus of left knee. Note hiatus for passage of popliteal tendon above tear. This tear has a propensity for extension, forming so-called "parrot beak," which concentrates stress, damaging overlying articular cartilage.

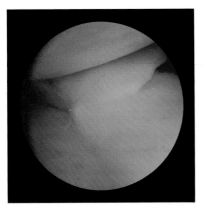
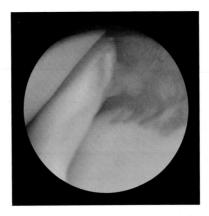

Fig. 15-19. Common flap tear of medial meniscus of right knee. This tear lacks mobility, and attempted manipulation even with heavy intraarticular instruments will not budge this tear. In my experience this type of tear has always been associated with damage of overlying articular cartilage.

and trimmed if necessary—a difficult procedure when performed through an arthrotomy incision. The morbidity is not much greater than that following diagnostic arthroscopy, and many patients have been able to resume limited work the next day.

Certain specific tears or situations are best handled by arthroscopic surgery.

1. The older patient with a horizontal cleavage tear and hyaline cartilage damage on the ipsilateral compartment or patellofemoral degeneration, whose primary complaint is pain, is an ideal candidate for partial excision. The pain relief is usually quite dramatic, and there is almost no risk of increasing the patient's symptoms.

2. The displaced bucket-handle tear is most advantageously handled by this technique. The peripheral rim may be studied after partial excision of a bucket, and if additional tears are found in the rim they may be excised as well.

3. Arthroscopic treatment of a minor tear in the otherwise normal meniscus of a young individual will allow years of normal meniscus function. If further tearing occurs that requires total meniscus excision later, the joint will be that much better for the additional normal meniscus function provided by the earlier partial excision.

4. Arthroscopic excision of meniscus tears in the athlete allows continued participation in sports until the end of a playing season, when total meniscectomy may be accomplished without sacrifice of playing time.

As experience with arthroscopic surgery has increased, the partial meniscectomy has proved to be quite satisfactory. Repeat meniscectomy is rarely necessary.

One of the difficulties in evaluating the technique of partial meniscectomy under arthroscopic control is the inability to repeat the arthroscopy at a later date except in patients with continuing complaints. The patient without symptoms is unwilling to

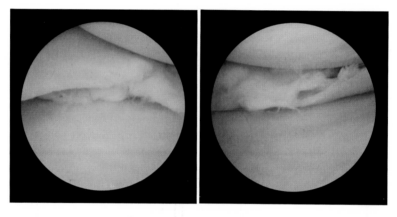

Fig. 15-20. Degenerative tear of medial meniscus of right knee. Note inferior flap on left.

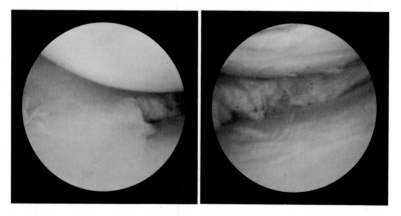

Fig. 15-21. Same medial joint line as in Fig. 15-20, seen through medial portal after partial excision, using operating arthroscope.

undergo arthroscopy and its expense just to satisfy his surgeon's academic interest. Arthroscopic follow-up has been obtained in patients with continuing complaints, or if the other knee becomes symptomatic. Several arthroscopic follow-ups have been quite instructive.

Case 1. A 63-year-old orthopedic surgeon had a typical horizontal cleavage tear of his left medial meniscus with a flap trapped beneath the meniscus (Fig. 15-20). The immediate postoperative result demonstrated the irregular thickened meniscus margin (Fig. 15-21). This man returned to strenuous downhill skiing within 48 hours and resumed racquetball and tennis shortly thereafter. The medial joint-line pain was alleviated, but an effusion persisted with discomfort, presumably due to his strenuous activities. Repeat arthroscopy 3 months later demonstrated that the meniscus rim had smoothed out (Fig. 15-22). The cause of the persistent effusion and discomfort was found to be in the synovium, with edema of the villi and occasional fibrotic capping (Fig. 15-23). Joint lavage, antiphlogistic agents, and rest have since allowed him to resume his active life.

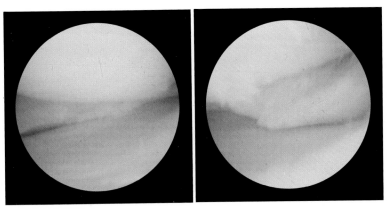

Fig. 15-22. Same knee (as in Fig. 15-20) 3 months later, as seen through lateral portal. Meniscus edges have smoothed out.

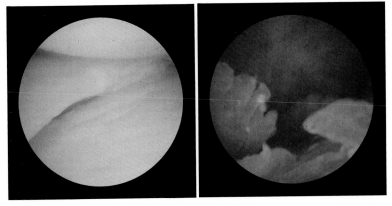

Fig. 15-23. On left, peripheral rim is seen closeup; thickened rim has almost triangulated. On right, cause of this patient's persistent complaints can be seen in synovium; villi are edematous, with dilatation of central vessel, and fibrotic capping is occurring.

Case 2. A 22-year-old college linebacker complained of nonlocalized popliteal pain. Physical examination and two arthrograms were unrewarding in establishing a diagnosis. Arthroscopy demonstrated a normal medial meniscus, a torn anterior cruciate ligament, and a thin but highly mobile flap tear of the posterior third of the lateral meniscus (Fig. 15-24). He was treated by excision of the flap tear. The immediate postoperative appearance is shown in Fig. 15-25. He returned to football, and at the end of the season he reinjured himself. Repeat arthroscopy demonstrated the smoothness of the peripheral rim of the lateral meniscus (Fig. 15-26). The medial meniscus, however, was found to be torn (Fig. 15-27). On the left of Fig. 15-27 a tear is seen in the inferior surface of the medial meniscus in its posterior one third; on the right (with the knee flexed 90° and anterior stress on the tibia) a tear dislocated beneath the medial femoral condyle can be seen. The anterior cut made with the operating arthroscope is shown on the right of Fig. 15-28. On the left (Fig. 15-28) the posterior attachment of the mobile fragments can be seen still affixed. Removal of these mobile fragments but not the entire meniscus enabled the patient to resume football this season (Fig. 15-29).

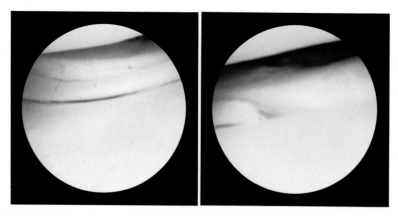

Fig. 15-24. Tear of lateral meniscus of right knee. This longitudinal rupture of posterior third has extended through inner edge near posterior tibial attachment and was observed flopping in and out of joint line.

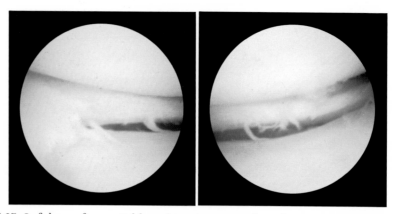

Fig. 15-25. Left knee after partial lateral meniscectomy through operating arthroscope. Site of attachment is visible at junction of posterior and middle thirds. Peripheral rim is thickened and ragged.

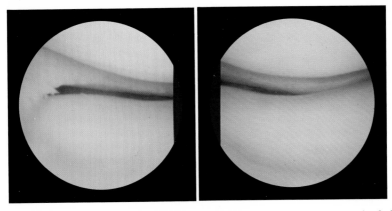

Fig. 15-26. Same patient (as in Fig. 15-25) 6 months later, following another football injury rupturing his medial meniscus. Opportunity was available to reexamine peripheral rim of lateral meniscus. Note that rim has triangulated and become smooth.

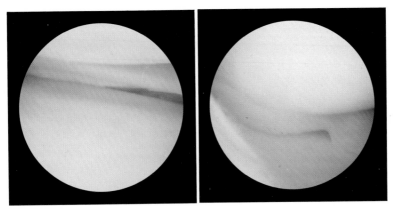

Fig. 15-27. On left, tear in inferior surface of right medial meniscus. On right, with knee in 90° flexion and application of anterior drawer test. Mobile fragment dislocated beneath medial femoral condyle centrally.

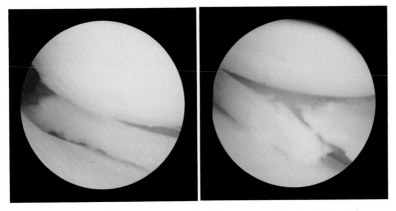

Fig. 15-28. The right medial meniscus tear has been severed anteriorly with operating arthroscope, as shown on right. Posterior attachment of mobile fragment is seen in slide on left.

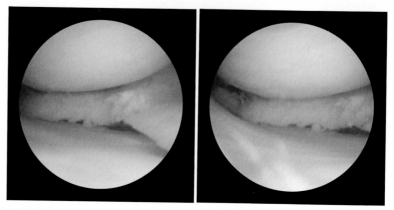

Fig. 15-29. Immediate postoperative appearance of peripheral rim of medial meniscus. Compare with Fig. 15-28.

SUMMARY

The results discussed in this chapter are reproducible, although considerable experience in diagnostic arthroscopy is necessary before the surgeon attempts to use this equipment therapeutically. The objective of arthroscopic surgery is to decrease morbidity and to preserve the joint. We are impressed with the former; how successful we are in achieving the latter will take years of follow-up to determine.

16. Joints other than the knee

Arthroscopy

Lanny L. Johnson

The value of arthroscopy in the knee joint is well accepted.[6] The ability to inspect other joints arthroscopically is not so well known. Burman first reported performing arthroscopy of various joints[2,3] on cadavers. His techniques were very similar to those performed today. His ability to inspect these joints exceeded the technology of his day. Certainly if he had had the quality of optics in the small-diameter endoscopes that have become available in the 1970s, these particular writings[2,3] would have been antiquated.

Watanabe[8] has inspected virtually every accessible joint, using a no. 24 Olympus Arthroscope* with the patient under general anesthesia. A number of arthroscopists have inspected other joints and have reported their findings.[1,4]

The purpose of this part of this chapter is to again draw attention to the possibility of using arthroscopy in body joints other than the knee and to present the arthroscopic technique. It is hoped that others will be encouraged to develop their arthroscopic skills in smaller joints. The shoulder, elbow, and ankle joint are easily inspected with a small-diameter endoscope even with the patient under only local anesthesia.

At this time the indications for arthroscopy of the various joints is limited. With experience in these other areas, a clear definition of the indications for arthroscopy will be possible. In addition exploration of the joints by this technique may well unfold new vistas in diagnosis and treatment of the various joint problems.

The indications and techniques of knee joint arthroscopy are well established.[6] The knee joint affords an opportunity to learn basic arthroscopic skills, that is, placement, palpation, redirection, cleansing, scanning the horizon, and pistoning. These skills then provide the arthroscopist with the basis upon which he can explore the other joints. These same basic arthroscopic techniques also apply to any other joints.

Attention will be given to the position of the patient, the position of the equipment, the position of the assistant, and the position of the arthroscopist in each of the subsequent specific joint techniques. The type of anesthetic used and the technical

---

*Manufactured by Olympus, Japan.

249

details, including the point of entry, will be outlined. The anatomic landmarks naturally differ from joint to joint. The important landmarks from which to work will be identified. Conditions in which arthroscopy may be of value are mentioned.

The Needlescope,* by virtue of its small diameter, provides ease of access to the smaller joints. It offers excellent optical clarity and good illumination. A 4.0 mm endoscope (Dyonics rod-lens system or the Storz-Hopkins rod-lens system) may be used for viewing the shoulder joint but only in a large person. This diameter (4.0 mm) will be too large for most patients' elbows or ankle joints. A 2.7 mm Storz arthroscope has been used in the hip of an obese person when a long endoscope was necessary. The best illumination for viewing and photographic work would be provided by the Dyonics Model 500 light source or the Storz xenon system.

THE SHOULDER

For examination of the shoulder joint the patient is placed on his side on an operating table (Fig. 16-1). He is best secured with a vacuum beanbag. The assistant stands in front of the patient. The arthroscopist stands behind the patient. The patient is prepared and draped in the customary fashion. The light source and the Mayo stand with the equipment are in front of the patient.

A posterior entry is preferred. A point immediately medial and inferior to the posterior angle of the scapula can be palpated as a sulcus. Lidocaine 1%, is infiltrated through the skin and directly into the joint (Fig. 16-2). No intraarticular anesthetic has been necessary. The skin is lacerated with a no. 11 blade. The cannula and trocar follow the path of the anesthesic, parallel and perpendicular to the long axis of the patient. The entry is sensed by palpation. Distraction of the arm by the assistant will increase the potential space of the joint. The arthroscopist may elect to distend the shoulder joint (from a superior position) with saline to facilitate penetration. The shoulder joint holds 15 to 35 ml of saline.

Intraarticular landmarks

The biceps brachii tendon and the horizon of the humeral head are the primary landmarks to identify (Fig. 16-3). From there it is possible to follow the biceps tendon to its insertion at the superior glenoid. The examiner may proceed to the entire glenoid fossae inferiorly or to the rotator cuff area superiorly. It is possible to see a labrum injury below, a dislocation of the shoulder, or a rotator cuff separation above, all with hemorrhage. The biceps tendon may be followed to the bicipital groove in the humerus if the arm is elevated and externally rotated. A ruptured biceps tendon will appear similar to an injured anterior cruciate in the knee. There will be fragmentation and miniature cross-hatching of the bundles. A subluxation of the biceps tendon will show considerable reaction and synovitis adjacent to the bicipital groove. If the examiner will retract the arthroscope gently and have the assistant externally

---

*Trademark of Dyonics, Inc., Woburn, Mass.

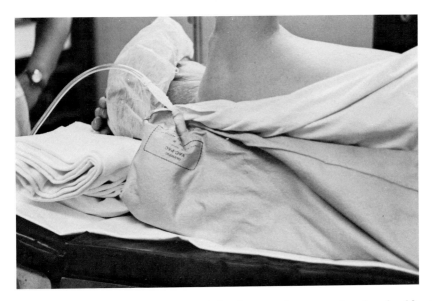

Fig. 16-1. Patient is secured in the lateral decubitus with vacuum bag for shoulder joint arthroscopy.

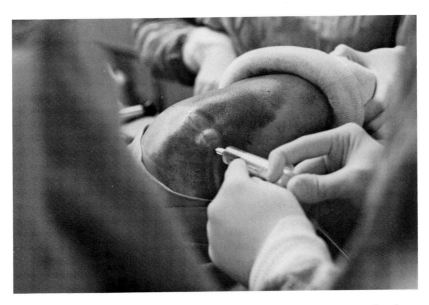

Fig. 16-2. Point of entry to shoulder is posterior and inferior to posterior angle of acromion. Local anesthetic is infiltrated along anticipated course of arthroscope.

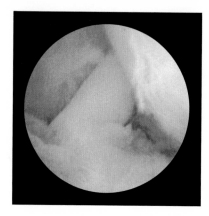

Fig. 16-3. Arthroscopic view of shoulder joint. Humeral head is between 12 o'clock and 3 o'clock. Biceps tendon courses obliquely from superior aspect of glenoid fossae to behind humeral head.

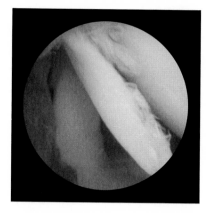

Fig. 16-4. Shoulder joint. Rotator cuff area is to left; a tag of ruptured rotator cuff tendon protrudes into glenohumeral joint. An elipse of humeral head is seen to right.

rotate the arm, it will bring a Hill-Sach lesion site into view on the posterior humeral head. A patient with diffuse synovitis may be difficult to examine arthroscopically because of limited space in the shoulder and villi blocking the examiner's view.

A simple dressing is used at the completion of the procedure.

Conditions in which arthroscopy is of value

Arthroscopy of an *acute dislocation* establishes the diagnosis and rules out loose bodies not seen at arthrotomy.

The diagnosis of *chronic dislocation* may be established by use of arthroscopy when other means of documentation have failed.

A *ruptured biceps tendon* as the cause of shoulder pain and swelling is easily identified arthroscopically.

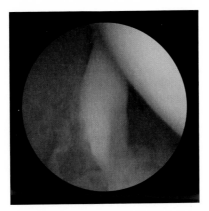

Fig. 16-5. Synovitis of shoulder joint. Reddened synovium is to left, biceps tendon is in middle, and humeral head is to right.

In a questionable clinical situation the arthroscopic examination can provide direct evidence of a *bicipital tendon subluxation*.

In a *rotator cuff injury* the acute incomplete lesion appears as a hemorrhagic separation beneath the synovium. A complete defect, although difficult to examine arthroscopically because of leakage of saline solution, is easily identified when in view with a tug of the tendon protruding through the defect (Fig. 16-4).

Arthroscopy provides direct visualization of the morphology associated with *synovitis* as well as access to culture and biopsy (Fig. 16-5).

Heretofore I thought *frozen shoulder* was related to capsular adhesions. Arthroscopy of the shoulder has shown many patients to have a very reactive vascular synovitis without fibrinoid exudate. Intraarticular cortisone injection without manipulation has resulted in rapid recovery from pain and loss of motion. I am now hesitant to manipulate this type of shoulder condition.

THE ELBOW

For examination of the elbow the patient is supine with his arm on a Boyes-Parker table. A 0.5% lidocaine intravenous regional anesthetic is preferred. It is possible to perform the examination with a simple infiltrative anesthetic under tourniquet control. I use regional anesthetic for increased patient comfort and ease of elbow manipulation. The assistant is on one side of the table and the arthroscopist on the other. It is important to place two folded towels under the patient's arm to elevate the elbow off the table. This permits a greater arc of excursion of the arthroscope. The equipment and the light should be at the end of the Boyes-Parker table.

The joint is first distended with saline through a hypodermic needle. This facilitates entry into the small joint. The medial side is inspected via a lateral puncture and vice versa. The lateral point of entry is superior and posterior to the radial head. Rotation of the forearm facilitates identification of this landmark. There will be a soft spot or sulcus just anterior to the humeroradial articulation. The coronoid process is identified by flexion and extension. The arm is taken into external rotation for the

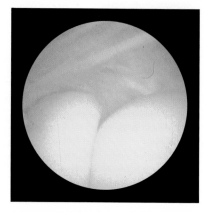

Fig. 16-6. Elbow joint. Radial head is to left and humeral head to right.

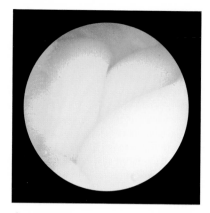

Fig. 16-7. Elbow joint. With retraction of arthroscope, entire humeroradial articulation is seen, as well as humeroulnar articulation.

medial approach. At a point immediately anterior and superior to the humeral medial epicondyle, the skin may be lacerated. The joint must be distended from this entry. It is possible to see the articulation between the humeral capitellum and the radial head (Fig. 16-6). Supination and pronation of the forearm will help identify this landmark. With retraction of the arthroscope the ulnar coronoid process comes into view (Fig. 16-7). It is possible to see the annular ligament.

The olecranon fossa is entered obliquely from the lateral side. The arm is internally rotated by the assistant, and with the joint distended it is possible to enter at the 30° angle toward posterior. The distended joint will actually bulge at this site. With an arthroscope of 1.7 mm diameter the examiner can enter the space between the humeral trochlea and the ulna. The olecranon may be seen posteriorly. There is a surprisingly large space posteriorly in a distended elbow joint.

A simple dressing is used at the close of the procedure.

Elbow conditions in which arthroscopy can be valuable are given below.

As with osteochondritis dissecans in the knee, the status of the lesion in *Panner disease* can be identified arthroscopically in a way not revealed by x-ray examination.

Often the exact amount of displacement in an *intraarticular fracture* cannot be determined by x-ray examination. Arthroscopy can show the separation and can influence clinical decisions.

It is possible to assess the extent of *degenerative arthritis* arthroscopically and to remove loose bodies.

Intraarticular inspection has shown synovitis about the radial head in "*tennis elbow.*" Also, many patients have synovial and articular debris. This is visualized arthroscopically, and removal is by vacuuming via the cannula. These patients' conditions have been improved by lavage. The arthroscope may be used to investigate this common condition.

THE WRIST

For examination of the wrist the patient is supine on the operating table with his arm placed on a Boyes-Parker table. A 0.5% lidocaine intravenous regional anesthetic is preferred. Local infiltrative anesthetic may be used under tourniquet control. We have used the regional anesthetic for increased patient comfort and ease of wrist manipulation. Local anesthetic also provides the patient with an opportunity for dynamic flexion and extension and ulnar or radial deviation, so that the arthroscopist might view these surfaces during actual compression and relaxation, or motion, or both. The patient's forearm will be held firmly by the assistant, and distraction may be placed upon the wrist in the metacarpal area.

The joint is first distended with saline through a hypodermic needle. This facilitates entry into the small joint. The joint between the radius and the carpal scaphoid is most easily entered obliquely just distal to the radial styloid. Care must be taken not to lacerate the superficial branches of the radial nerve, which can be palpated over the actively extended extensor pollicis longus tendon. Other points of entry or inspection, with less well-defined landmarks, can be helped by radiologic monitoring.

With an arthroscope of 1.7 mm diameter it is possible to enter a variety of these spaces to inspect the articular surfaces and the synovial walls. There are surprisingly large spaces especially between the distal radius and carpal scaphoid.

A simple dressing is used at the close of the procedure.

The following are wrist conditions for which arthroscopy can be valuable.

Often the exact amount of displacement in an *intraarticular fracture* cannot be determined by x-ray examination, or the presence of a small articular incongruity in a small joint can produce relatively greater symptoms; in these instances arthroscopy can be helpful.

Arthroscopy can be used to assess the extent of articular changes and presence of small loose bodies seen in *degenerative arthritis*.

Some patients have complained of *synovial thickening* about their wrists even on an undetermined basis. Arthroscopy can provide a means of inspection and biopsy.

Often patients have complained of well-localized *pain of undetermined origin* in the wrist joint. The x-ray films would be normal. Arthroscopic inspection can establish the exact status of the articular cartilage and the synovial tissues.

THE FINGER

For examination of the finger joints the patient is supine on an operating table with his arm on a Boyes-Parker table. A tourniquet is utilized. The preparation and draping are performed in a standard manner. The arthroscopist and the assistant sit across from one another. The equipment on the Mayo stand is at the end of the table, and the light source is beyond.

A digital or wrist regional block is preferred. The joint is distended with a no. 25 needle. The skin is carefully lacerated to restrict the opening to a tight fit for the 2 mm–outer diameter cannula of the Needlescope. The joint is entered obliquely dorsal to the collateral ligaments, and the Needlescope is aimed volarward. This is best accomplished by careful palpation with the cannula and trocar.

Visualization is surprisingly easy (Fig. 16-8). Distension may be maintained by forcing saline adjacent to the endoscope via a K-52 catheter as in knee joint arthroscopy.

Finger conditions in which arthroscopy can be valuable are given below.

The question of a juxtaarticular ossification versus a *loose body* in the finger joint may be determined arthroscopically and without an arthrotomy.

The extent of *articular cartilage damage* in the finger joint may be assessed. It may dictate opening the joint during reconstruction. The prognosis can better be established with the use of arthroscopy.

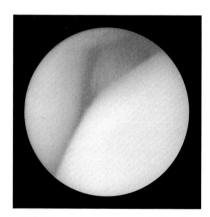

Fig. 16-8. Interphalangeal joint of thumb. Indented contour of the proximal phalanx is superior and to left. Matching prominence of distal phalanx is to right.

Arthroscopy can be used to accurately determine in an *intraarticular fracture* the actual amount of displacement in certain cases of difficult judgment.

THE HIP

For examination of the hip the patient is placed in the supine position on a fracture table. A peroneal post is utilized for countertraction. A general anesthetic is required. The assistant is on the opposite side of the patient from the hip to be examined. The arthroscopist also stands adjacent to the hip in question. The patient is prepared and draped in the customary fashion. The Mayo stand and equipment are on the assistant's side of the table, as is the light source.

The approach to the hip joint can be either anterior or posterior. The most satisfactory is the anterolateral approach familiar to orthopedists who have performed hip joint needle aspirations. With the endoscopic cannula entering lateral to the neurovascular femoral bundles and aimed superior and medially 45° the hip joint can be identified. Radiologic control can be of benefit.

Distension of the joint with an 18-gauge spinal needle initially will distend the joint with saline and facilitate entry. After entry has been achieved, continued instillation of the joint via the arthroscope with continued traction on the extremity provides the best view of the acetabulum. Pure manual traction will not suffice in an adult. A child's hip can be distracted manually. With mechanical means of distraction and internal and external rotation the anterior, medial, and lateral portions of the hip can be inspected as well as the labrum and acetabular dome. Inspection for articular abnormality or synovitis is possible.

A rod-lens arthroscope of 2.7 or 4.0 mm diameter has been utilized when a large patient required the greater length telescope.

The points of reference that are looked for are internal and external rotation of the femoral head, which identifies it in juxtaposition to the joint space and the anterior labrum of the acetabulum.

The following are hip conditions in which arthroscopy can be valuable.

Shneider[7] has investigated arthroscopically a series of patients with *Legg-Perthes disease*, either established or inspected, and demonstrated the articular compression fracture of the femoral head. In addition some of these patients had a compression fracture of the acetabular side as well.

Gross[5] has reported a chondrolysis in a patient with *slipped capital-femoral epiphysis* in which aspiration of the joint and lavage rendered the patient asymptomatic.

Gross has studied *congenital dislocation* of the hip arthroscopically and has reported his preliminary experience.

Arthroscopy of the hip in a patient with *osteochondritis dissecans* can establish the extent of the lesion or the existence of its articular separation.

Some patients with *aseptic necrosis of the femoral head* have sequestration on the articular cartilage and immediate subchondral bone. An arthroscopy of the hip can make this determination. If indeed there is a sequestration or convolution of the

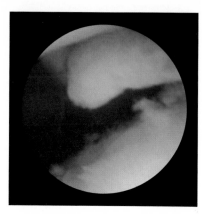

Fig. 16-9. Hip joint. Degenerative surface of femur is inferior, and a large loose body is at 2 o'clock, just below the superior elipse of acetabular rim.

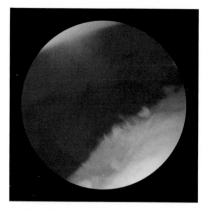

Fig. 16-10. Hip joint. Femoral head is between 3 and 6 o'clock. There is a loss of articular surface. With distraction of femur on a traction table, femur is moved away from acetabular lip above.

articular surface the patient would not be a candidate for a bone graft in that there had already been permanent alteration in the articular surfaces.

Arthroscopy of the hip in patients with *synovial disease* affords direct inspection of the extent of the articular damage as well as access to synovial biopsy for diagnostic purposes.

Acute hip pain may be secondary to early changes resulting from *degenerative arthritis* (Figs. 16-9 and 16-10). Loose bodies may be in the joint, producing a synovitis pain. X-ray films and tomograms may be normal. An arthroscopy will establish the diagnosis and vacuuming the loose bodies will relieve the symptoms.

THE ANKLE

For examination of the ankle the patient is supine on an operating table. The assistant stands to the side of the table to secure the extremity. The arthroscopist stands at the end of the table. The patient is prepared and draped in a customary fashion. The Mayo stand and equipment is to the side of the table and in front of the assistant.

The approach to the ankle may be direct anterior, anteromedial, or anterolateral. The puncture site should be opposite the area of the ankle to be viewed. It is helpful to insert an 18-gauge needle initially in order to distend the joint with saline. The ankle will hold 10 to 20 ml of saline. In some instances where the ankle capsule is very lax or ruptured, maintenance of this needle for continued saline distension will facilitate viewing.

Another important technical point is distraction of the ankle. This is accomplished by traction with the arthroscopist's free hand cupped around the patient's heel and pulling distally. This maneuver is more effective than forceful plantar flexion of the foot and ankle. Maximum arthroscopic visibility is provided by combined continuous saline distension and joint distraction.

A small stab wound lacerates the skin, and the cannula with trocar is placed into the distended joint.

Inspection of the ankle, including the underside of the distal tibia, that is the tibial plafond, and the inner surface of the medial malleolus may be accomplished. The entire dome (Fig. 16-11) of the talus is visible, including the medial and lateral vertical sides. On the lateral side of the talus, the articular facet of the distal fibula can be visualized (Fig. 16-12). Also the facet of the medial malleolus may be documented.

Ankle conditions in which arthroscopy can be valuable are given below.

Arthroscopy has been valuable in examining *osteochondral fractures* of the dome of the talus. After injury to the ankle mortise, the examiner can assess the progress of healing and evaluate the articular surfaces from a prognostic standpoint.

Ligament injury in the ankle can also be delineated with the use of arthroscopy. The transverse deep portion of the deltoid ligament is visible directly in the ankle if the puncture is made in the anteromedial side. The arthroscope can also be placed down the inner side of the talus. This will give direct access to the deltoid ligament. The extent of injury to the deltoid ligament can be determined. If a lateral puncture is selected, it is also possible to see the ends of the fibular collateral ligament where they attach to the distal fibula. Arthroscopy has been useful in evaluating acute ligament injuries to the ankle.

Arthroscopic evaluation of the articular surfaces can be important if there is loss of motion after a *healed fracture* of the ankle. There is some prognostic value. The loss of motion may be the scar of the injury or surgery or both, rather than intraarticular changes.

There may be a medicolegal value as well.

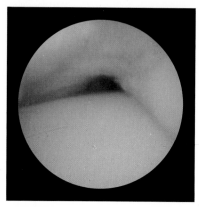

Fig. 16-11. Ankle joint. Dome of talus is in mid field. Distal tibia is between 9 and 3 o'clock. Fibular articulation is to left.

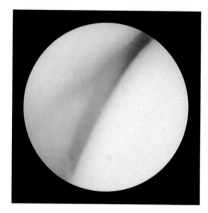

Fig. 16-12. Ankle joint. Arthroscope penetrates into talofibular articulation. This is a normal joint appearance.

Arthroscopy of the ankle makes possible direct observation of the *synovial morphology* as well as access to synovial culture and biopsy.

SUMMARY

Arthroscopy of the various joints and its potential has been known since Burman's work in the 1930s. Watanabe has established a technique for a variety of joints. This work has been duplicated by others. Still the clinical indications and benefits are limited. On the other hand I have outlined the techniques that make this type of tool available to the orthopedist in selected cases. The small-diameter arthroscopes provide access to virtually every joint.

With the technology now available, providing photographic documentation of our observations of the various joints should increase the indications and benefits of arthroscopy.

References

1. Aignan, M.: Arthroscopy of the hip. In International review of rheumatology: Arthroscopy (special edition), 1976.
2. Burman, M.: Arthroscopy or direct visualization of joints: an experimental cadaver study, J. Bone Joint Surg. 13:669-95, 1931.
3. Burman, M.: Arthroscopy of the elbow joint: a cadaver study, J. Bone Joint Surg. 14:349-50, 1932.
4. Cheng, Y.: Arthroscopy of the ankle joint. In International review of rheumatology: Arthroscopy (special edition), 1976.
5. Gross, R. H.: Arthroscopy in hip disorders in children, Orthop. Rev. September 1977.
6. Johnson, L. L.: Comprehensive arthroscopic examination of the knee, St. Louis, 1977, The C. V. Mosby Co.
7. Shneider, D.: Personal communication, 1976.
8. Watanabe, M.: Recent advances in arthroscopy. In International review of rheumatology: Arthroscopy (special edition), 1976.

Arthrography

Murray K. Dalinka

THE SHOULDER

Arthrography of the shoulder is a common, well-accepted diagnostic procedure in the evaluation of chronic shoulder pain. Its main use is in the diagnosis and documentation of complete tears of the rotator cuff musculature, but it can also be used to document adhesive capsulitis, that is, frozen shoulder, or to demonstrate the location and severity of soft tissue damage in patients with recurrent dislocations.[12,13]

Shoulder arthrography is safe and relatively easy to perform. Positive-contrast arthrography demonstrates the integrity, shape, and capacity of the glenohumeral joint.

Method

The shoulder is prepared with povidone-iodine (Betadine), and a keyhole drape is placed over the joint. All studies are performed under fluoroscopic control with image intensification. I use a sterilizable lead grid for localization of the injection site. The shoulder is infiltrated with local anesthetic with the patient in an anteroposterior projection. A 20-gauge spinal needle is then directed into the glenohumeral space under fluoroscopic control; when the contrast is injected into the joint it flows away from the needle tip. I use 12 to 15 ml of an equal mixture of 1% procaine and Renografin 60%. Dilution of the Renografin decreases the hypertonicity of the contrast agent, and therefore there is less postarthrographic pain. Routine roentgenograms are taken in internal and external rotation and the axillary projection. If these films are normal, delayed films are obtained after exercise, because with some small

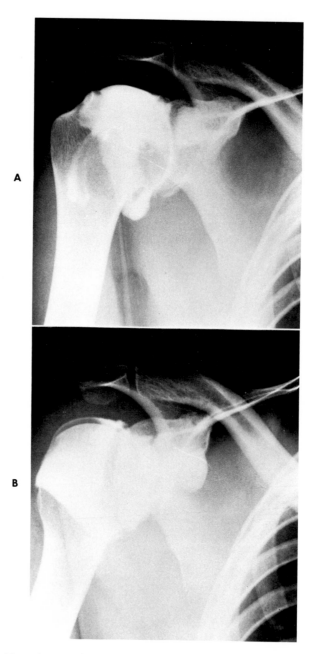

Fig. 16-13. A, Normal external rotation view. Tendon sheath of long head of biceps is well seen as are axillary and subscapularis bursae. **B,** Normal internal rotation view. Subscapularis bursa is well seen. Joint capsule is projected laterally. Area beneath acromion is free of contrast.

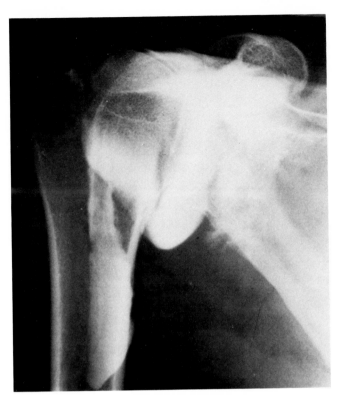

Fig. 16-14. Normal arthrogram with contrast leaking along bicipital tendon sheath after exercise.

cuff tears the examiner may not see filling of the subacromial-subdeltoid bursa on the initial study.[12]

Normal arthrograms

The normal shoulder arthrogram outlines the smooth regular articular cartilage over the humeral head (Fig. 16-13). The long head of the biceps muscle is frequently observed within its recess at the superior aspect of the shoulder joint. Its synovial sheath is almost always visible within the bicipital groove. Occasionally, particularly in the postexercise films, contrast material is noted to leak across the course of the tendon into the upper arm (Fig. 16-14). I agree with Killoran and associates[12] that this is a normal finding and probably is secondary to distension or increased intra-articular pressure.

The subscapularis recess is seen extending beneath the coracoid process deep to the muscle. Occasionally dissection of contrast is seen adjacent to this bursa, which is also thought to be secondary to overdistension. An axillary recess or fold is seen at the inferior margin of the shoulder joint with an indentation between it and the sub-scapularis recess. The subscapularis recess is prominent in internal rotation but is

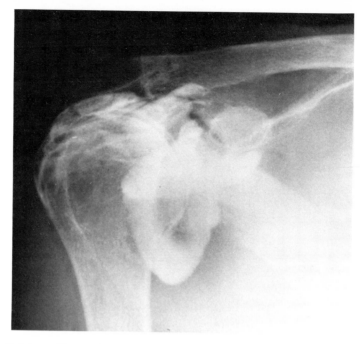

Fig. 16-15. Rotator cuff tear. Contrast material has entered subacromial-subdeltoid bursa and is seen beneath acromion process and lateral to greater tuberosity of humerus.

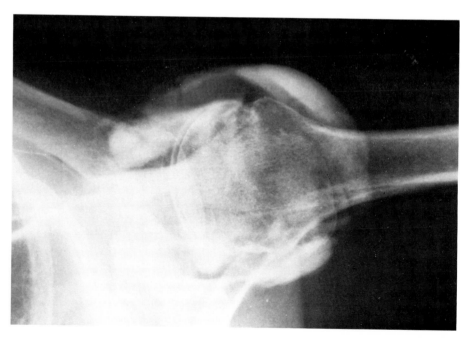

Fig. 16-16. Axillary view of patient with rotator cuff tear, demonstrating subdeltoid bursa projecting across surgical neck of humerus.

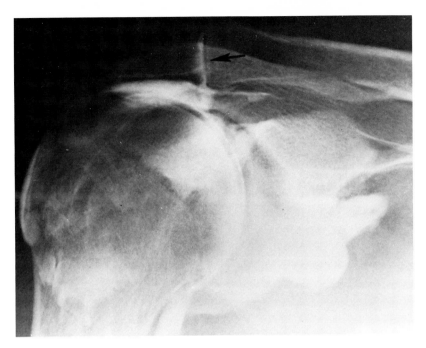

Fig. 16-17. Complete tear of rotator cuff and communication with acromioclavicular joint (*arrow*).

taut in external rotation. In external rotation, contrast extends only to the anatomic neck of the humerus. In the axillary view, the glenohumeral space is usually well seen as are the cartilaginous margins of the glenoid labrum. The bicipital tendon is well seen anteriorly as is the subscapularis recess.

Abnormal arthrograms

In complete tears of the rotator cuff there is filling of the subacromial-subdeltoid bursa (Fig. 16-15). Contrast material is present beneath the acromial process and above and lateral to the greater tuberosity of the humerus. Normally the rotator cuff separates this bursa from the glenohumeral joint, and hence communication can only occur with a complete tear. In the axillary view the bursa projects across the surgical neck of the humerus, which normally is devoid of contrast media (Fig. 16-16). The size of the bursa does not indicate the size of the tear. Occasionally with complete cuff tears, there is also communication with the acromioclavicular joint[11] (Fig. 16-17).

Partial rotator cuff tears may only be visualized if the partial tear is in the under-surface of the tendon, and a collection of contrast media is visible within the tendon itself. No communication with the bursa exists.[12]

In patients with adhesive capsulitis, the joint capacity is decreased, injection is under pressure, and the recesses are small and partially obliterated. The biceps tendon sheath is poorly visualized or not seen at all.[12]

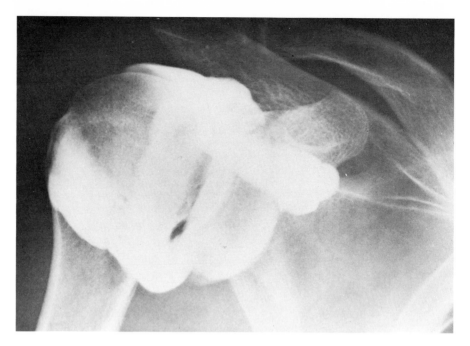

Fig. 16-18. Large medial convex pouch where capsule has been detached from glenoid labrum in patient with recurrent anterior dislocations of shoulder.

In recurrent anterior dislocations, the examiner sees a large medial pouch consisting of the continuous subscapularis and axillary pouches where the capsule has been detached from the glenoid (Fig. 16-18). The size of the pouch indicates the degree of capsular disruption and is best seen on internal rotation. The loss of the triangular appearance of the glenoid labrum on the axillary view, described by Reeves[19], has not been of value in our experience. Recently Preston and Jackson[17] have used double-contrast shoulder arthrography to demonstrate the thickness of the rotator cuff as well as the integrity of the glenoid labrum.

ANKLE

Ankle arthrography is of value in the precise diagnosis of ligamentous injury.[2] It has also been used in the diagnosis of adhesive capsulitis[7] and loose bodies.[9]

Method

The technique of ankle arthrography varies with the indication. In patients with acute ankle injuries, I inject 5 to 8 ml of a mixture of Renografin 60% and 1% procaine. In patients with a suspected loose body or osteochondritis dissecans, 1 to 2 ml of Renografin 60% and sufficient room air to distend the ankle joint are used. In acute ankle injuries, the injection is performed on the medial aspect of the joint for lateral symptomatology and vice versa. I use an anteroposterior approach under fluoroscopic control.

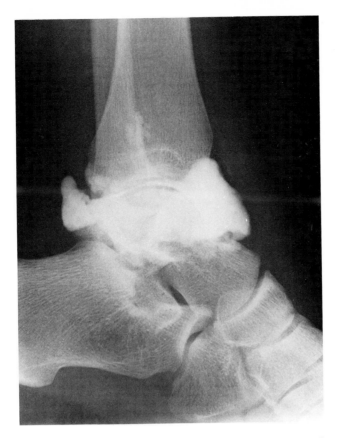

Fig. 16-19. Normal lateral view of ankle arthrogram, demonstrating anterior and posterior recesses.

Normal arthrogram

The normal ankle arthrogram demonstrates small anterior and posterior recesses (Fig. 16-19) and medial and lateral pouches. The flexor longus and flexor hallucis tendon sheaths may communicate with the ankle joint as may the posterior subtalar joint.[2,9] The contrast material outlines the smooth, regular articular cartilage over the talar dome and a syndesmotic recess between the tibia and fibula.

Abnormal arthrogram

The presence of extraarticular contrast media, except in the medial tendons or along the injection site, is abnormal.

With tears of the anterior talofibular ligament contrast material is seen lateral to the fibula and extending anterosuperiorly to the joint capsule[4] (Fig. 16-20). When the calcaneofibular ligament is torn, there is filling of the peroneal tendon sheaths[2,6] (Fig. 16-21). The strongest lateral ligament is the posterior talofibular ligament, which is

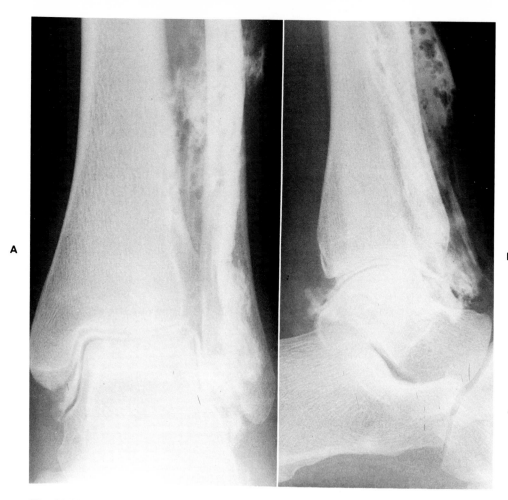

Fig. 16-20. A, Anteroposterior view of ankle arthrogram, demonstrating extravasated contrast media overlying tibia. **B,** Lateral view, showing that extravasation is anterior, which indicates a tear of anterior talofibia ligament.

rarely torn without associated tears of the other lateral ligaments. When the distal tibiofibular ligament is torn, the contrast will extend into the syndesmotic recess.[8] Combined tears are frequent and the roentgenographic findings usually additive. Staples[23] stated that patients with combined anterior tibiofibular and calcaneofibular ligament tears may show leakage anteriorly only. He felt that the large amount of leakage and lack of resistance of the injection were significant indications of double-ligament injury in these cases.

With tears of the strong deltoid ligaments, medial extravasation will occur.

In patients with adhesive capsulitis the joint capacity will be decreased and the recesses small to obliterated. Only a small amount of contrast material can be injected.[7]

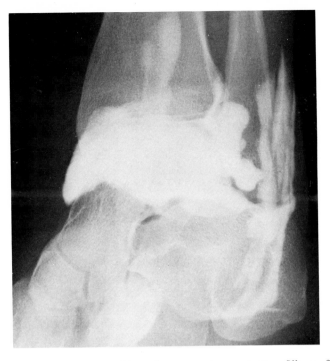

Fig. 16-21. Oblique view during ankle arthrogram, demonstrating filling of flexor tendon sheaths medially and peroneal tendon sheaths laterally. Filling of flexor tendons is a normal variation, but filling of peroneal tendons indicates a tear of calcaneofibular ligament.

I have used double-contrast arthrography, using 1 to 2 ml Renografin 60% and 3 to 6 cc of room air in four cases of osteochondritis dissecans of the talus to look for loose bodies and to evaluate the status of the articular cartilage. The articular cartilage was normal in all four cases, and no loose bodies were found. In one case the periarticular lymphatics were filled. This is thought to be a nonspecific sign of inflammation.

HIP

Arthrography of the hip has been used to demonstrate the capsular, muscular, ligamentous, and cartilaginous components of the hip joint, particularly in children.[15,16] The status of the overlying articular cartilage may be demonstrated in patients with osteoarthritis[24] and aseptic necrosis. Tanaka and associates[24] found arthrography to be a helpful adjunct in determining the method of treatment in selected patients with osteoarthritis. Hip arthrography has also been used following prosthetic hip surgery to demonstrate loosening of the prosthesis.[3,14,22]

Method

The hip is prepared with povidone-iodine (Betadine) in an aseptic manner. A keyhole drape is placed over the hip joint, and a sterile radiopaque grid is then

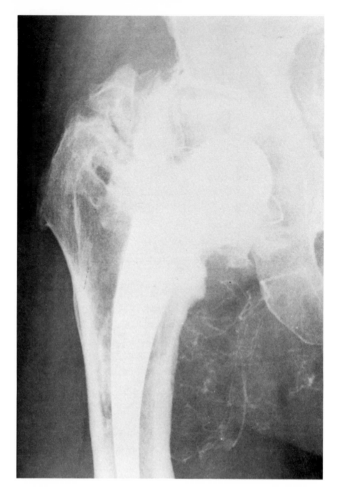

Fig. 16-22. Hip arthrogram in patient with Charnley-Mueller prosthesis. Contrast material is seen parallel to lateral femoral stem at bone-cement interface, indicating loosening of prosthesis. There is extensive filling of lymphatics medially, indicating inflammation. Slight periosteal changes are evident along femoral shaft secondary to low-grade osteomyelitis.

placed over the hip. The skin and subcutaneous tissue are anesthetized with 1% procaine and a 21-gauge spinal needle is directed to the superolateral aspect of the femoral neck or the comparable area of the metallic prosthesis. Aspiration of the joint or pseudojoint is attempted. If the patient has a prosthesis, and no fluid is obtained, then irrigation of the joint with 2 to 3 ml of sterile saline followed by aspiration is done. When evaluating a prosthesis, I inject up to 15 ml of 30% Renografin (Renografin 60% and 1% procaine in equal parts) and obtain films with and without traction in the anteroposterior projection. In children Ozonoff[15,16] advocates 1.5 to 5 ml of Renografin-60, depending upon the joint capacity. He[15,16] obtains films in neutral rotation, frog-leg lateral, abduction with internal rotation, adduction with neutral rotation, 25° abduction, 25° flexion, and occasionally he uses a true lateral with a horizontal beam or stereoscopic exposures.

Abnormal arthrogram

Hip arthrography in children helps differentiate congenital subluxations from dislocations. Subluxations demonstrate the underformed cartilaginous femoral head inferior to the glenoid labrum. The capsule is large, and there is mobility with stress. In dislocations the cartilaginous head is flat, and the acetabulum is small with synechiae. The limbus is inferior to the femoral head, the round ligament is hypertrophied, and the isthmus is contracted.[15]

The cartilaginous outline can be demonstrated in aseptic necrosis and after femoral head and neck fractures. Early aseptic necrosis usually demonstrates a normal or minimally flattened femoral head, but in late cases the contour of the cartilage may not follow the bony outline.

In our institution, which has essentially no pediatric inpatients, the most common indication for hip arthrography is pain after prosthetic hip replacement. The arthrogram is of value in the diagnosis of loosening and infection. The hip is aspirated, and if no fluid is obtained the joint is irrigated with sterile saline and then aspirated and sent for culture. The pseudojoint is injected with 8 to 15 ml of 30% Renografin, and films are taken in the anteroposterior projection with traction. Contrast media extending along the bone-cement interface indicates loosening (Fig. 16-22). In patients with radiopaque cement, subtraction films are frequently necessary.[22] Cavities communicating with the joint usually indicate infection. Lymphatic filling is sometimes seen; this is an indirect sign of inflammation about the pseudojoint.[5]

Murray and Rodrigo[14] stated that arthrographic evidence of loosening was not confirmed surgically in 5 of 12 cases and was demonstrated in more than one fifth of asymptomatic hips.

WRIST

Arthrography of the wrist has been used to evaluate soft tissue injury caused by trauma and the early soft tissue changes preceding the osseous abnormalities in the arthridities.[20] Wrist arthrography has also been used in the evaluation of ganglions; two thirds of the ganglions studied communicated with the wrist joint. Direct injection into the ganglion did not demonstrate the connections.[1]

Method

The injection of 2 ml of Renografin 60% is made into the radiocarpal joint under aseptic conditions. This outlines the radiocarpal joint, but communications with the midcarpal and distal radioulnar joint are not infrequent. The synovium is smooth, and a prestyloid recess and volar excrescences are common.

I believe that although arthrography of the wrist may graphically demonstrate soft tissue abnormalities, it is rarely of diagnostic value. The compartmental analysis, advocated by Resnick,[20] is extremely helpful, but arthrography is not usually necessary for its demonstration. The filling of periarticular lymphatics and synovial corrugations are found in inflammatory arthritides and are not specific. Trentham and associates[25] found frequent intercarpal communications between the joint compartments and tendon sheaths in random volunteers. This was at variance with the findings of Ranawat and associates,[18] but they worked with cadavers.

ELBOW

Elbow arthrography is occasionally used to demonstrate capsular abnormalities, cartilaginous defects, or the identification of nonopaque loose bodies. Three to 4 ml of Renografin 30% is injected into the olecranon fossa, outlining the joint capsule, articular cartilage, and annular ligament of the radius.

SUBTALAR JOINT

Resnick[21] has described the arthrographic anatomy of the talocalcaneal articulations. Twenty percent of his cases showed communication with the ankle joint. Kaye and associates[10] have used subtalar arthrography in the evaluation of tarsal coalition and have demonstrated nonfilling of the sustentacular talocalcaneal joint with a cartilaginous bar.

MISCELLANEOUS

Weston of New Zealand has written and described the arthrographic anatomy of the acromioclavicular,[26] pisi-cuneiform,[33] metacarpophalangeal, interphalangeal,[32] and midtarsal joints.[31] He has also injected many normal bursae and described their roentgenographic appearances.[27-30] The interested reader should refer to his articles for a detailed description.

References

1. Andren, L., and Eiken, O.: Arthrographic studies of wrist ganglions, J. Bone Joint Surg. [Am.] **53**:299-302, 1971.
2. Brostrom, L., Liljedahl, S. O., and Lindvall, N.: Sprained ankles. II. Arthrographic diagnosis of recent ligament ruptures, Acta Chir. Scand. **129**:485-499, 1965.
3. Brown, C. S., and Knickerbocker, W. J.: Radiologic studies in the investigation of the causes of total hip replacement failures, J. Can. Assoc. Radiol. **24**:245-253, 1973.
4. Callaghan, J. E., Percy, E. C., and Hill, R. O.: The ankle arthrogram, J. Can. Assoc. Radiol. **21**:74-84, June 1970.
5. Coren, G. S., Curtis, J., and Dalinka, M. K.: Lymphatic visualization during hip arthrography, Radiology **115**:621-623, 1975.
6. Fordyce, A. J. W., and Horn, C. V.: Arthrography in recent injuries of the ligaments of the ankle, J. Bone Joint Surg. [Br.] **54**:116-121, 1972.
7. Goldman, A. B., Katz, M. C., and Freiberger, R. H.: Posttraumatic adhesive capsulitis of the ankle: arthrographic diagnosis, Am. J. Roentgenol. Radium Ther. Nucl. Med. **127**:585-588, 1976.
8. Gordon, R. B.: Arthrography of the ankle joint. Experience in one hundred seven studies, J. Bone Joint Surg. [Am.] **52**:1623-1631, 1970.
9. Kaye, J. J.: Ankle arthrography, Bone and Joint Radiology Course, Harvard Medical School, October 25-27, 1976.

10. Kaye, J. J., Ghelman, B., and Schneider, R.: Talocalcaneonavicular joint arthrography for sustentacular-talar tarsal coalitions, Radiology **115**:730-731, 1975.
11. Kernwein, G. A.: Roentgenographic diagnosis of shoulder dysfunction, J.A.M.A. **194**:179-183, 1965.
12. Killoran, P. J., Marcove, R. C., and Freiberger, R. H.: Shoulder arthrography, Am. J. Roentgenol. Radium Ther. Nucl. Med. **103**:658-668, 1968.
13. Kummel, B. M.: Arthrography in anterior capsular derangements of the shoulder, Clin. Orthop. **83**:170-176, 1972.
14. Murray, W. R., and Rodrigo, J. J.: Arthrography for the assessment of pain after total hip replacement, J. Bone Joint Surg. [Am.] **57**:1060-1065, 1975.
15. Ozonoff, M. B.: Hip arthrography in children, Bone and Joint Radiology Course, Harvard Medical School, October 25-27, 1976.
16. Ozonoff, M. B.: Controlled arthrography of the hip: a technic of fluoroscopic monitoring and recording, Clin. Orthop. **93**:260-264, 1973.
17. Preston, B. J., and Jackson, J. P.: Investigation of shoulder disability by arthrography, Clin. Radiol. **28**:259-266, 1977.
18. Ranawat, C. S., Harrison, M. O., and Jordan, L. R.: Arthrography of the wrist joint, Clin. Orthop. **83**:6-12, 1972.
19. Reeves, B.: Arthrography of the shoulder, J. Bone Joint Surg. [Br.] **48**:424-435, 1966.
20. Resnick, D.: Arthritic disorders of the adult radiocarpal joint: anatomic considerations and an evaluation of fifty consecutive abnormal cases, J. Can. Assoc. Radiol. **26**:104-111, 1975.
21. Resnick, D.: Radiology of the talocalcaneal articulations, Radiology **111**:581-586, 1974.
22. Salvati, E. A., Freiberger, R. H., and Wilson, P. D.: Arthrography for complications of total hip replacement, J. Bone Joint Surg. [Am.] **53**:701-709, 1971.
23. Staples, O. S.: Ruptures of the fibular collateral ligaments of the ankle. Result study of immediate surgical treatment, J. Bone Joint Surg. [Am.] **57**:101-107, 1975.
24. Tanaka, S., Ito, T., and Yamamoto, K.: Arthrography in osteoarthritis of the hip, Am. J. Roentgenol. Radium Ther. Nucl. Med. **124**:91-95, 1975.
25. Trentham, D. E., Hamm, R. L., and Masi, A. T.: Wrist arthrography: review and comparison of normals, rheumatoid arthritis and gout patients, Semin. Arthritis Rheum. **5**:105-120, 1975.
26. Weston, W. J.: Arthrography of the acromio-clavicular joint, Aust. Radiol. **18**:213-214, 1974.
27. Weston, W. J.: The deep infrapatellar bursa, Aust. Radiol. **17**:212-218, 1973.
28. Weston, W. J.: The bursa deep to tendo achillis, Aust. Radiol. **14**:327-331, 1970.
29. Weston, W. J.: The bursae deep to gluteus medius and minimus, Aust. Radiol. **14**:325-326, 1970.
30. Weston, W. J.: The olecranon bursa, Aust. Radiol. **14**:323-324, 1970.
31. Weston, W. J.: Positive contrast arthrography of the normal mid-tarsal joints, Aust. Radiol. **13**:365-367, 1969.
32. Weston, W. J.: The normal arthrograms of the metacarpo-phalangeal, metatarso-phalangeal and inter-phalangeal joints, Aust. Radiol. **13**:211-218, 1969.
33. Weston, W. J., and Kelsey, C. K.: Functional anatomy of the pisi-cuneiform joint, Br. J. Radiol. **46**:692-694, 1973.

17. Role of the assistant in arthroscopy

Ruth L. Becker*
Lanny L. Johnson

Arthroscopy is no less than a surgical procedure. To be performed correctly, with satisfactory results, the same preparation, organization, and execution that one would consider for open surgery should be a part of every arthroscopy.

The arthroscopist, no matter how skilled, should find that a well-coordinated and disciplined operating room staff, including a skilled assistant, will facilitate his ability to perform arthroscopy. The capacity to perform arthroscopy with the patient under local anesthesia is related to the skill and speed of the arthroscopist. Coordinated effort on the part of the assistant is absolutely essential for this to be accomplished with minimal discomfort to the patient. And last but not least it ought to make the arthroscopist's life more pleasant to receive excellent help.

For purposes of this discussion the details for performing arthroscopy with the patient under local anesthesia will be emphasized in that there are less details and more time available than when arthroscopy is performed with the patient under general anesthesia.

The individuals involved in arthroscopy in addition to the physician arthroscopist are the assistant and the circulating nurse. Arthroscopic technique has been covered in Chapter 6. Our own preference has been documented in other publications.[1] Therefore we will not emphasize the role of the arthroscopist. The following discussion describes our routine, which may be modified to suit individual needs.

ARTHROSCOPIC ASSISTANT

After a surgical scrub, the assistant enters the operating room and prepares the back table. We should emphasize that no matter which method one uses it is important to do each step in the same manner each time. Each instrument ought to be placed in the same position on the table in the room, so as to provide an inherent check of any omissions in instrumentation.

The back table has been opened by the circulating nurse. In the right-hand lower corner against the table is an apron, a suction tube, gloves, a gown, and a towel (Fig. 17-1). The right upper corner has the paper sheets and the cloth drapes, plus towels. In the central area above, there is the dressing, and a no. 18, 38 mm (1½ inch), needle. In the center is the stockinette wrap for the leg, a K-52 catheter, and a no.

---

*Licensed Practical Nurse, East Lansing, Mich.

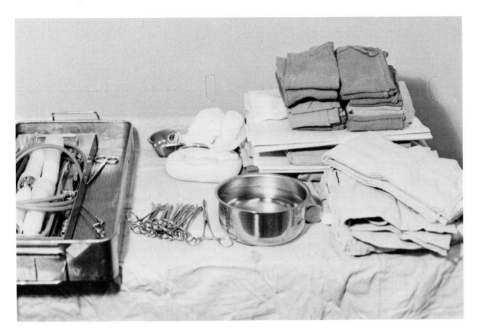

Fig. 17-1. Back table.

21, 38 mm (1½ inch) needle. In the lower portion of the center is a basin for saline. To the right of that are the 12 ml syringe for local anesthetic and the 60 ml syringe for saline. To the left are towel clips. Sponge sticks for skin preparation are in front.

The entire left-hand side of the table remains free for the instrument tray that will be delivered from the autoclave by the circulating nurse.

After the back table is set up, attention is turned to the Mayo stand. The arthroscope is removed from Cidex, rinsed with saline, and dried (Fig. 17-2). The Mayo stand is set up the same way each time (Fig. 17-3) with the arthroscope suspended on two sterile towels in the most superior corner away from the patient. The towel where the ocular rests is considered contaminated. Every attempt is made to avoid touching that area other than with the ocular. In the superior corner adjacent to the patient rests the saline in a bowl. At the inferior corner away from the patient is the syringe with lidocaine (Xylocaine) and sponge used to protect the gloved finger during palpation. The inferior pole adjacent to the patient is the cannula; the sharp and blunt trocar, the K-52 catheter, and the syringe that holds the saline are also shown in Fig. 17-3.

Paper barrier draping is used because it avoids soaking of the patient and provides a barrier to any discomfort the patient might have, especially if he is under local anesthesia. It also provides a barrier against bacteria. The assistant takes his position at the superior aspect lateral to the patient. The foot of the table is dropped. During most of the examination the assistant stabilizes the thigh, which wants to naturally roll into external rotation. The assistant holds the thigh with his arm or elbow. During inspection of the medial side, he provides a fulcrum against the distal femur

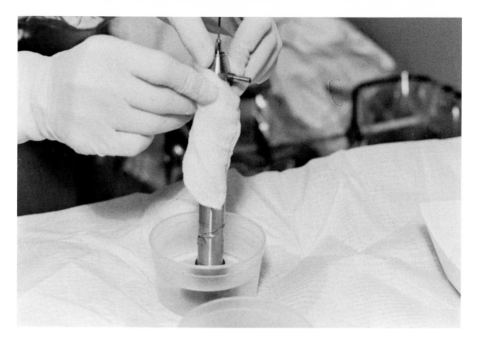

Fig. 17-2. Assistant rinsing arthroscope.

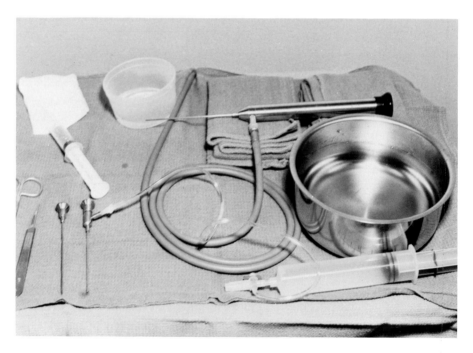

Fig. 17-3. Mayo stand.

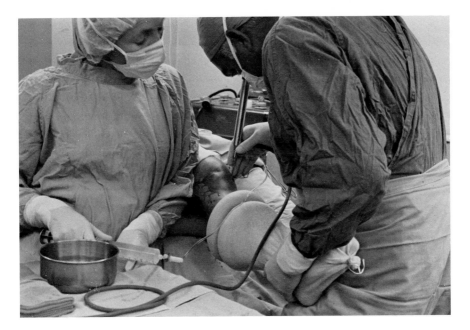

Fig. 17-4. Fulcrum provided by assistant's elbow.

(Fig. 17-4), and during inspection of the lateral compartment he provides a fulcrum with his hand or wrist or both against the medial distal femur (Fig. 17-5).

During the procedure, the assistant hands the local anesthetic in the syringe, the knife handle with the no. 11 blade, and the cannula with the sharp and then the blunt trocar. This is performed in a manner similar to handing surgical instruments. It allows the arthroscopist to keep his eye on the topographic landmarks.

The joint is distended or vacuumed or both throughout the procedure, preferably without moving from the compartment where the vacuuming has been carried out.

The assistant may force a stream of saline from the syringe via the K-52 catheter and about the arthroscope through the cannula; it will either cleanse proteinaceous material at the end of the arthroscope or cleanse the compartment immediately in front of the viewing ocular (Fig. 17-6).

This participation requires a disciplined assistant. With no opportunity for visualization unless the procedure is being documented on television, his reward has to be in the benefit to the patient and the service to the arthroscopist in facilitating the procedure.

The role of the assistant becomes even more important and necessary during operative arthroscopy. The assistant may hold the television camera that is documenting the intraarticular surgery (Fig. 17-7) or may provide manipulation of the extremity necessary for exposure for condylar or meniscal cutting.

If the inflow and outflow system is utilized, then the assistant may have to regulate the flow.

At the close of the procedure, the assistant again follows a routine. The first duty

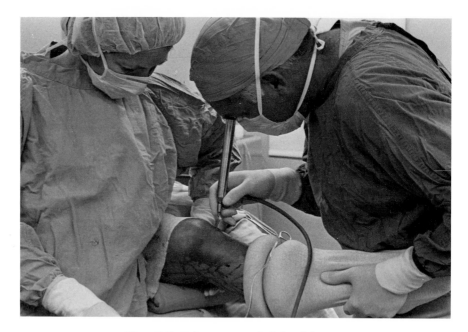

Fig. 17-5. Fulcrum to medial distal femur.

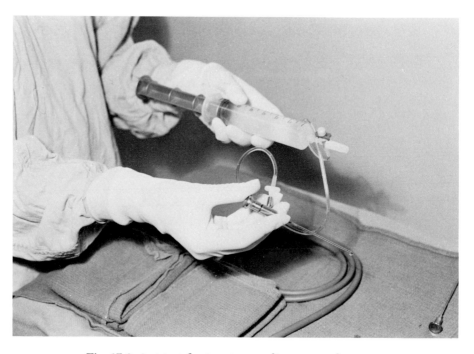

Fig. 17-6. Assistant forcing stream adjacent to arthroscope.

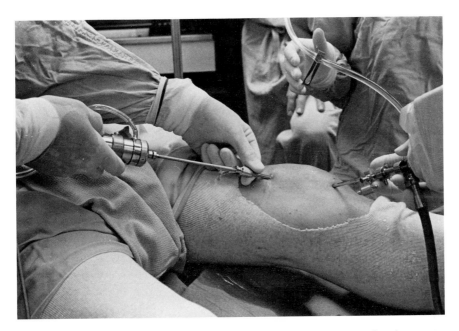

Fig. 17-7. Assistant holding television on arthroscope (right) as motorized arthroscopic tool is placed in cannula by surgeon.

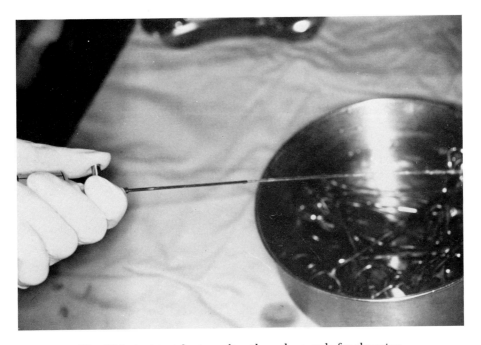

Fig. 17-8. Assistant forcing saline through cannula for cleansing.

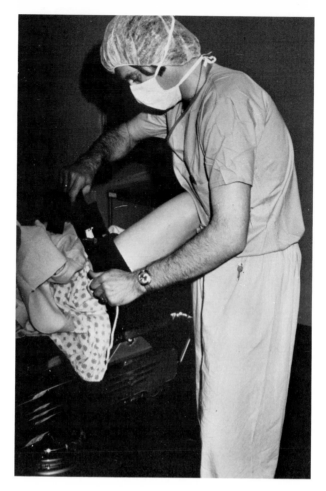

Fig. 17-9. Circulating nurse placing tourniquet.

is to cleanse the arthroscope with saline, dry it, and place it in the Cidex solution. Then the cannula is cleaned by forcing saline through it (Fig. 17-8). The drapes are removed and placed in the appropriate receptacle. The cable is cleansed with saline and dried. The equipment is placed in the instrument tray for steam autoclaving. The arthroscopes are placed in the Cidex disinfectant solution.

CIRCULATING NURSE

The circulating nurse tests and prepares the suction apparatus. He tests and prepares the pneumatic tourniquet (Fig. 17-9). The autoclavable instruments are delivered to the back table (Fig. 17-10). He assists the patient to the operating table and reassures him.

It is important that he establish rapport with the patient, especially when the arthroscopy is done with the patient under local anesthesia. He may engage in a comforting conversation to reduce any anxiety the patient may experience.

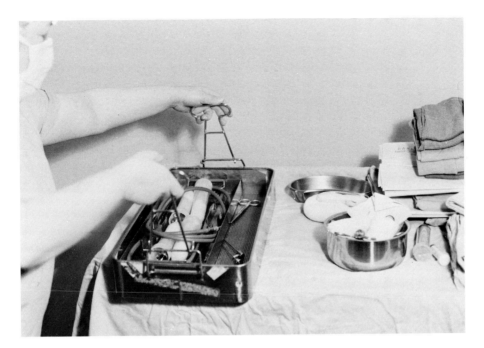

Fig. 17-10. Autoclavable instruments delivered to back table.

When inflow and outflow drainage of saline is utilized for therapeutic arthroscopy, the circulating nurse also would place and replace the saline bags and maintain the gravity flow system.

At the close of the procedure, he manages the necessary administrative paper work, assists in removing the drapes from the table, and secures the dressing on the patient's extremity. He removes the drainage tubes and suction device and assists the patient to the recovery room.

The circulating nurse then is prepared to assist in subsequent cases. When this type of organization and coordination is adhered to, it is possible to perform diagnostic arthroscopy on an outpatient basis and to have a turnaround time of 30 minutes. This improves the physician's efficiency, and the organization promotes confidence in the patient and pride within the operating personnel.

Handling and storage of the arthroscopes and all the equipment is preferably performed by one individual. When this is adhered to, the breakage or loss of this expensive equipment is minimized. In fact our team has not experienced any arthroscopic loss or breakage in more than 2,000 cases over 5 years. We attribute this to the organization and the compulsiveness of the arthroscopist, the assistant, and the operating room personnel.

Reference

1. Johnson, L. L.: Comprehensive arthroscopic examination of the knee, St. Louis, 1977, The C. V. Mosby Co.

18. Photography in arthroscopy

John B. McGinty

As soon as a surgeon has mastered the technique of arthroscopy and established his own routine, and as soon as he has become familiar with the pathologic lesions seen with the arthroscope, he will be eager to make a permanent record of these visual impressions. A written or oral report of visual observations becomes very hazy as time passes and is a poor substitute for photographic documentation. Clinical documentation and medical education are the main reasons why a photographic record is necessary.

Clinical documentation must be extremely accurate, as the physician refers to his record in the continuing management of his patient. It is the only way to accurately recall pertinent findings as time passes and the pathogenesis of disease continues or new factors occur. For example, if the surgeon sees a small meniscus tear and concludes that it is not responsible for the presenting symptoms, he may elect not to remove the damaged meniscus. If, at a later time, symptoms change or a new injury occurs, the only basis for comparison is a good photographic record.

Documentation of arthroscopic findings is extremely helpful if not essential in planning for subsequent surgery. Diagnostic arthroscopy frequently precedes definitive intraarticular surgery by weeks if not months. I frequently review my arthroscopic photographs on the evening before a scheduled surgical procedure. There is no better way to plan and execute surgical approaches than to know precisely what the surgical lesion is and where it is located. When a physician is consulting on a clinical problem or seeking a consultation, the photographic record is far superior to the written word.

In our society the practice of orthopedic surgery frequently brings the surgeon into the medicolegal arena or the often compromising field of compensation liability. Decisions in this area, which may be economically disastrous to the individual or extremely expensive to the society, are usually made by nonphysicians: individuals, juries, and boards who have little familiarity with pathologic entities and medical terminology. When the physician is called to testify in a courtroom as an expert witness or to appear before a workmen's compensation board, no oral description can adequately substitute for a well-exposed and well-presented photograph.

Most physicians who gain experience in the endoscopic world inside joints will want to share this expertise with their colleagues and students. It is impossible to present arthroscopic material, whether to small conferences or large audiences, without clear, well-exposed photographs. Educational credibility is far better established by concrete graphic evidence than by verbose descriptive narration. Finally in education in arthroscopy, I have found the television camera to be the most effective tool for one-on-one teaching of technique.

HISTORICAL BACKGROUND

The first significant development leading to endoscopic photography was in 1840 when Alfred Donné presented microscopic daguerreotypes, obtained by artificial light, to the French Academy in Paris. These were followed in 1845 by a microscopic atlas illustrated by Léon Foucault, a physicist, with copper engravings from daguerreotypes. One of the first textbooks in medical photography was published by Joseph Gerlach in 1863 and was titled *Photography as an Aid to Microscopic Research*. In 1882 Thomas R. French of New York developed an effective method of photographing the larynx and nasopharynx by indirect laryngoscopy.

The first successful photographic endoscope was developed by Max Nitze in 1882 (Fig. 18-1). He used a rotating disk containing a glass plate with sensitized areas, which could be selectively placed in front of the cystoscope by moving a prism while viewing through an offset eyepiece. Nitze produced some rather astonishing photographs in his *Cystophotographic Atlas* published in 1894.

Kenji Takagi, after developing the first arthroscope in Tokyo in 1918, proceeded to produce the first black and white photographs in 1932, followed by color photographs and moving pictures in 1936. Photography in arthroscopy was further refined with the development of the no. 21 arthroscope and its 35 mm camera system by Masaki Watanabe in 1957, thereby making easy photographic documentation available to anyone eager to learn the technique of arthroscopy (Fig. 18-2).

In the 1970s photography was further expanded by the introduction of closed-circuit television, first in black and white and shortly thereafter in color, when a camera of practical size was developed (Fig. 18-3). This advance permitted a photographic record to be made on videotape, which could later be edited to be used in conferences or with small audiences. The concurrent development of videobeam projectors permitted large audience visualization with 4 × 6 foot and larger screens (Fig. 18-4). As the electronics industry develops more innovations, such as the videodisc with its ability to store large quantities of photographic images with instant recall, it does not take a great deal of imagination to project the potential for understanding the long-term pathogenesis of many intraarticular problems by sequential photographic imagery in skillful hands.

OPTICAL PRINCIPLES

It is important to look at certain optical principles in order to appreciate the variables that are involved in the production of a satisfactory photograph with an arthroscope. These principles are discussed in Chapter 3.

The most important optical concept in determining the brightness of the image

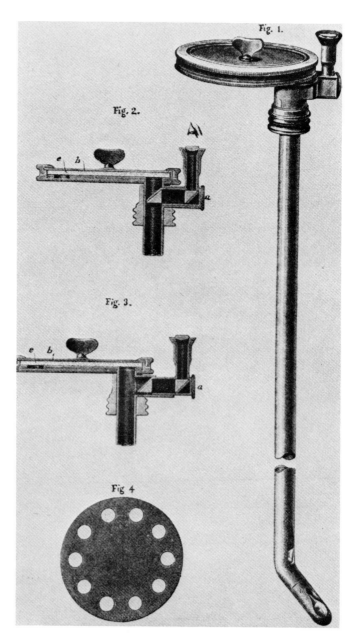

Fig. 18-1. Nitze's photographic cystoscopy (1894). *1*, Instrument as a whole. *2*, Cross-sectional view, showing optical arrangement for focusing instrument. *3*, Focusing apparatus shifted upward to permit photograph to be taken. *4*, Perforated disk of the camera. (From Ciba Found. Symp., vol. 4, nos. 5 and 6, p. 1351, August-September, 1942.)

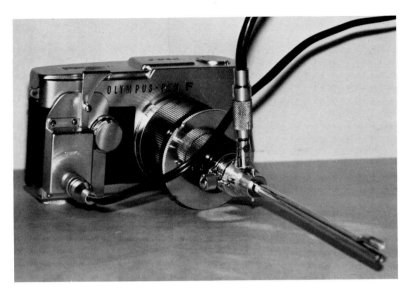

Fig. 18-2. Watanabe no. 21 arthroscope attached to Olympus half-frame 35 mm camera. Note cable running from shutter release to relay in transformer to double voltage and therefore brightness of light as shutter is tripped.

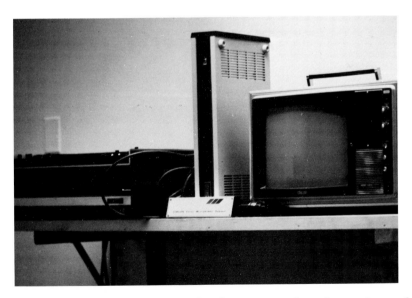

Fig. 18-3. Circon color television system with video tape recorder, color monitor, and small camera weighing only 20 ounces capable of direct connection to an endoscope.

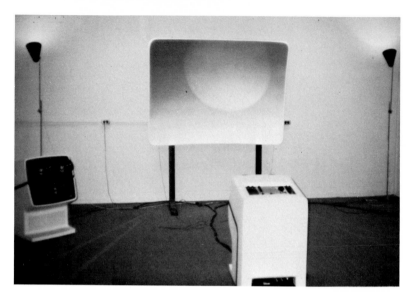

Fig. 18-4. Advent Video-Beam projector capable of projecting 4 × 6 foot image, adequate for audiences up to 200 people.

and consequently the exposure latitude of the photograph is the *exit pupil.* The brightness of the image to be photographed is determined at the exit pupil. The pupil of a camera lens system is usually located somewhere behind the front element of the lens in the general location of the iris diaphragm. In the ideal arthroscopic-photographic system the camera pupil and the exit pupil are in the same plane. This is rarely the case, the camera pupil usually being some distance behind the exit pupil of the arthroscope. The solution to this problem, which unresolved results in vignetting of the photographic image, is to leave the camera lens wide open and allow the ultimate diameter or f-stop to be controlled by the exit pupil of the arthroscope. For example, if the exit pupil is 2 mm, and the photographer is using a 50 mm lens, the f-stop will be

$$\text{f-stop} = \frac{\text{focal length of lens}}{\text{diameter of lens}} = \frac{50}{2} = 25$$

As any amateur photographer knows, f/25 is a very small aperture, with the disadvantage of severe limitation on the quantity of light reaching the film plane. However, this is compensated for by the nearness of the light source to the object to be photographed, for example, 1 candlepower at 1 inch equals 144 footcandles. Also the very small aperture has the advantage of a large depth of field, resulting in a fixed-focus system and thereby eliminating the necessity of focusing.

PHOTOGRAPHIC VARIABLES

There are essentially five variables to be considered in obtaining a sharp, well-exposed, final photographic image (Fig. 18-5). They are the light source, the re-

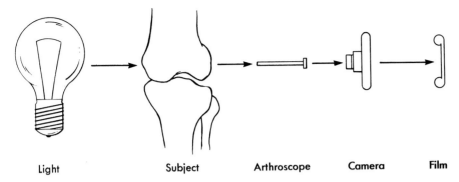

| Light | Subject | Arthroscope | Camera | Film |

Fig. 18-5. Variables in obtaining well-exposed photographic image.

flective properties of the subject, the endoscopic instrument, the camera and its lens, and the film. For the purposes of this discussion, we are referring to 35 mm still photography. The same principles apply to large format photography, Polaroid prints, or cinematography. Each of these variables will be considered independently; finally a workable system that is relatively inexpensive and can be reliably used by any experienced arthroscopist will be presented.

Light source

The Watanabe no. 21 system provides illumination with a tungsten lamp on the end of the instrument inside the joint. This lamp is powered by a transformer with a 16-V output for viewing. By means of a relay in the power source coupled to the camera shutter release the voltage is doubled to temporarily increase illumination when the shutter is tripped, without significantly decreasing the life of the lamp. However, the system requires a specially adapted Olympus half-frame camera, resulting in smaller though adequate images on the film.

The use of a bulb on the end of the arthroscope has been virtually completely replaced by fiber optic systems. There is a loss of light in the fiber optic bundles when the source is remote from the instrument. This loss represents 5% per foot of fiber optic cable and 30% at each connection. Therefore the connections must be kept to a minimum and the cable as short as practical to allow sufficient illumination for photography.

Most standard fiber optic viewing light sources use a 150 W tungsten lamp focused by a parabolic mirror and, in some instances, a condenser (Fig. 18-6). This lamp requires slow shutter speeds and therefore must be used with extreme care to prevent camera movement. It also has a lower color temperature, resulting in a warmer or more yellow quality to the final image.

There are high-intensity light sources available at considerable expense, which provide intense white light for fiber optic systems, light that has a color temperature of 5,000 kelvin or the equivalent of daylight (Fig. 18-7). Most of these sources make use of xenon lamps. These lamps have special filters to eliminate ultraviolet and in-

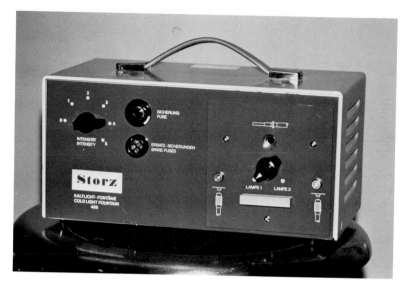

Fig. 18-6. Standard 150 W fiber optic light source.

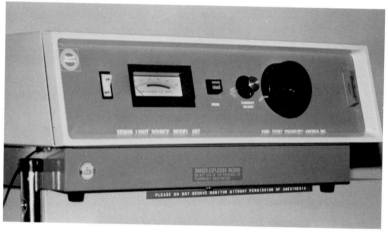

Fig. 18-7. High-intensity xenon light source capable of producing light at 5,000 kelvin.

frared radiation (thereby reducing heat) and must be specially housed, since some have been known to explode. These high-intensity sources are essential for cinematography and television through the arthroscope.

For excellent color photographs with superb color balance, fully predictable on every exposure, strobe lighting is available (Fig. 18-8). An electronic flash generator with a rheostat to vary intensity can be purchased at considerable expense. This is connected to a flashtube placed directly on the fiber optic outlet of the arthroscope

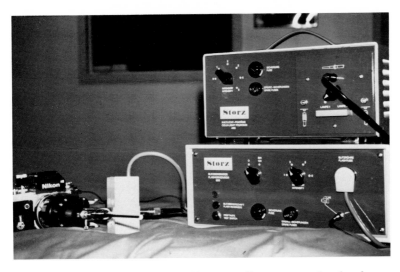

Fig. 18-8. Camera with strobe unit attached between fiber optic cord and arthroscope, standard light source for viewing, and strobe generator.

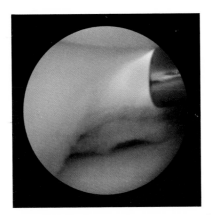

Fig. 18-9. Arthroscope probing undersurface of meniscus. Note different reflective properties of meniscus, articular cartilage, and synovium.

(to minimize fiber optic connections and therefore light loss). The generator is in turn connected to and synchronized with the camera shutter. The duration of the flash is 2 to 5 msec (0.002 to 0.005 second), fast enough to prevent any blurring from camera motion. I believe that this light source, combined with Kodachrome ASA 64 film, gives the best color 24 × 36 mm slides if cost is no object.

Subject

The reflective properties of the subject affect the amount of light ultimately reaching the film and therefore the exposure (Fig. 18-9). Articular cartilage is more reflective than meniscus, which is considerably more reflective than synovium. If a picture of synovium is metered for articular cartilage, it will be underexposed. This variable can be controlled by through-the-lens metering, averaging the exposure, or by bracketing the exposure (taking several exposures at different shutter speeds).

Arthroscope

The significant variable of the arthroscope is its diameter. I have shown that the f-stop is inversely proportional to the diameter of the arthroscope; or, to put it in another way, the diameter of the exit pupil is directly proportional to the diameter of the arthroscope. Therefore with smaller arthroscopes either brighter light sources or longer shutter speeds must be used.

Camera

Almost any 35 mm single lens reflex camera can be adapted to the arthroscope. The camera must be single lens reflex so that the image viewed is the image photographed. Some manufacturers provide cameras specifically adapted to their systems, usually at greater expense. Some of the cameras are adapted without lenses, using the optics of the telescope to focus the image; some use simple supplementary lenses. Some use motor-driven film transports so that the photographer can concentrate on the subject and not even have to advance the film. However, any 35 mm camera can be used. The manufacturers of arthroscopes will provide an adapter to couple the lens of any standard 35 mm camera rigidly to the arthroscope (Fig. 18-10). The coupling must be rigid so that the instrument can be manipulated, using the camera as a handle. If the photographer is going to use the viewing light source, it is advisable to use through-the-lens metering to get proper exposures. When the telescope is coupled to the camera, a circular field is seen in the viewfinder, and the edges of the rectangular field in the viewfinder are black, usually blacking out the meter scale.

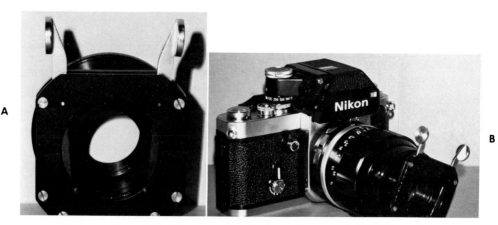

Fig. 18-10. A, Adapter obtainable from endoscope manufacturers to couple arthroscope to 35 mm camera. **B,** Adapter in place in 35 mm camera ready to receive arthroscope.

Certain cameras (e.g., Nikon and Contarex) obviate this problem with a small window that illuminates the meter scale independently of the lens.

Film

For color slides color reversal film is essential. With strobe or high-intensity light sources, Kodachrome ASA 25 or Kodachrome ASA 64 is recommended because of the excellent color balance. However, if the surgeon is developing a system based on ordinary fiber optic viewing light sources (tungsten lamp), high-speed film is essential. Super Ektachrome daylight film (ASA 160) will give color pictures balanced slightly to the warm side with emphasis on browns and yellows. This film can be pushed in developing to ASA 400. Super Ektachrome tungsten film (ASA 125) will give color pictures balanced slightly to the cool side with emphasis on greens and blues. This film can be pushed in developing to ASA 320. With this system shutter speeds are necessarily slow (1/4 to 1/15 second) but not impossible. By practice, bracing the camera against the forehead, and multiple exposures the arthroscopist can obtain perfectly adequate pictures.

SUMMARY

Once the arthroscopist has chosen a light source, this variable is fixed; the arthroscope fixes the f-stop; focusing is unnecessary because of the extreme depth of field. The only remaining variables are the shutter speed and the reflective properties of the subject. Therefore the only variable controlled by the photographer is the shutter speed, and this can be determined by through-the-lens metering or by bracketing exposures. I recommend the following system (Figs. 18-11 to 18-13):

Fiber optic viewing light source
Large-diameter arthroscope
35 mm single lens reflex camera (preferably with through-the-lens metering)
Super Ektachrome daylight film (shot at ASA 400)

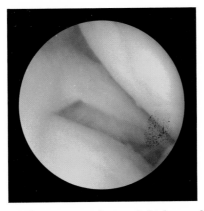

Fig. 18-11. Regenerated medial meniscus taken with high-speed Ektachrome daylight film ASA 160 and exposed and processed at ASA 400.

Fig. 18-12 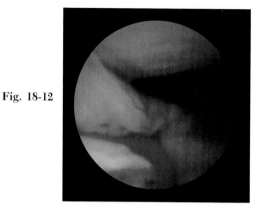 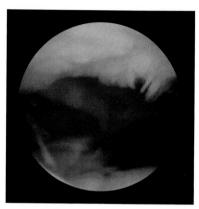 Fig. 18-1

Fig. 18-12. Bucket-handle tear of medial meniscus, taken with strobe lighting on Kodachrome 64.

Fig. 18-13. Chondromalacia patellae, taken with strobe lighting on Kodachrome 64.

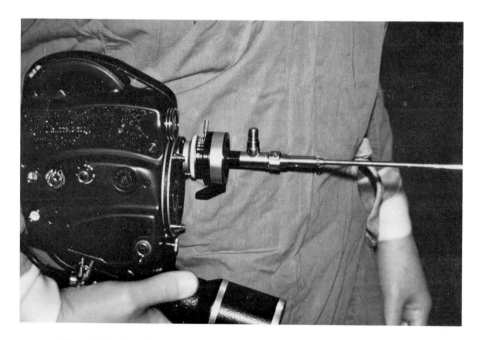

Fig. 18-14. Beaulieu 16 mm movie camera with arthroscope attached.

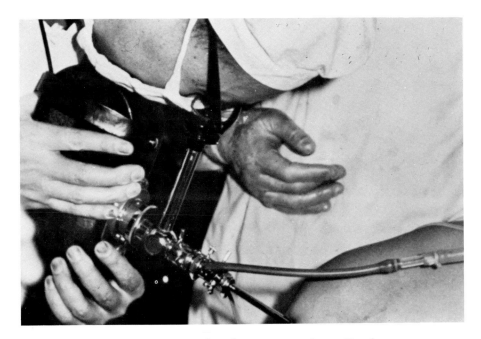

Fig. 18-15. Dr. M. Watanabe taking movies with no. 21 arthroscope.

CINEMATOGRAPHY

The choice of making movies with an arthroscope varies with the purpose of making the movies. If the purpose is purely documentation, super-8 format is adequate. However, if large audience projection is anticipated, 16 mm format is essential. Most projection facilities in lecture halls provide 16 mm projectors but not super-8. Detail at a distance in super-8 is frequently inadequate. An optical sound track can be easily added to 16 mm film.

The light source must be high intensity and balanced for 5,000 kelvin color temperature. The camera must have through-the-lens viewing and metering. The 16 mm Beaulieu has proven to be an excellent camera for this purpose (Figs. 18-14 and 18-15). Although somewhat heavy, it can be handled quite skillfully with practice.

TELEVISION

I am of the opinion that television far outperforms movies as a means of complete documentation. Circon of Santa Barbara, California has developed a microvideo camera with a 1-inch vidicon tube that weighs only 20 ounces. This camera can be connected to the arthroscope, either directly or with a beam splitter, and then attached by a 20-foot cable to the amplification circuits, which in turn, are connected to a videotape recorder and monitor (Fig. 18-16). Therefore by pushing a foot switch the arthroscopist can record any image he desires at any time. The tape can be stored as a record or edited into presentable form. Television also provides a unique method of one-on-one teaching. At the conclusion of the examination, the arthroscopist can

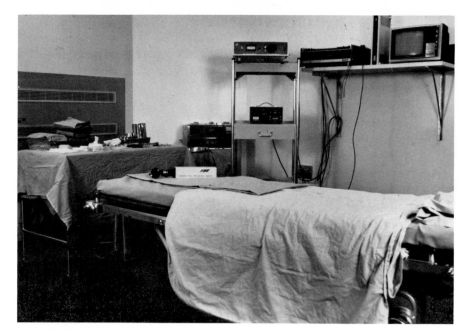

Fig. 18-16. Operating room with television system ready to function. Note size of camera on operating table.

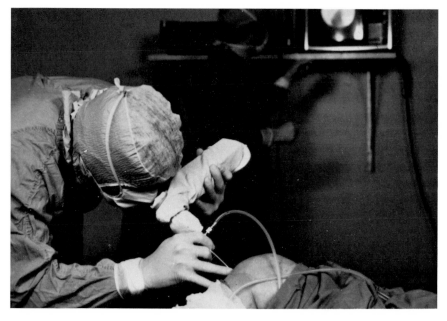

Fig. 18-17. Resident doing arthroscopy with television camera attached to arthroscope through beam splitter. Surgeon is at monitor, directing resident.

give the arthroscope with the camera attached by a beam splitter to his student. With the beam splitter (15% of the light going to the eye of the examiner and 85% going to the camera) the student can directly perform the examination while the arthroscopist directs him from the remote location of the monitor (Fig. 18-17). There is no better way to learn a psychomotor skill such as arthroscopy than to be able to do it with your own hands, while being directed from another location.

SUMMARY

In summary some methods and techniques of photography as applied to arthroscopy have been outlined. As experience is gained the arthroscopist-photographer will develop many more methods and techniques, some of which will represent improvements. However, he will also be engaged in the communication of observations and ideas, the only way that this fascinating field will continue to grow.

Suggested readings

Berci, G.: Endoscopy, New York, 1975, Appleton-Century-Crofts, pp. 242-279.
Ciba Symposia: Medicine and early photography, vol. 4, nos. 5 and 6, August-September, 1942.
McGinty, J. B.: Closed circuit television in arthroscopy, Rheumatology 33:45-50, 1976.
Prescott, R.: Optical principles of endoscopy, J. Med. Primatol. 5:133-147, 1976.
Time-Life Books: Life library of photography, New York, 1971, Time Inc.

19. Diagnostic aids in arthroscopy

Robert C. Bechtol

In the overall attempt to solve clinical problems relating to the knee, arthroscopy itself should be thought of as a diagnostic aid. It is used after the more basic diagnostic measures, including a complete history of the problem, careful clinical examination, and roentgenographic studies of the knee have been used judiciously and have been found wanting.

From the time the patient is brought into the operating room for arthroscopy, through the actual arthroscopy procedure, and into the follow-up period, there are a number of factors that can aid in arriving at, adding to, or refining a diagnosis. The present discussion of these aids will necessarily overlap some areas of technique. Some of these techniques can be easily overlooked because they only indirectly aid in diagnosis, but careful attention to detail will make arthroscopy the valuable diagnostic procedure it should be.

OPERATING ROOM ENVIRONMENT

The first consideration is the operating room environment, which should be conducive to thoughtful observation on the part of the arthroscopist. This cannot be the case when the arthroscopist is being urged to finish quickly in order that the room can be made ready for the next operation, or when the anesthesiologist is trying to get away to another hospital. Under these circumstances, the arthroscopic examination may well be sketchy. An unrushed examination is much more apt to be a thorough one. Ample time, allowing for the occasional delay, should be scheduled for each arthroscopic examination. Most often it is the overly optimistic arthroscopist who repeatedly schedules too short an operating time for himself, thereby destroying the operating room schedule and engendering ill will on the part of the nurses and his colleagues. A serious attempt to avoid this state of affairs should be made.

Operating room personnel who are well versed in the details of arthroscopic examination are invaluable. During the procedure there is no substitute for an experienced assistant who can keep track of and check all instruments and equipment, thereby freeing the arthroscopist for concentration on diagnostic matters.

INSTRUMENTS AND EQUIPMENT

Trouble-free equipment is essential. The arthroscopist must be able to concentrate on the creative solving of diagnostic problems at hand—not on maintenance of equipment. This means that all instruments should be checked before use. All electrical connections in instruments using tungsten bulbs should be working properly. Light generators for glass fiber light cables should be tested, and spare bulbs must be available. The cables should have the proper connectors for the light generator and the arthroscope. When other glass fiber light cables are being used for various endoscopy instruments, the wrong cables have been known to be offered to the arthroscopist during the procedure. The arthroscope itself should be checked for optical and mechanical function. Instruments used with the arthroscope, such as scissors, grasping forceps, and basket punches, should be checked for bent parts, missing parts, and especially for loose parts. The small hinge pins of these instruments have been known to fall out while in use.

It is advisable to have extra instruments and equipment available. Extra light bulbs, light cords or cables, and arthroscopes are the insurance that a given arthroscopy procedure, once begun, can be successfully completed.

Accessory equipment such as cameras (including closed circuit television cameras) should be tested and set properly before arthroscopy to avoid delays when documentation is desirable or necessary. Cameras should be checked to make sure the proper lens is being used, and the correct film has been loaded. Video tape recorders should be checked out to make sure the equipment is operating, and that the recording is a good facsimile of sound and color.

CLINICAL EXAMINATION

When arthroscopy is done with the patient under general anesthesia, the first opportunity to gain additional information is after muscular relaxation has occurred. This is an excellent time to check the stability of the knee with respect to its ligament supporting structures (Fig. 19-1). The collateral ligaments and capsule as well as the anteroposterior stability of the knee can be tested and compared with the opposite knee. A better idea of the resting ligament stability is often obtained when the patient is not awake and resisting. Awareness of the amount of ligament laxity may prevent possible misinterpretation later when abnormal meniscus dynamics are seen with the arthroscope, or when too much of the meniscus is seen and a peripheral tear is assumed. The stability of the patella can be checked from a position of full extension through several positions in flexion and compared with the preanesthesia examination.

The knee should be manipulated in an effort to obtain meniscus signs that perhaps were not obtained when the patient was awake and tense. Meniscal crepitus or thrusting may indicate an arthroscopic search in an area unsuspected heretofore. This is also an ideal time to check carefully the range of motion of the knee, which the patient often resists when he has a painful knee and is awake. A stiff knee or one with extensive adhesions can limit the arthroscopic procedure severely. On the other

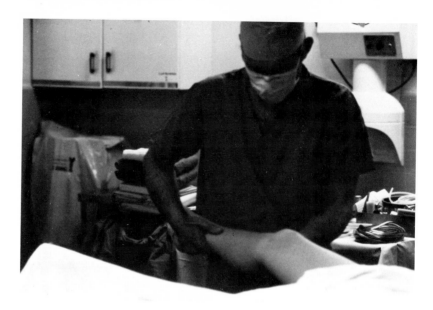

Fig. 19-1. Clinical examination of knee with patient under anesthesia is done as part of arthroscopic procedure when general anesthetic is used.

hand a so-called "locked knee" will be found at times to extend completely with no force at all being applied by the operator. Examination of the knee with the patient under anesthesia as a part of the arthroscopic procedure can be easily overlooked, but if it is developed as a regular routine, the operating room staff will be expecting this, and the extremity will not be already prepared or dripping with antiseptic solution at the time the arthroscopist wishes to do the examination.

SYSTEMATIC ARTHROSCOPIC EXAMINATION

An orderly arthroscopic examination aids greatly in diagnosis because it results in a complete examination. If arthroscopy of the knee is done routinely in a systematic way, no areas of the knee will be inadvertently skipped or forgotten. The order in which areas of the knee are examined is not so important as the routine itself—so that no areas will be missed. However, a definite plan of examination should be well in mind before starting. Repeated observation, that is, coming back several times to a given area in question, is often a valuable diagnostic aid.[1]

IRRIGATING SOLUTION

During observation of the interior of the knee through the arthroscope, anything contributing to good "seeing" is an essential diagnostic aid. Keeping the irrigating fluid clear is most important. At times this can be trying because the knee has loculated areas where cloudy fluid can collect and be extruded into the area under vision, either by external pressure on the knee or by knee motion. If continuous

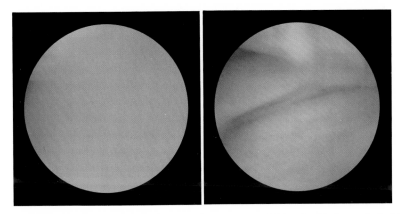

Fig. 19-2. On left, arthroscopic field obscured by a few red blood cells from slight bleeding. On right, same arthroscopic field clearing as saline irrigation proceeds.

irrigation is used through a needle or an arthroscope sheath in the suprapatellar pouch, the outflow should be adjusted to keep the knee distended by saline from the inflow. This can aid seeing by keeping synovial tissue from collapsing over the lens of the arthroscope.

Another way to keep fluid clear is alternately to fill the knee with saline and drain it through the arthroscope itself, thereby removing cloudy fluid from the knee and replacing it with clear fluid each time. In this case it is sometimes faster to have a suction tube attached to the outflow stopcock on the arthroscope sheath. Even a small amount of bleeding will result in poor visibility, and the beginner may interpret this "out of focus" appearance as an optical defect in the arthroscope. A few red cells in the irrigating solution result in blurring without any red coloration (Fig. 19-2). From a diagnostic point of view, it is better to start the arthroscopy without the use of a tourniquet, so the structures, especially the synovium, can be viewed in their normal states. However, if there is even a small amount of persistent bleeding it is sometimes better to use a tourniquet rather than to spend too much time not being able to see with diagnostic clarity.

When the irrigating solution is crystal clear, observation of the hydrodynamics of structures in the fluid stream can be a diagnostic aid. Normal synovial villi and fronds display their seaweedlike flexibility. If they are edematous or fibrotic, their rubbery firmness is indicated by their behavior in the fluid stream exiting from the end of the arthroscope. In like manner the irrigating fluid is sometimes useful in examining the menisci. At times the fluid stream will lift the meniscus for a good view of the undersurface and occasionally will open up a heretofore unseen horizontal cleavage lesion. Often a meniscus flap will be betrayed by its motion in the stream. To accentuate these effects a 60 ml syringe can be attached to the inflow connection of the arthroscope, and while the structure under question is being viewed, a bolus of saline can be firmly injected and the structures observed at that time (Fig. 19-3). This is also a good way to clear the irrigating fluid in case of turbidity when photographic

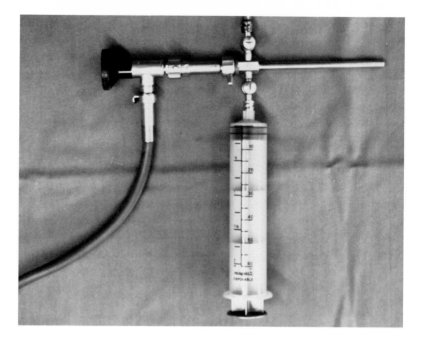

Fig. 19-3. A 60 ml syringe attached directly to sheath of arthroscope for instilling a saline bolus in order to clear field of view or to observe hydrodynamics of structures in fluid stream. Three-way stopcock can be used on syringe connecting to bottle of saline for repeated refill of syringe.

documentation of a lesion is needed. A pedicled synovial nodule often can be easily distinguished from a loose body by its behavior in the fluid stream, whereas observation under static conditions may be deceptive. If suction is being used, the knee can be deliberately emptied of saline, and the meniscus will be sucked farther into the knee. At times this will reveal more of the meniscus surface; this is especially true on the lateral side. Ordinarily the synovium does not collapse over the end of the arthroscope if it is placed deeply within the joint.

ARTHROSCOPE MOTION

Movements of the arthroscope are important as diagnostic aids; first, by scanning areas thoroughly to bring lesions into view and to show comparative sizes, and second, by advancing and retracting motions to give a better three-dimensional interpretation of the structures under observation. The latter motion also helps one to judge the size of structures, as the magnification of the arthroscope varies, depending on the distance of the structures from the lens.

LIGHT

The observing light can be used in several ways as a diagnostic aid. If color absorption filters are available, at times they can be used to advantage at the eyepiece

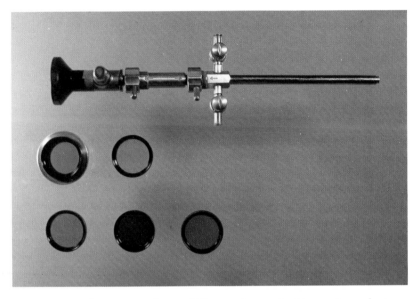

Fig. 19-4. Arthroscope with set of filters to be used with eyepiece adapter.

Fig. 19-5. Arthroscopic view through green filter, showing transverse meniscus tear.

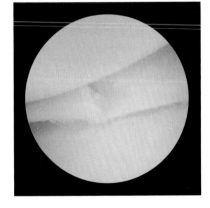

(Fig. 19-4). Filters transmitting only the colors near the center of the visual spectrum (greens and greenish yellows) often seem to give the best contrast and image definition through the arthroscope (Fig. 19-5). This is in part an individual subjective phenomenon and in part due to the fact that the two extremes of the visual spectrum (reds and blues) do not focus at the same point and are both absorbed by the green filter.

Varying the intensity of the light and changing the position of the light by rotating the arthroscope are helpful, particularly in observing closely the surface of articular cartilage.

A polarizing filter in the eyepiece is sometimes helpful in giving increased visual contrast when the examiner is looking toward a light source that is being used to transilluminate the articular cartilage.

Transillumination of articular cartilage and the synovium with a separate light source can give an additional visual dimension to areas of chondromalacia of the articular cartilage or areas of increased villous formation with fibrosis and thickening in the synovium.

Magnification of the viewed image such as may be obtained through the viewfinders of certain cameras attached to the arthroscope is another way that light can be used to advantage. Some arthroscopists have found that magnification improves the image so significantly that they have used the arthroscope with camera attached to obtain this effect.[1]

Innocuous dye has been used to change the reflectivity of tissue in the knee, thereby causing lesions that pick up the stain to be more easily seen.[2] Small amounts of sterile methylene blue introduced during observation will sometimes stain and emphasize the borders of chondromalacia and tears or attritional lesions of the menisci. Articular cartilage, synovium, and meniscus tissue can pick up a small amount of stain and give a light blue appearance. In cases of chondrocalcinosis, unstained punctate areas of crystal deposition may stand out against a more or less homogeneous light blue background. A red filter accentuates these areas by passing the longer wavelengths of light and cutting out the blue light—making the lightly stained areas appear almost black and the areas of calcinosis a contrasting bright red

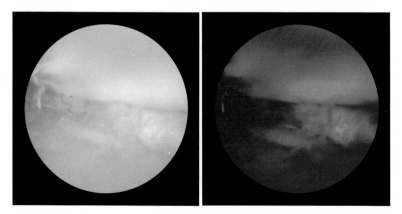

Fig. 19-6. On left, degenerative changes in medial meniscus and medial femoral condyle associated with deposits of calcium pyrophosphate crystals (chondrocalcinosis) with methylene blue stain. Areas of chondrocalcinosis do not stain. On right, same area through no. 25 red filter. Areas of chondrocalcinosis stand out as deep red; uninvolved areas are black.

(Fig. 19-6). Biopsy of these areas will show typical calcium pyrophosphate crystals when the sections are viewed with a microscope using polarized light.

EXTERNAL MANIPULATION OF KNEE

Under conditions of good "seeing" within the knee, there are some external manipulations of the knee that may aid in diagnosis. When the arthroscopist is examining the undersurface of the patella with the arthroscope, his free hand can be used to tilt or rock the patella from side to side, and it can also be pushed medially and laterally (Fig. 19-7). Each of these maneuvers often gives a different or a better view of the patellar articular surface. Lifting the patella is also often helpful. In instances where the patella is hypermobile, almost the entire articular surface can sometimes be seen. The knee can be manipulated into flexion in order to observe the action of the patella in the trochlear groove of the femur. Bringing the knee into 30° flexion should result in the patella beginning to settle down in the trochlear groove. If by 60° flexion the medial facet of the patella is not in good congruous contact with the trochlear groove, the examiner must consider the possibility of a laterally subluxating patella.[1] While the patella is being tested in this way, the tip of the arthroscope must not be deep enough to interfere with patellar position. In questions of patellar function, it is often useful to view the patella and the patellofemoral joint also from a lateral suprapatellar portal. This view of the patellofemoral joint, from above and

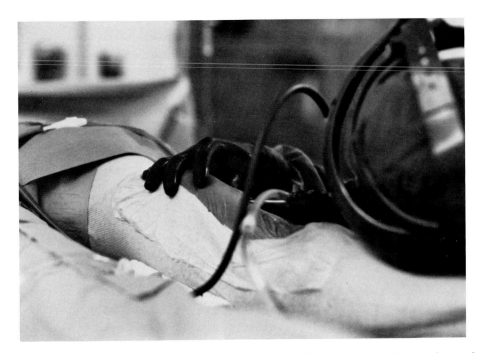

Fig. 19-7. Patella of left knee is externally manipulated while articular surface is observed with arthroscope.

lateral, gives another perspective of the patella and its function, which is not seen from below. Manipulation of the patella with the free hand can also be carried out while the patellofemoral joint is examined from this second viewpoint.

Observation of the menisci is enhanced at times by the examiner's using his free hand to apply pressure to the periphery of the meniscus along the meniscal attachments (Fig. 19-8). At times this will bring more meniscus surface into better view. Manipulation of the knee into flexion and extension, combined with internal and external rotation of the tibia, may not only bring more of the meniscus into view but also may reveal abnormal meniscus dynamics as these motions occur.

When observing the medial meniscus, in addition to the above maneuvers, valgus stress is applied, whereas the lateral meniscus is viewed with the knee forced into varus position (Fig. 19-9). When there is a tear in the substance of the meniscus, manipulation of the knee may bring it into view simply by extending the area of the meniscus that is visible. A horizontal cleavage lesion with a flap on the undersurface of the meniscus may cause obvious disturbance in the motion of the meniscus when the leg is internally or externally rotated, and the knee is placed under varus or valgus stress. Peripheral tears of moderate length either in the substance of the meniscus or in the extraperipheral area may often cause bulging or pouting of the inner edge of the meniscus so that the normal, smooth, even concave edge of the meniscus shows an area of straightness or even convexity.[4,14] This distortion may be accentuated by manipulation of the knee. Longer peripheral tears, particularly of the medial meniscus, will allow the inner edge of the meniscus to be extruded farther centrally beneath the medial femoral condyle, when the tibia is externally rotated and the knee placed under valgus stress. Even without complete displacement of the inner limb of a bucket-handle tear, the thin edge of the meniscus may appear to turn upward and climb up the surface of the medial femoral condyle in an abnormal manner, giving the meniscus a twisted appearance (Fig. 19-10).

An area of redundant, edematous, or hyperemic synovium at the meniscosynovial border may be the clue to a peripheral tear outside the substance of the meniscus. A wisp of tissue appearing under the medial meniscus may point to a tear in the meniscotibial portion of the deep capsular ligament (Fig. 19-11).[9,14] More extensive tears of the medial collateral ligament produce laxity of the inner edge of the meniscus and transverse "kinking" across the middle segment, as well as central displacement of the meniscus on external rotary stress of the knee.[9] Extraperipheral tears, although at times not seen directly, may result in these indirect manifestations of their presence, and manipulation of the knee helps to bring out these findings.

If there is a question of a peripheral tear in the posterior segment not seen from an anterior approach, the arthroscope can be inserted posteromedially or posterolaterally as needed. The posterior approaches are more easily done with one of the small-diameter arthroscopes and with the flexed knee well distended with saline.

When the examiner is observing the anterior cruciate ligament, manipulation of the knee by forcing the tibia anteriorly and posteriorly helps to assess the stabilizing

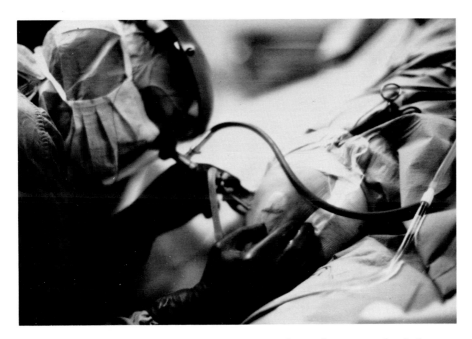

Fig. 19-8. Free hand is used to apply pressure to periphery of meniscus of right knee to increase visible surface.

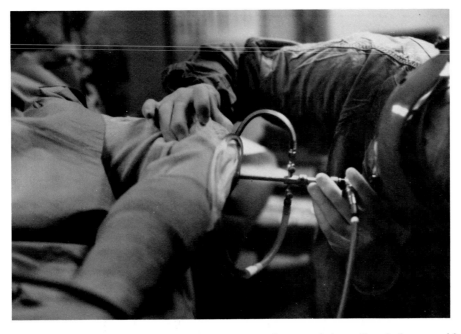

Fig. 19-9. Arthroscopist viewing lateral meniscus with patient's knee flexed, foot on table, and knee forced into varus position. Arthroscope is in lateral infrapatellar site of left knee.

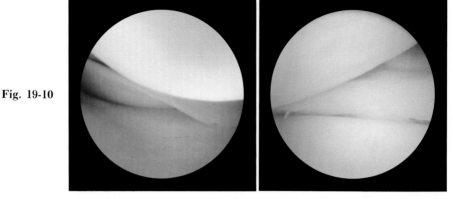

Fig. 19-10

Fig. 19-11

Fig. 19-10. Right medial meniscus with indirect evidence of peripheral tear in posterior segment and part of middle segment. Note abnormal dynamics with external rotary stress of knee. Posterior segment tends to turn up or "climb" medial femoral condyle, giving meniscus twisted or "propeller" appearance. Actual tear is not seen but was confirmed at meniscectomy.
Fig. 19-11. Wisp of tissue appearing under medial meniscus may be clue to tear of meniscotibial deep capsular ligament.

function of this ligament. A tear in continuity may be misinterpreted as an intact ligament unless the knee is manipulated; this is especially true if the knee was not examined clinically with the patient under anesthesia at the beginning of the procedure. Occasionally the ligamentum mucosum masquerades as an intact synovium-covered anterior cruciate ligament, so that careful observation here is required (Fig. 19-12). When the anterior cruciate is intact, the posterior cruciate is usually not seen except for its area of attachment on the lateral surface of the medial femoral condyle in the intercondylar notch region.

Simple flexion and extension of the knee must not be forgotten while the examiner observes the status of the articular cartilage, as it is chiefly these motions that bring more of the articular cartilage surfaces into view and make it possible to assess the contact areas.[3] While observing the contact areas during motion, the examiner is frequently able to see where areas of cratering or of deep fissuring of the articular cartilage are causing the "catching" of which the patient complains and which interfere with the smooth uniform motion of the bearing surfaces. An area of articular cartilage that shows minimal damage or attritional change may afford a clue to a meniscus tear. For example, in a young adult with otherwise smooth articular-bearing surfaces, attritional surface abrasion of the posterolateral area of the medial femoral condyle may point to a posterior segment tear in the medial meniscus.

Manipulation of the knee is also helpful when the synovium is being observed, particularly in examination of any areas of adhesions that may appear more innocuous under static observation than when the knee is placed in motion. In a similar manner the so-called "medial shelf" may be completely innocuous, or if thickened and fibro-

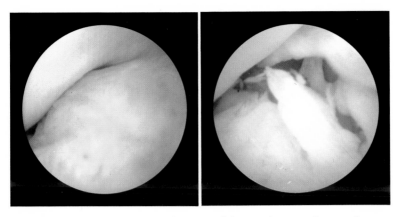

Fig. 19-12. On left, arthroscopic view of intercondylar notch area, showing how attachment of ligamentum mucosum may masquerade as intact anterior cruciate ligament with its synovial covering. On right, in same arthroscopic view, but with ligamentum mucosum pushed aside to show complete disruption of anterior cruciate ligament.

tic, may show actual "catching" and grooving of the medial femoral condyle when it is observed with the knee in motion.

The infrapatellar fat pad is another area worthy of observation while the knee is being manipulated. Smillie has described the pathologic anatomy of various fat pad lesions and their clinical significance.[12] Occasionally a tongue of fat pad that shows suspicious hyperemia, or even an old hemorrhagic area, may be seen to be trapped by the femoral condyle, usually on the medial side, when the knee is moved into extension. The lateral fat pad area is at times well seen with the arthroscope in the lateral suprapatellar portal where it can be moved down through the lateral pouch so the examiner can view part of the posterior surface of the fat pad in the lateral compartment.

Finally external manipulation of the knee is helpful in bringing loose bodies into view. Manipulation of the knee in the various planes as noted above for viewing the menisci may bring loose bodies into view coincidentally. Sudden pushing in the popliteal area with the flat of the free hand in a concussive manner, or on the posterior areas of the medial and lateral pouches of the knee, will at times bring loose bodies forward into the field of view. Under influence of the fluid stream from the arthroscope, loose bodies may tend to circle from the lateral pouch up into the suprapatellar pouch, down under the patella into the intercondylar notch, and continue circling in this manner. Under these conditions a loose body, thought lost to view, will often return shortly if the arthroscope is held in the same position.

Movement of the saline-filled knee during arthroscopy can cause filling of a popliteal cyst if it is connected with the knee joint. It is now that careful palpation in back of the knee may reveal the discrete borders of a tensely filled cyst that otherwise could be detected only with difficulty if at all.[13]

INTRAARTICULAR MANIPULATION OF STRUCTURES IN KNEE

Some of the maneuvers used in external manipulation of the knee have been discussed as diagnostic aids. In a similar manner intraarticular manipulation can be used as an aid to diagnosis. One simple way to do this is to use the end of the arthroscope as a probe. This can be helpful in roughly determining the consistency of articular cartilage, but here the examiner must be careful not to score the surface. With an arthroscope of small diameter (usually 2.5 cm or smaller), it is possible to gain information by probing meniscus surfaces as well as observing under the meniscus for areas of attritional change or actual tears in the substance of the meniscus. If arthroscopy is being done with a small arthroscope, with the patient under local anesthesia, probing of specific areas under question for elicitation of pain can be done. The location and type of pain that is produced may be identified by the patient as the area causing clinical symptoms.[5,11] The end of the arthroscope can be useful at times in distinguishing whether a cartilaginous body is truly a loose body or whether it is tethered in place by a pedicle. This may have some bearing as to whether it is to be removed or not.

The use of instruments through a second portal for intraarticular manipulation can be an extremely helpful diagnostic aid. The simplest form of this is to use the drainage needle, which may be in the suprapatellar pouch. A Verres needle works well

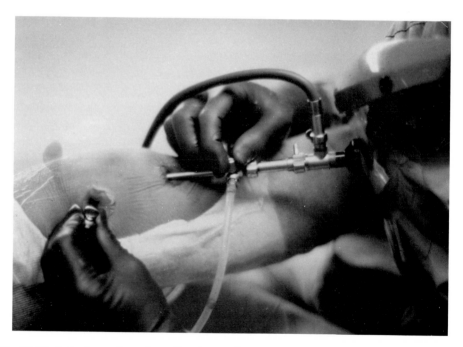

Fig. 19-13. Articular surface of patella is being observed while a blunt-ended Verres drainage needle is used to test firmness of articular cartilage.

here because of the blunt, rounded end. This needle, which is already well positioned, can be used to probe the articular surface of the patella, testing the firmness of the articular cartilage; it can also be used to palpate the synovium in the suprapatellar pouch (Figs. 19-13 and 19-14). By dropping it down into the lateral pouch, it can be used to palpate structures in that area, including the popliteal tendon. Another method that is sometimes used, particularly in examining the menisci, is to penetrate the knee from the outside with an 18-gauge needle in the area of question.[4] The meniscus can then be probed or lifted with the needle for better visibility and to observe the meniscus as it is being moved. An undisplaced bucket-handle tear may be opened up and made visible by this means.

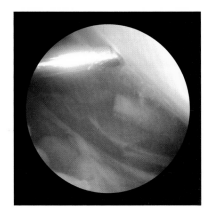

Fig. 19-14. Arthroscopic view of undersurface of patella as articular cartilage is being tested with blunt-ended Verres needle.

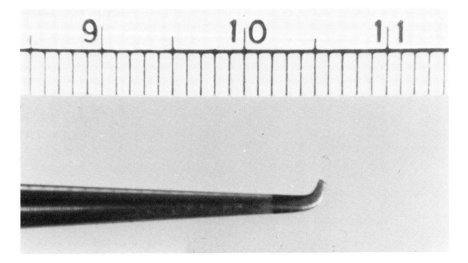

Fig. 19-15. Instrument with small right-angled end for exploring meniscus surfaces under arthroscopic observation. Scale is in centimeters.

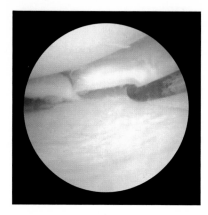

Fig. 19-16. Arthroscopic view of instrument being used to explore tear in medial meniscus of right knee.

Introducing an instrument through a second portal probably allows more flexibility in the use of intraarticular manipulation as a diagnostic aid. The instrument that is used through the second portal can be one with a blunt crochet hook–type end or one that has approximately a right-angle curve on its tip (Fig. 19-15). Instruments with full hooks on the end are apt to become caught. The end of the instrument should be such that it can always be easily retracted out of the knee. When the medial meniscus is being examined with the arthroscope in the lateral infrapatellar portal, the instrument portal can be at the medial infrapatellar site. With the instrument under arthroscopic observation, it is used to explore both surfaces of the meniscus with its curved end (Fig. 19-16). Instruments can be used in a similar manner to explore the lateral meniscus. In this way the most common types of meniscus tears can be sorted out and a more refined diagnosis made. If the arthroscopist makes a rough diagram of the meniscus lesion at this time, it will aid in diagnostic precision. Sterile paper and marking pen should be available for each case.

The anterior cruciate ligament is another area in which intraarticular manipulation is helpful. The previously mentioned tear in continuity is more easily recognized by probing in this manner with an instrument, as redundant synovium can be shunted aside, allowing better visibility and testing of the ligament. If an operating arthroscope is being used, instruments can be inserted through the arthroscope and used in a similar manner.

When the examiner is confronted with an unexpected diagnostic problem during arthroscopy, it is often very helpful to take a moment to review the patient's history, physical findings, and roentgeongrams and then to return again to any suspected areas for further observation. Sometimes a second or third look at an area will make the diagnosis.

MEASUREMENTS

The measurement of structures and lesions in the knee can be considered as a part of the complete diagnosis, since it may give some indication as to whether the treatment should be surgical or nonsurgical. Furthermore if it is possible to measure lesions, the measurements may show progress or regression on repeated arthroscopy. Rough measurements may be made by comparing the size of the lesion to one of the instruments that is inserted in the knee under observation. A hook-type scissors with an attached dial indicator can be used to advantage as a caliper for measuring. Serial photographs can be used, but care must be exercised in order to obtain the same field of view relative to the knee each time a measurement is made. The same focal-length camera lens must be used on the same type of arthroscope for the measurements to be comparable. In the future perhaps reticle eyepieces will be developed for routine measurement.

PHOTOGRAPHY

Documentation by means of photography can be a definite diagnostic aid, particularly in borderline cases. To assure the identity of the film when returned from processing, the first photograph can be that of the patient's name and the date as previously printed on the sponge-count board in the operating room. When taking still pictures, camera orientation is important. If a 35 mm camera is being used, it should be placed with the long axis of the film format at right angles to the leg (parallel to the tibial articular surface) for consistent orientation. When the fluid is cloudy, but it is important to obtain a documentary picture, the use of a saline bolus pushed through the arthroscope with a syringe will clear the fluid, as mentioned previously. Then the picture can be taken, thus perhaps saving a good deal of time. Occasionally study of projected and enlarged color photographs taken at arthroscopy can help to clarify the diagnosis.

As an interesting sidelight, photography with infrared color film has been used and appears to show the depth of the articular cartilage better than visible light. Some of the photographs suggest changes in the articular cartilage well beyond the lesions shown by visible light (Fig. 19-17). This may be found to be of some value in diagnosis and prognosis of articular cartilage lesions. Since interpretations of findings with infrared films are not settled as yet, this is not being recommended as a routine procedure.

Movies have been important diagnostic aids in arthroscopy, especially in teaching. They give a three-dimensional rendition of the structures as a result of the motion of the arthroscope or of the knee while the pictures are being taken. The same advantage comes from closed circuit television viewing and repeat viewing by videotape. In addition, motion of the structures in the knee can be well seen during palpation, under fluid stream effects, and during manipulation.

LABORATORY TESTS

During arthroscopy, specimens can be taken for laboratory tests. Synovial fluid is obtained at the initial puncture. Here it is important to avoid contaminating the synovial fluid with particulate matter.[10] Talc particles are one of the common contaminants and can be very confusing when an attempt is made to identify crystals in the synovial fluid specimen. Another source of error can be the injection, within

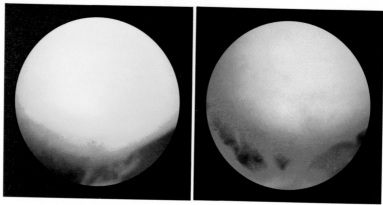

Fig. 19-17. On left, chondromalacia of articular cartilage of medial femoral condyle in right knee. Area of osteonecrosis in medial femoral condyle seen on roentgenogram. On right, infrared photograph of same area, showing apparent changes in articular cartilage beyond lesion seen with visible light.

a month previously, of microcrystalline steroids.[6] If there is any question of an inflammatory lesion, or if there was a previous arthrotomy, the synovial fluid can be cultured. A differential cell count is obtained routinely. At times it is useful to wash the knee out with saline and have the washings centrifuged down for a button, which can be stained and sectioned (Fig. 19-18). Lavage itself may be therapeutic in cases of crystal-induced synovitis.[8] The synovial fluid samples should be sent to the pathology laboratory immediately after collection.

In most arthroscopic examinations a synovial biopsy is taken for routine study. It is best to place this specimen in absolute alcohol because formalin tends to dissolve the types of crystals that are being sought. This is quite important if a crystal-induced synovitis is suspected. Care should be taken not to crush the tissue. Specimens should go directly to the laboratory since tissue placed in absolute alcohol becomes dehydrated and hard when kept too long before processing. Synovial biopsy may be taken either blindly or under arthroscopic observation. It is better to take the biopsy under observation so that a definite area under suspicion can be obtained. This is almost essential if rheumatoid arthritis is suspected because of the often patchy areas of affected synovium, other areas being normal. A bit of articular cartilage in an area of chondromalacia, for example, is easily obtained as a biopsy specimen under direct observation and should be handled in the same manner as a synovial specimen.

PATIENT'S POSTARTHROSCOPY RESPONSE

A feeling for the normal early response to arthroscopy is developed by the examiner after he has done a number of these procedures. Usually the postarthroscopy morbidity is minimal. Immediate ambulation without crutches is the rule. Any marked variation from this (Fig. 19-19), without apparent due cause, may give the arthroscopist some insight into the patient's possible postsurgical course if a surgical procedure on the knee is contemplated.

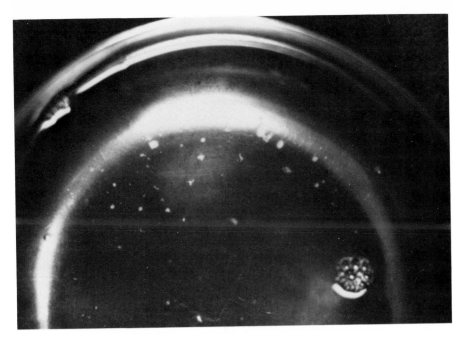

Fig. 19-18. Debris washed from knee during arthroscopy.

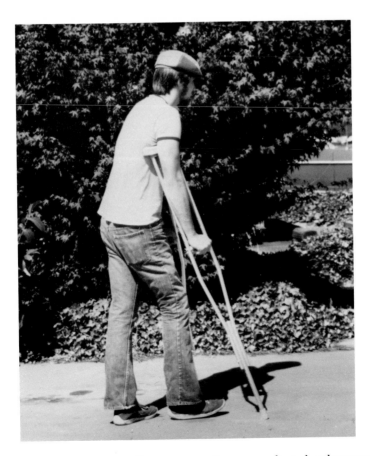

Fig. 19-19. Crutches are not usually necessary after uncomplicated arthroscopy. Minimal postarthroscopy pain is normal response.

Some anxiety will be felt by the surgeon who comes up with a negative arthroscopic examination in spite of the patient's complaint of knee pain. Under these circumstances it is not unusual, particularly in adolescents, to see gradual disappearance of the patient's knee symptoms later in the postarthroscopy follow-up period. The patient's late response is welcome confirmation of the original arthroscopic diagnosis.

Occasionally the examiner encounters a structural variation difficult to classify as normal or abnormal, but the patient continues to have symptoms in the later postarthroscopy period that could logically result from the questionable lesion. If remedial surgery results in lessening or elimination of symptoms, the correlation of these follow-up findings is significant.

The above examples are sufficient to illustrate the necessity of follow-up and its importance in developing diagnostic skill in arthroscopy.

References

1. Casscells, S. W.: Arthroscopy of the knee joint, J. Bone Joint Surg. [Am.]**53:**287, 1971.
2. Guten, G.: Staining articular cartilage with methylene blue during arthroscopy. Paper read before the International Arthroscopy Association, Copenhagen, July 10, 1975.
3. Jackson, R. W., and Abe, I.: The role of arthroscopy in the management of disorders of the knee, J. Bone Joint Surg. [Br.] **54:**310, 1972.
4. Jackson, R. W., and Dandy, D. J.: Arthroscopy of the knee, New York, 1976, Grune & Stratton.
5. Johnson, L. L.: Personal communications, 1976.
6. Kahn, C. B., Hollander, J. L., and Schumacher, H. R.: Corticosteroid crystals in synovial fluid, J.A.M.A. **211:**807, 1970.
7. McGinty, J. B.: Closed circuit television in arthroscopy, R Rev. Internat. Rheumatol. **33:**45, 1976.
8. O'Connor, R. L.: Arthroscopy in the diagnosis and treatment of acute ligament injuries of the knee, J. Bone Joint Surg. [Am.] **56:**333, 1974.
9. O'Connor, R. L.: The arthroscope in management of crystal-induced synovitis of the knee, J. Bone Joint Surg. [Am.] **55:**1443, 1973.
10. Phelps, P., Steele, A. D., and McCarty, D. J., Jr.: Compensated polarized light microscopy. Identification of crystals in synovial fluids from gout and pseudogout, J.A.M.A. **203:**166, 1968.
11. Poehling, G. G., Bassett, F. H., III, and Goldner, J. L.: Arthroscopy: its role in treating nontraumatic and traumatic lesions of the knee, South. Med. J. **70:**465, 1977.
12. Smillie, I. S.: Diseases of the knee joint, Edinburgh, 1974, Churchill Livingstone.
13. Thompson, R. W., Jr.: Personal communication, 1977.
14. Watanabe, J., Takeda, S., and Ikeuchi, H.: Atlas of Arthroscopy, ed. 2, Tokyo, 1969, Igaku Shoin Ltd.

20. Laboratory aids in the teaching of arthroscopy

Robert E. Eilert

Arthroscopy is a new technique for most orthopedic surgeons, since it has not been a routine part of the training program in the past. Advances in instrumentation, particularly in optics and fiber optics, have made arthroscopic examination of joints practical. In order to familiarize the orthopedic surgeon with the technique of arthroscopy as well as the equipment that is necessary to perform it, a laboratory situation was developed in which the student could practice on a model of the knee joint under supervision of an experienced instructor.

CONCEPT

The basic concept of the laboratory is to provide individual instruction in a small group with one-on-one supervision. A second part of the philosophy is to have the student handle the arthroscope so as to familiarize himself with the mechanics, construction, and care of the instrument. A third concept of the laboratory is to provide a joint to examine so that the instruments can actually be inserted and manipulated just as the surgeon would do for his patient.

INDIVIDUAL TEACHING

Instructors are chosen based on adequate personal experience in performing arthroscopy and their willingness to teach.

A table equipped with arthroscopic instruments is provided for each instructor. The number of students is limited to four or five per instructor. With this number each person can be instructed individually without having an excessive waiting time for the other members of the group. Seating the group helps to make the waiting easier and more comfortable. A round table is useful in that the group can circulate, with each member being successively in the position of the examiner. The teacher is immediately available for questions and feedback. In the small-group environment this type of exchange takes the form of a conversation rather than being simply a one-way communication from the instructor.

315

FAMILIARIZATION

In order to present the student with all the possible combinations of equipment, voluntary support was obtained from all the manufacturers of arthroscopic instruments. These manufacturers provide light sources, fiber optic cables, and various sizes of arthroscopic telescopes and sheaths in order that the student can examine a variety of equipment. One type of instrumentation is set up on each table, and during the laboratory there is time allotted to rotate to the various tables. Having all of this equipment available as well as having technicians from the company to explain the different features as requested presents a logistic problem but is well worth the effort. A model of the knee joint with simulated pathology is provided for each table (Figs. 20-1 to 20-6). Each model is made with different lesions so that students can see different types of meniscus tears, for example. The model is clamped to the table to allow easy manipulation by the instructor and students. The mainstay of the familiarization is the guided psychomotor activity, in which the student is expected to go through an arthroscopic examination on the model in a rehearsal for the same type of examination that he would do on his own patient.

KNEE JOINT MODEL

There are advantages of a knee joint model over the use of a cadaver specimen. The first of these is flexibility. If specimens are obtained from the morgue, rigor mortis often limits the amount of flexibility. Cadaver specimens may not be available in sufficient number, require freezing, and can only be used once. The model is portable and can be easily transported in a case or box. Another advantage is that the models have no odor or offensive drainage of blood and greasy fluid. The main advantage is the fact that the models can be constructed with various designated abnormalities, such as torn meniscus, free bodies, torn anterior cruciate ligament, cartilaginous lesions, or synovitis. In cadaver specimens the examiner usually sees either degenerative arthritis or a completely normal knee joint. The models can be used repeatedly for various courses. They are also useful for review by residents in anticipation of a procedure.

PROCEDURE

The format for the beginner's laboratory requires about 90 minutes of program time. The first phase is familiarization with the equipment. The various components of the arthroscopic system are demonstrated, including the sheath, the obturators that are used within the sheath, the telescope itself, the light cable, and the light source. The optical characteristics of the arthroscope are demonstrated, as well as the advantages of various sizes and angles of arthroscopes.

The second phase is to review the operating room setup, with the instructor pointing out that the examiner may or may not use a sterile mask. The type of irrigation flow may be either intermittent through the arthroscope or continuous, using a type of drainage needle. General or local anesthesia may be used, depending on whether the examination is simply diagnostic or further surgery is planned.

Text continued on p. 323.

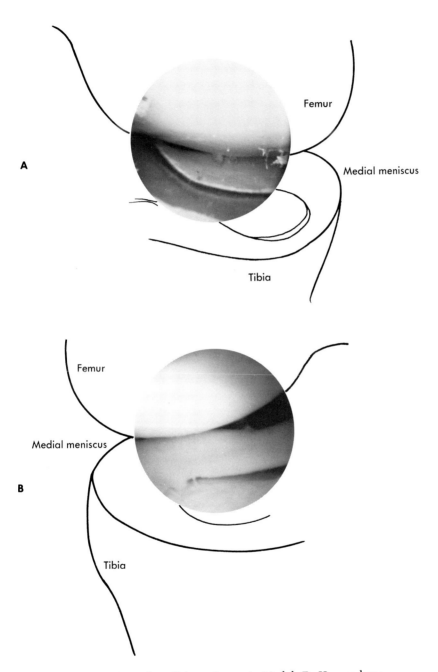

Fig. 20-1. Normal medial meniscus. **A,** Model. **B,** Human knee.

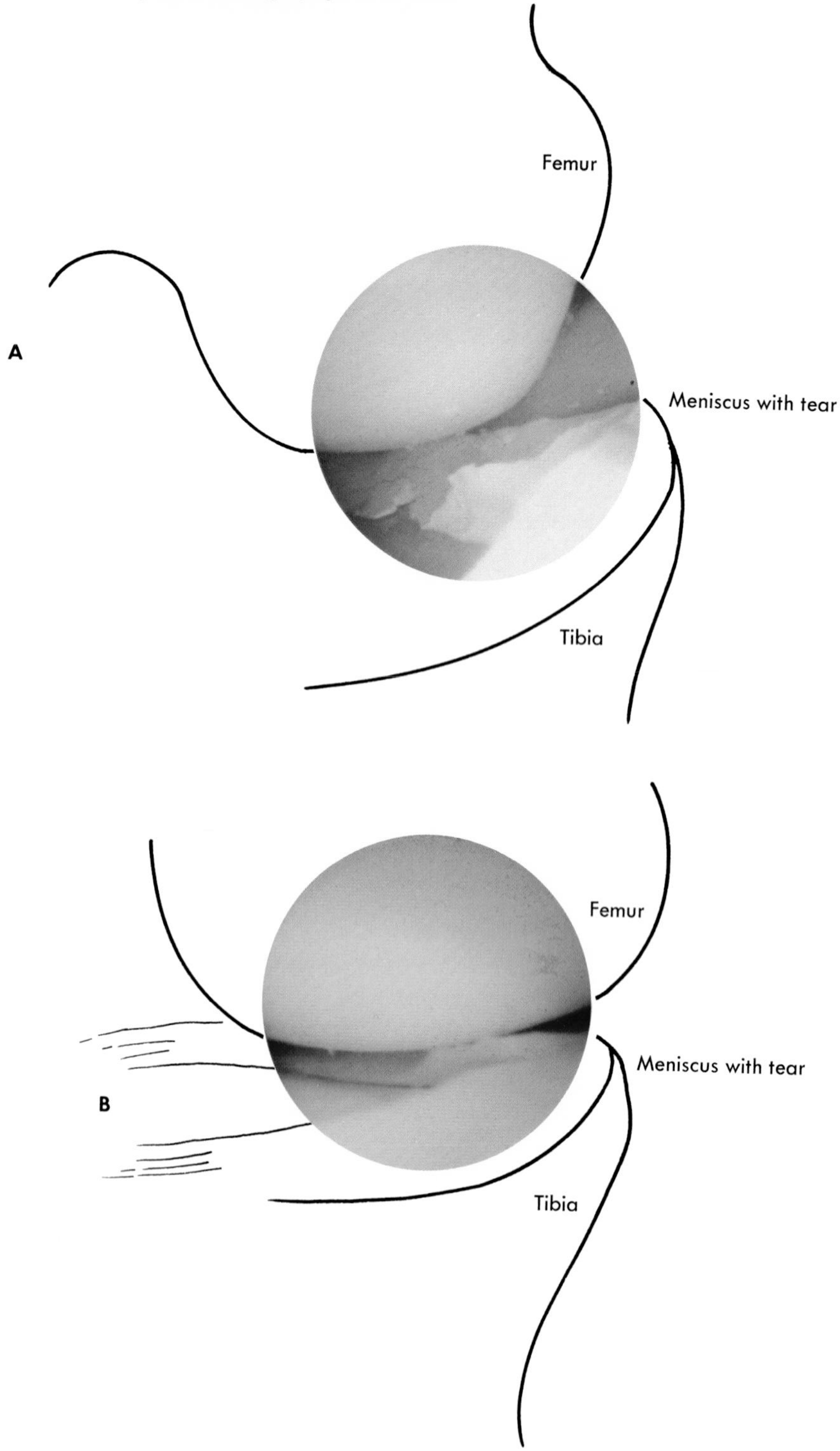

Fig. 20-2. Torn lateral meniscus. **A,** Model. **B,** Human knee.

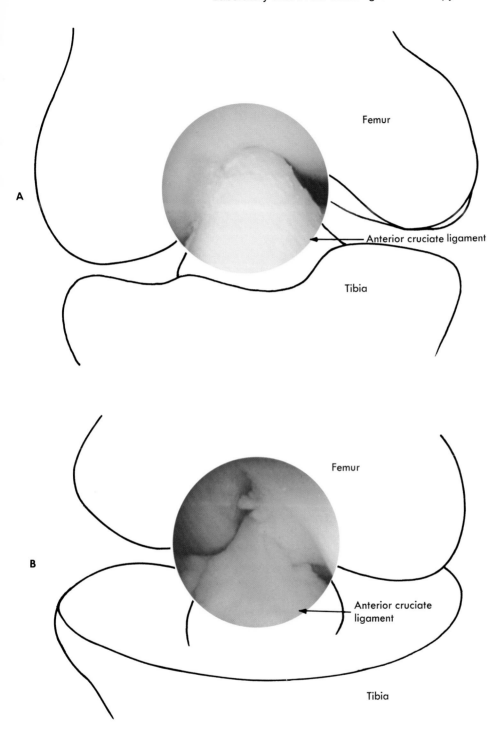

Fig. 20-3. Normal anterior cruciate ligament. **A,** Model. **B,** Human knee.

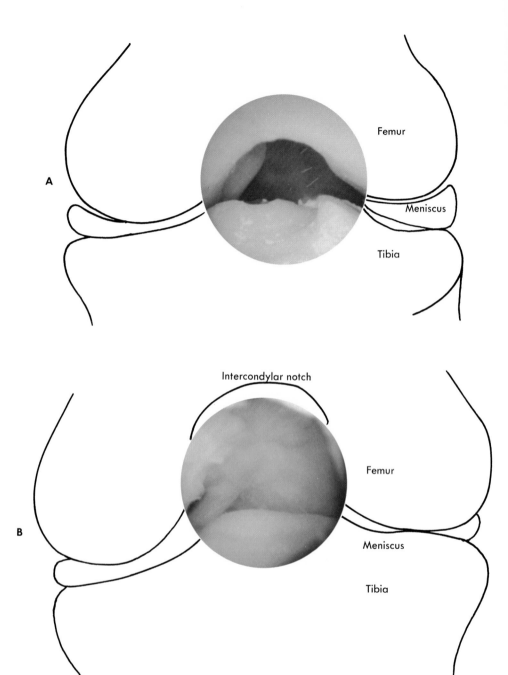

Fig. 20-4. Absent anterior cruciate ligament. **A,** Model. **B,** Human knee.

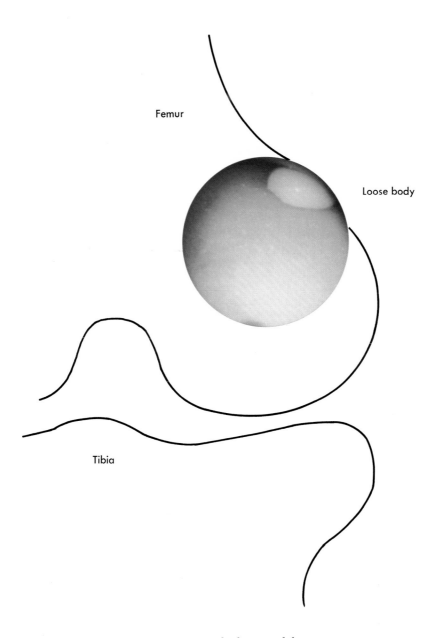

Fig. 20-5. Loose body in model.

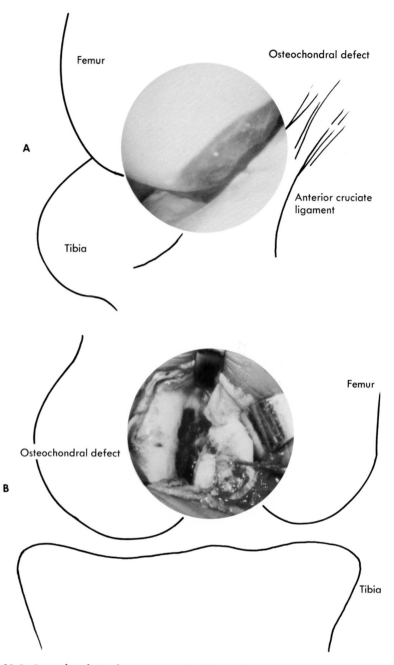

Fig. 20-6. Osteochondritis dissecans. **A,** Model. **B,** Human knee, intraoperative view.

Choice of anesthesia may also be influenced by the age of the patient and his equanimity. The use of a tourniquet is also optional and may be an advantage for certain cases, such as acute hemarthrosis, whereas blanching in the synovium may be a disadvantage at other times. This presentation of how to set up in the operating room nearly always stimulates discussion with a chance for each student to question or contribute, which is the great asset of a small group in a practical laboratory.

After this introduction the landmarks for insertion of the arthroscope are pointed out on the model, being either medial or lateral to the patellar ligament, posterior to the collateral ligaments, or superior to the patella. These landmarks can be identified on the model both visually and by palpation. Insertion using the sheath and obturators is then demonstrated and experienced by the participants. They are taught how to direct the arthroscope toward the notch, using the blunt obturator to protect against damage to the cartilage. They palpate the intercondylar notch to confirm that the arthroscope is indeed intraarticular, and the technique for passing the arthroscope past the patella into the suprapatellar pouch is practiced by each student in turn.

The next phase of examination is to identify in succession the five areas of the joint, that is, the medial compartment, the lateral compartment, the intercondylar notch area, the patellofemoral joint, and the suprapatellar pouch. The instructor supervises as the student practices moving the arthroscope from compartment to compartment (Fig. 20-7). He demonstrates how to recover when visualization is lost and how to get the best exposure of each area of the joint by manipulation in flexion and extension with lateral and rotatory stress. The instructor may use a teaching attachment to view simultaneously in order to guide the student (Fig. 20-8).

The next exercise is interpretation of pathology. For this phase the students in turn analyze each compartment of the model, describing the structures within it, such as the femoral condyle, the menisci, the tibial plateau, and the adjacent synovium. During this phase the techniques of following the horizons within the joint, pistoning to gain better depth percpetion, and scanning to go from known to unknown are pointed out and practiced. After this description of each compartment, the diagnosis is confirmed by any participant who may have missed an important finding on his initial observation.

The final phase is for the student to switch tables and instructors in order to examine different types of arthroscopic equipment and to see various pathologic lesions within the different knee models.

ANATOMIC SPECIMENS

It has been a popular part of the laboratory session to show anatomic variations in the knee. This has been done by an anatomy professor who has a table with a number of dissected cadaver knee specimens that can be examined by the participants. These cadaver specimens are used to demonstrate such things as the attachment of the ligaments to the menisci, the folds within the synovium itself, and the relationship of the fat pad to the internal structure of the joint. This exercise helps make the transition from the facsimile model to the living patient.

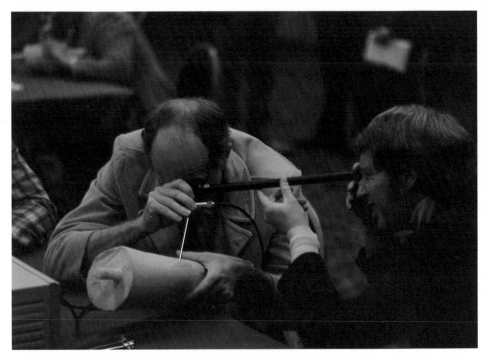

Fig. 20-7. Teaching with model. Instructor looks through viewing piece while student moves telescope within knee.

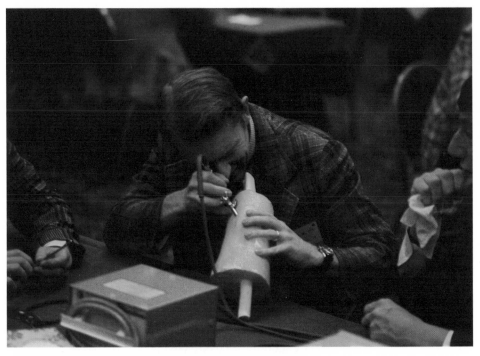

Fig. 20-8. Teaching with model. Model is transilluminated between student's fingers as he moves arthroscope into suprapatellar pouch for full visualization.

Another technique that has been used on occasion is to examine the joint model using a television camera attached to the arthroscope. This technique is valuable for teaching in the operating room and allows the student to move the arthroscope completely on his own, with the instructor being able to follow the whole procedure on the television monitor.

FABRICATION OF THE KNEE JOINT

The knee joint is fabricated from various plastics and rubber products in order to simulate the anatomic knee. Epoxy resins are used to make castings of the bones taken from cadavers. The menisci are made of RTV silicone rubber based upon clay sculptures of various meniscus and cruciate lesions. The skin is simulated with latex rubber and the subcutaneous tissue by polyurethane foam. The model is held together by ligaments made of synthetic fiber as well as suturing of the anterior cruciate in place as one would do in a surgical repair. The synovium is attached by stitching it posteriorly in the midline, and the simulated skin and soft tissues are placed over the capsule and bone assembly. The total construction requires about 20 man-hours of time in addition to the drying time for the various stages.

SUMMARY

A practical laboratory for teaching arthroscopy was designed around the philosophy of small-group instruction and use of a model of the knee joint. The concept has been useful in teaching about 3,000 surgeons in courses in the United States and Europe.

21. Correlation of arthroscopy and arthrography

Benjamin E. Bierbaum

To correlate the message from these chapters, which is to describe, illustrate, and define the role of arthroscopy and arthrography of the knee, has been delegated to me. I have had personal experience in performing several hundred examinations of each type. There is no question that each procedure offers significant, helpful diagnostic information for the management of knee problems. Although it need not be said that every patient needing knee surgery must have one or the other examination prior to operation, with greater use and interpretation of these tests more information is gained, and thus their role is necessarily expanded. Clinical acumen alone may not reveal the full answer in evaluation of the knee either by the rheumatologist or by the surgeon, and it is for these situations that arthrography or arthroscopy provides invaluable assistance. No experienced knee surgeon can afford to be without the availability of the arthroscopist or the arthrographer.

Why do we need diagnostic tests such as those provided by arthrography or arthroscopy? To be sure, there has been a broadening of the knowledge of knee function and anatomy. A greater demand has been placed on the surgeon to restore the injured knee to as functional a state as possible, whether in a high-performance athlete or in the more casual performer. The age of consumerism has influenced our patients to expect these refinements and to demand the highest performance levels. Not only has the physician become more sophisticated but so has the consumer. No longer is there a rule for "exploratory" surgery of the knee. The objective evidence obtained by the impartial arthrogram and the special aspects of arthroscopy that can be photographed gives precision in diagnosis and aid in management for workmen's compensation, disputed injury, and medicolegal situations.

There is useful information common to both examinations. This includes the ability to retrieve and examine synovial fluid. Not only should the character and the fibrin clot of the fluid be observed, but also cellular, crystal, bacteriologic, and chemical analysis should be performed when indicated. The integrity of both articular and meniscus cartilages can be largely determined by either examination. The definition and location of cartilaginous loose bodies not apparent on plain x-ray examination is possible. Instability and joint displacement are readily identifiable as the examiner is performing the test.

Arthroscopy offers unique advantages over arthrography. The character of the synovium can be determined, and synovial biopsy is easy to perform at the conclusion of the procedure. Chronic arthritidies can be evaluated by serial arthroscopy. The character of articular cartilage is more easily demonstrated, especially as to the depth of the articular cartilage erosion and as to the character of the base. Follow-up evaluation after debridement of articular cartilage surfaces can help determine rate of healing and activity levels for the patient. The demonstration of cruciate ligaments, although extrasynovial, is best delineated with the arthroscope. Attenuated ligaments can be identified by the examiner placing stress on the joint, whereas torn or absent cruciates can be seen in spite of an intact ligamentum mucosum or other synovial reflections, which trap arthrographic dye. Finally arthroscopy allows a unique role for joint lavage of debris and for endoscopic surgery. Loose bodies can be removed, synovial plica resected, lateral retinacular release performed and abnormal menisci resected, or articular cartilage erosions debrided through endoscopic surgery. In no other area of medicine can the diagnosis and treatment of certain conditions be correlated so easily in one procedure as in diagnostic arthroscopy and associated endoscopic surgery.

Information unique to the arthrographer includes the identification and location of synovial and meniscus cysts. Any communication with the synovial lining allows for clear delineation of cystic walls as well as the character of their lining. In addition any capsular abnormality including the disruption of the capsule by recent injury or abnormal reflection to bony attachment is easily identified. Peripheral meniscus tears may be better discerned by the arthrogram, particularly those incomplete horizontal tears in the posterior horn of the medial meniscus whose cleavage begins at the periphery. The congruity of the tibial femoral articulation, especially with weight-bearing x-ray films, is better demonstrated arthrographically.

How can the practicing physician decide which diagnostic test to turn to and in what sequence? Many variables influence his decision. Certainly the availability of the tests and the proximity and ease of scheduling of the patient are of great importance. Relative costs should be considered by comparing information obtained with dollars invested. Patient acceptance must be considered, in that arthrography is a relatively noninvasive technique whereas arthroscopy is invasive. For those arthroscopists who can perform in an outpatient ambulatory surgical center with the patient under local anesthesia, the complexity of arthroscopy more clearly parallels that of arthrography. Either examination can be learned and performed with reliable results by any physician interested to take the time and effort to become proficient in the procedure. The expertise of the examiner usually closely parallels the amount of enthusiasm, carefulness, and experience invested. This book has been prepared by those with great expertise in their respective fields.

Potential complications need to be considered in choosing when to perform arthrography or arthroscopy. For arthrography an allergy to local anesthetic or the iodine-containing contrast media negates the use of either product. Infection is always a possibility, although reported incidences are rare. A postinjection synovitis may develop and mimic an acute attack of gout, low-grade sepsis, or any nonspecific synovitis. The examination itself may be painful when the joint is stressed to obtain a more clear delineation of the meniscus cartilage. This may aggravate a recent injury, with resultant swelling and local tenderness. The persistence of air within the synovial lining may lead to the production of unsocial noises, and the patient should be warned that this might occur for 2 to 3 days after the examination.

The threat of infection and postinstrumentation synovitis is as real with the arthroscope as with the arthrogram. Contamination of the endoscopic eyepiece or sterile field can lead to direct invasion of bacteria within the knee unless the examiner adheres to strict precautions of aseptic technique. A subcutaneous hematoma or hemarthrosis may develop, especially in those patients with a deficit in clotting mechanisms. Damage to articular cartilage from the trocar or overzealous use of the arthroscope may yield additional knee difficulty. There is always a possibility of fragmentation of instruments within the joint, necessitating immediate arthrotomy.

When should neither test be utilized? Active infection is a relative contraindication. Presence of a total-joint prosthesis is a relative contraindication for arthroscopy and should be approached with great care in arthrography. The acutely injured locked knee with a flexion contracture of 35° or greater restricts the amount of information obtainable and makes the examination futile. Patients with blood coagulation defects should be exposed to the examination only after restoration of the clotting mechanism.

How soon can arthrotomy be safely performed after diagnostic evaluation? If strict attention to detail and aseptic technique is followed, an arthrotomy within the same 24-hour period is reasonably safe. However, our institution does not recommend surgery if both arthrography and arthroscopy have been performed within the same day. Arthroscopy is best preceded by arthrography to avoid confusion of capsular punctures, although a frothy synovium greets the arthroscopist. If the availability and expertise of those persons performing the two techniques are comparable, the clinical diagnosis should best determine which test to perform first. For example, if a synovial or meniscus cyst or a posterior horn tear of the medial meniscus is suspected, arthrography is probably the first test to perform. In those patients with suspected lateral meniscus tears, synovial disease, or articular cartilage erosion, the arthroscope may yield the most information.

As in all fields of medicine, a fundamental knowledge of anatomy is essential to understand the subtleties of either examination. Likewise, the role of arthrography and arthroscopy is an adjunct for the best possible care of the patient. In no instance should either procedure be substituted for the thoughtful history and careful physical examination of the patient. As Ward Casscells so aptly stated, "Seeing is no substitute for thinking."

Bibliography

Aglietti, P., and Pimpinelli, P.: Arthrography of the knee with fluoroscopic technique, Ital. J. Orthop. Traumatol. 2(1):89-102, 1976.

Aglietti, P., and Pimpinelli, G.: Double contrast arthrography of the knee, Chir. Organi. Mov. 62(6):617-631, 1975.

Alm, A., Gillquist, J., and Liljedahl, S. O.: The diagnostic value of arthroscopy of the knee joint, Injury 5(4):319-24, 1974.

Alm, A., Gillquist, J., and Strömberg, B.: The medial third of the patellar ligament in reconstruction of the anterior cruciate ligament. A clinical and histologic study by means of arthroscopy or arthrotomy, Acta. Chir. Scand. [Suppl.] 0(suppl. 445):5-14, 1974.

Ambanelli, U., Manganelli, P., Nervetti, A., and Ugolotti, U.: Demonstration of articular effusions and popliteal cysts with ultrasound, J. Rheumatol. 3(2):134-139, 1976.

Andersen, R. B., and Rossel, I.: Arthroscopy of the knee joint in rheumatic diseases, Ugeskr. Laeger 135(2):71-73, 1973.

Anderson, P. W., and Maslin, P.: Tomography applied to knee arthrography, Radiology 110(2):271-275, 1974.

Angell, F. L.: Fluoroscopic technique of double contrast arthrography of the knee, Radiol. Clin. North Am. 9(1):85-98, 1971.

Arthroscopy of the knee joint, Injury 5(4):318, 1974.

Ashby, M. E., Shields, C. L., and Karmy, J. R.: Diagnosis of osteochondral fractures in acute traumatic patellar dislocations using air arthrography, J. Trauma 15(11):1032-1033, 1975.

Aube, L., Dionne, G., and Tardif, A.: Study of the meniscus in arthrography of the knee, Laval. Med. 37(10):1056-1062, 1966.

Aube, L., and Fortin, B.: A support used for knee arthrography, J. Can. Assoc. Radiol. 24(2):128, 1973.

Axer, A., Segal, D., Hendel, D., Shikiar, S., Rabinowitz, J., Halperin, N., Rzetelny, V., and Gershuni, D.: Arthrography and arthroscopy in the diagnosis of internal derangement of the knee, Harefuah 91(3-4):61-63, 1976.

Baars, H. G.: Arthrography of the knee joint with "visotrast" (VEB Fahlberg-list), Radiol. Diagn. (Berl.) 7(3):307-313, 1966.

Barlow, J. B.: Radiologic seminar LXXXIV: arthrography of the knee, J. Miss. State Med. Assoc. 10(5):207-208, 1969.

Baumann, D., and Kremer, H.: Arthrography and ultrasound scanning for the detection of Baker cysts (author's transl.), R.O.E.F.O. 127(5):463-466, 1977.

Bernageau, J., Guedj, P., and Bourdon, R.: Radiologic study of ligamanta cruciata genus during gas arthrography (normal and pathologic aspects), J. Radiol. Electrol. Med. Nucl. 50(6):558-559, 1969.

Bernhard, J., and Trefftz, F.: Does arthrography of the knee joint support the indication for meniscectomy, Beitr. Orthop. Traumatol. 15(4):246-251, 1968.

Bessler, W.: Arthrography of the knee joint, Roetigenpraxis 19(7):169-182, 1966.

Betts, W. E., Jr.: Trenery memorial lecture 1975. Arthrography of the knee for meniscal tear: clinical, surgical and pathologic correlations, J. Am. Osteopath. Assoc. **75**(5):475-485, 1976.

Betts, W. E., Jr.: Double contrast arthrography of the knee, J. Am. Osteopath. Assoc. **67**(6):637-642, 1968.

Bidaut, C.: Apparatus of contention for knee-arthrography (gaseous or mixed), J. Radiol. Electrol. Med. Nucl. **58**(3):237-238, 1977.

Bierbaum, B. E.: Double contrast knee arthrography. A safe and reliable aid to diagnosis of "internal derangement," J. Trauma **8**(2):165-176, 1968.

Björk, L., Erikson, U., Ingelman, B., and Stenport, G.: Clinical experience with a new contrast medium used in angiography, arthrography, orography, etc., Nord. Med. **85**(20):632, 1971.

Borgan, D. W.: Positive-contrast knee arthrography, Am. Fam. Physician **5**(1):92-94, 1972.

Bots, R. A.: Knee joint arthroscopy, Ned. Tijdschr. Geneeskd. **119**(49):1938-1942, 1975.

Bowerman, J. W., and Muhletaler, C.: Arthrography of rheumatoid synovial cysts of the knee and wrist, J. Can. Assoc. Radiol. **24**(1):24-32, 1973.

Bradley, N. E., Lockwood, W. B., and Hicks, M. C.: Double contrast arthrography of the knee, J. Okla. State Med. Assoc. **67**(6):253-256, 1974.

Bramson, R. T., and Staple, T. W.: Double contrast knee arthrography in children, Am. J. Roentgenol. Radium Ther. Nucl. Med. **123**(4):838-844, 1975.

Brase, A., Hesse, W., and Bockslaff, H.: Xerographic diagnosis of lesions of the cruciate ligaments of the knee-joint (author's transl.), Roentgenblaetter **29**(3):142-147, 1976.

Brinckmann, W., and Frahm, W.: Persistent ache caused by a residual meniscus (author's transl.), Zentralbl. Chir. **102**(2):99-102, 1977.

Brown, C. D., and Thomas, D. P.: Knee arthrography, a diagnostic aid in internal derangement of the knee, J. Ky. Med. Assoc. **74**(10):507-511, 1976.

Brunelli, G., and Gadda, E.: Arthrography in the diagnosis of total prosthesis mobilization, Clin. Ortop. **23**(4):271-274, 1971-72.

Bryan, R. S., DiMichele, J. D., and Ford, G. L., Jr.: Popliteal cysts. Arthrography as an aid to diagnosis and treatment, Clin. Orthop. **50**:203-208, 1967.

Butt, W. P., and McIntyre, J. L.: Double-contrast arthrography of the knee, Radiology **92**(3):487-499, 1969.

Camerlain, M.: Arthroscopy and its rheumatologic perspectives, Union Med. Can. **103**(7):1262-1265, 1974.

Carpenter, J. R., Hattery, R. R., Hunder, G. G., Bryan, R. S., and McLeod, R. A.: Ultrasound evaluation of the popliteal space. Comparison with arthrography and physical examination, Mayo Clin. Proc. **51**(8):498-503, 1976.

Casscells, S. W.: Arthroscopy of the knee joint. A review of 150 cases, J. Bone Joint Surg. [Am.] **53**(2):287-298, 1971.

Channon, B. T.: Arthrography of the knee joint, Radiography **39**(465):246-249, 1973.

Clark, J. M.: "Arthrography diagnosis of synovial cysts of the knee," Radiology **115**(2):480-481, 1975.

Czekala, Z.: Double-contrast arthrography technic of the knee joint using the horizontal x-ray beam, Pol. Przegl. Radiol. **30**(1):11-17, 1966.

Dalinka, M. K., Brennan, R. E., and Canino, C.: Double contrast knee arthrography in children, Clin. Orthop. (125):88-93, 1977.

Dalinka, M. K., Coren, G., Hensinger, R., and Irant, R. N.: Arthrography in Blount's disease, Radiology **113**(1):161-164, 1974.

Dalinka, M. K., Coren, G. S., and Wershba, M.: Knee arthrography, CRC Crit. Rev. Clin. Radiol. Nucl. Med. **4**(1):1-59, 1973.

Dalinka, M. K., Lally, J. F., and Gohel, V. K.: Arthrography of the lateral meniscus, Am. J. Roentgenol. Radium Ther. Nucl. Med. **121**(1):79-85, 1974.

Dandy, D. J., and Jackson, R. W.: The diagnosis of problems after meniscectomy, J. Bone Joint Surg. [Br.] **57**(3):349-352, 1975.

Dandy, D. J., and Jackson, R. W.: The impact of arthroscopy on the management of disorders of the knee, J. Bone Joint Surg. [Br.] **57**(3):346-348, 1975.

Dashefsky, J. H.: Arthroscopy of knee, N.Y. State J. Med. **74**(6):1049-1053, 1974.

Debnam, J. W., and Staple, T. W.: Arthrography of the knee after meniscectomy, Radiology **113**(1):67-71, 1974.

DeHaven, K. E., and Collins, H. R.: Diagnosis of internal derangements of the knee. The role of arthroscopy, J. Bone Joint Surg. [Am.] **57**(6):802-810, 1975.

Dick, W., Henche, H. R., and Morscher, E.: The cartilage-damage after fracture of the patella, Arch. Orthop. Unfallchir. **81**(1):65-76, 1975.

Dorfmann, H., and Dreyfus, P.: Arthroscopy of the knee joint. Methods and results, Munch. Med. Wochenschr. **114**(13):611-614, 1972.

Dorfmann, H., and Dreyfus, P.: Arthroscopy of the knee (methods and results), Cah. Med. **12**(7):561-564, 1971.

Dorfmann, H., and Dreyfus, P.: Arthroscopy of the knee. Methods and results, Minerva Med. **62**(51):2621-2624, 1971.

Dorfmann, H., and Dreyfus, P.: Arthroscopy of the knee. Methods and results, Rev. Clin. Esp. **121**(6):545-548, 1971.

Dorfmann, H., Figueroa, M., and Sèze, S. de: Value of arthroscopy in isolated monoarthritis of the knee, Sem. Hop. Paris **50**(3):179-188, 1974.

Dorfmann, H., and Sèze, S. de: Filarial monoarthritis. Apropos of a case diagnosed by arthroscopy. Nouv. Presse Med. **1**(15):1013-1016, 1972.

Dorfmann, H., and Sèze, S. de: Further observations on knee arthroscopy. Results of a personal experience, Sem. Hop. Paris **48**(46):3011-3019, 1972.

Drugov, A. B.: Arthrography of the knee. Possibilities—limits—perspectives, Sb. Lek. **74**(1):19-25, 1972.

Drugov, A. B., Kolar, J., and Babick, Y. A.: 133 XE-arthrography in synovitis of the knee, Sb. Lek. **75**(3):65-71, 1973.

Duncan, A. M.: Arthrography in rupture of the suprapatellar bursa with pseudocyst formation, Am. J. Roentgenol. Radium Ther. Nucl. Med. **121**(1):89-93, 1974.

Edelstein, M. M.: An aid to knee arthrography, J. Can. Assoc. Radiol. **28**(2):162-163, 1977.

Edgar, M. A., and Lowy, M.: Arthroscopy of the knee: a preliminary review of fifty cases, Proc. R. Soc. Med. **66**(6):512-515, 1973.

Edgren, W., Heikel-Laurent, U., and Riska, E. B.: Arthrography of the knee in the diagnosis of torn semilunar cartilage, Acta Orthop. Scand. **38**(2):235-246, 1967.

Eikelaar, H. R.: Looking inside, gaining insight. Aspects of arthroscopy of the knee, Ned. Tijdschr. Geneeskd. **119**(48):1882-1890, 1975.

Eubanks, R. G., and Nelson, C. L.: Arthroscopy of the knee, J. Arkansas Med. Soc. **73**(5):205-208, 1976.

Fehér, M., Magyar, E., den Oudsten, S. A., and Wouters, H. W.: Deep vein thrombosis in the differential diagnosis of knee joint capsule changes in rheumatoid arthritis, Z. Rheumatol. **35**(3-4):164-172, 1976.

Ficat, P., Philippe, J., and Belossi, J.: Opaque arthrography of the knee, J. Radiol. Electrol. Med. Nucl. **52**(6):337-347, 1971.

Firodznia, H., Seliger, G., Baruch, H., and Weathers, R.: Tomographic technique for visualization of the cruciate ligaments in double contrast arthrography, Radiol. Technol. **47**(6):385-389, 1976.

Fischedick, O.: Significance of arthrography of the knee joint, Z. Orthop. **106**(4):759-765, 1969.

Fischer, J., Mollowitz, G., and Thiemann, K. J.: Frequency of degeneration and fissures in the residual meniscus (results of double-contrast arthrography in 141 meniscectomized patients), Hefte Unfallheilkd. **107**:259-262, 1970.

Fleming, M. A., Murray, J. A., and Jensen, K. M.: Knee arthrography, Tex. Med. **69**(3):63-71, 1973.

Fluckiger, A., and Aazam-zanganeh, F.: Diagnostic limits in knee arthrography (a retrospective study) (author's transl.), Praxis **64**(16):491-495, 1975.

Fordham, S. D., and Turner, A. F.: Arthrography in penetrating injuries, J.A.C.E.P. **5**(4):265-267, 1976.

Forrest, J., and Staple, T. W.: Synovial hemangioma of the knee. Demonstration by arthrography and arteriography, Am. J. Roentgenol. Radium Ther. Nucl. Med. **112**(3):512-516, 1971.

Frahm, W., and Rinke, W.: Value of positive contrast–media arthrography in the diagnosis of meniscus injuries, Zentralbl. Chir. **98**(41):1463-1467, 1973.

Franken, T., Frommhold, H., and Klammer, H. L.: Xeroradiographic examination of the capsule and ligaments of the knee joint. II. Demonstration of injuries to the cruciate and lateral ligaments and menisci (author's transl.), R.O.E.F.O. **126**(4):381-386, 1977.

Freiberger, R. H.: Arthrography of the knee for diagnosis of torn meniscus, J. Sports Med. **1**(1):24, 1972.

Freiberger, R. H., Killoran, P. J., and Cardona, G.: Arthrography of the knee by double contrast method, Am. J. Roentgenol. Radium Ther. Nucl. Med. **97**(3):736-747, 1966.

Frommhold, H., Franken, T. H., and Klammer, H. L.: Xeroradiographic studies on the capsule and ligaments of the knee joint. I. Anatomy of the cruciate and lateral ligaments in the xerotomogram, R.O.E.F.O. **125**(2):140-145, 1976.

Fuchs, G., Dau, W., Stankovic, P., and Schuster, R.: Experiences with arthrography in meniscus surgery, Monatsschr. Unfallheilkd. **74**(5):228-231, 1971.

Gallannaugh, S. C.: Arthroscopy of the knee [letter], Br. Med. J. **1**(6058):445, 1977.

Gallannaugh, S. C.: Arthroscopy of the knee joint, Br. Med. J. **3**(874):285-286, 1973.

Gelman, M. I., and Dunn, H. K.: Radiology of knee joint replacement, Am. J. Roentgenol. Radium Ther. Nucl. Med. **127**(3):447-455, 1976.

Gerson, E. S., and Griffiths, H. J.: A simple marking device for knee arthrography, Am. J. Roentgenol. Radium Ther. Nucl. Med. **127**(6):1057-1058, 1976.

Gillquist, J., and Hagberg, G.: A new modification of the technique of arthroscopy of the knee joint, Acta Chir. Scand. **142**(2):123-130, 1976.

Gillquist, J., and Hagberg, G.: Arthroscopy of knee joint—a useful method? Lakartidningen **72**(38):3545-3547, 1975.

Gillquist, J., Hagberg, G., and Oretorp, N.: Arthroscopy in acute injuries of the knee joint, Acta Orthop. Scand. **48**(2):190-196, 1977.

Gillquist, J., Hagberg, G., and Oretorp, N.: Therapeutic arthroscopy—a case report, Lakartidningen **73**(21):2039, 1976.

Gilula, L. Z.: A simplified stress device for knee arthrography, Radiology **122**(suppl. 2):828-829, 1977.

Gjori, C. Z.: Importance and possibilities of arthroscopy in the diagnosis of knee injuries and knee diseases, Acta Med. Iugosl. **21**(2):103-110, 1977.

Glinz, W.: Arthroscopy diagnosis of the traumatic cartilage lesion of the knee joint, Hefte Unfallheilkd. (129):242-246, 1977.

Glinz, W.: Diagnosis of chondral injury in trauma of the knee joint (author's transl.), Langenbecks Arch. Chir. **345**:423-429, 1977.

Glinz, W.: Arthroscopy in injuries meniscus, Z. Unfallmed. Berufskr. **69**(3-4):106-115, 1976.

Glinz, W.: Arthroscopy in cartilage lesions of the knee joint, Hefte Unfallheilkd. (127):46-57, 1975.

Glinz, W.: Diagnostic importance of arthroscopy in prearthroses of the knee joint, Z. Unfallmed. Berufskr. **67**(4):260-265, 1974.

Goldstein, W. B.: Dysplasia epiphysialis hemimelica with confirmation by knee arthrography, Br. J. Radiol. **46**(546):470-472, 1973.

Goodyear, M.: Arthroscopy, Ona J. 3(6):190, 1976.

Gorgerino, F.: Advantages of peridural anesthesia in arthrography for meniscal lesions of the knee, G. Batteriol. Virol. Immunol. [Microbiol.] 58(11):617-621, 1965.

Grepl, J.: Contribution of positive arthrography to the differential diagnosis of pathological changes of popliteal bursae (author's transl.), Cesk. Radiol. 28(1):20-26, 1974.

Grepl, J.: Suggestion for the new method of aimed picturing of knee joint arthrography (author's transl.), Cesk. Radiol. 28(4):233-237, 1974.

Grepl, J.: Positive arthrography for the demonstration of pathological changes in the popliteal bursa, R.O.E.F.O. 119(1):84-90, 1973.

Haage, H., and Watanabe, M.: Arthrography and arthroscopy. An assessment of the value of these techniques (author's transl.), Z. Orthop. 111(2):178-183, 1973.

Hall, F. M.: Buckled meniscus, Radiology 126(1):89-90, 1978.

Hall, F. M.: Pitfalls in knee arthrography, Radiology 118(1):55-62, 1976.

Hall, F. M.: Radiographic diagnosis and accuracy in knee joint effusions, Radiology 115(1):49-54, 1975.

Hall, F. M.: Epinephrine-enhanced knee arthrography, Radiology 111(1):215-217, 1974.

Hanssens, J. F.: Indications for knee arthrography (author's transl.), J. Belge Radiol. 60(1):77-81, 1977.

Harvie, K. W., Faerber, G. O., Smith, D. W., and Neufeld, C. L.: Double contrast arthrography of the knee joint, J. Am. Osteopath. Assoc. 68(1):84-90, 1968.

Henche, H. R.: Arthroscopy of the knee joint, Beitr. Orthop. Traumatol. 24(4):217-220, 1977.

Henry, A.: Arthroscopy of the knee joint, Guy's Hosp. Rep. 121(1):25-30, 1972.

Henry, A. N.: Arthroscopy in practice, Br. Med. J. 1(6053):87-88, 1977.

Hermann, G., Alvarez, E., and Lavine, L. S.: Value of knee arthrography in nonmeniscal damage, N.Y. State J. Med. 77(6):916-920, 1977.

Hertel, E.: Possibilities and limits of arthroscopy of rheumatic joints, Z. Orthop. 113(4):798-801, 1975.

Horns, J. W.: The diagnosis of chondromalacia by double contrast arthrography of the knee, J. Bone Joint Surg. [Am.] 59(1):119-120, 1977.

Horns, J. W.: Single contrast knee arthrography in abnormalities of the articular cartilage, Radiology 105(3):537-540, 1972.

Iakovets, V. V.: Symptoms of injuries of the knee joint menisci in contrast arthrography, Ortop. Travmatol. Protez. 34(12):25-29, 1973.

Iakovets, V. V.: Diagnosis of injuries of the knee joint menisci using contrast arthrography, Voen. Med. Zh. 9:81-82, 1972.

Imbert, J. C., Bolze, O., and Mouilleseaux, B.: Value of arthroscopy for the diagnosis and treatment of intra-articular disorders of the knee, Rev. Chir. Orthop. 62(suppl. 2): 137-141, 1976.

Jackson, R. W.: The role of arthroscopy in the management of the arthritic knee, Clin. Orthop. 101:28-35, 1974.

Jackson, R. W., and Abe, T.: The role of arthroscopy in the management of disorders of the knee. An analysis of 200 consecutive examinations, J. Bone Joint Surg. [Br.] 54(2):310-322, 1972.

Jackson, R. W., and DeHaven, K. E.: Arthroscopy of the knee, Clin. Orthop. (107):87-92, 1975.

Jayson, M. I., and Dixon, A. S.: Arthroscopy of the knee in rheumatic diseases, Ann. Rheum. Dis. 27(6):503-511, 1968.

Jelaso, D. V.: Positive contrast arthrography of the knee, Am. J. Roentgenol. Radium Ther. Nucl. Med. 103(3):669-673, 1968.

Johansesn, J. G., Lilleas, F. G., and Nordshus, T.: Arthrography of the knee joint with amipaque, Acta Radiol. [Diagn.] (Stockh.) 18(5):523-528, 1977.

Johnson, P. H.: Arthrography of the knee (a follow-up study), J. Arkansas Med. Soc. **72**(12):493-497, 1976.

Johnson, P. H.: Arthrography of the knee, J. Arkansas Med. Soc. **71**(9):283-289, 1975.

Kallwett, H., Ott, J., and Ludwig, G.: Results with double contrast arthrography in meniscus lesions of the knee joint, Monatsschr. Unfallheilkd. **73**(7):320-324, 1971.

Kamprad, F., and Hasert, V.: Tomography of the cruciate ligament in double contrast arthrography of the knee joint, R.O.E.F.O. **112**(4):449-504, 1970.

Kannangara, P. N., and Kirk, J. A.: Synovial fluid in the calf, Rheumatol. Rehabil. **15**(3):136-137, 1976.

Katz, R. S., Zizic, T. M., Arnold, W. P., and Stevens, M. B.: The pseudothrombophlebitis syndrome, Medicine (Baltimore) **56**(2):151-164, 1977.

Kaye, J. J., and Freiberger, R. H.: Arthrography of the knee, Clin. Orthop. (107):73-80, 1975.

Kellermann, S., and Abesser, E. W.: Our experiences in arthrography using visotrast, with special reference to the knee joint, Dtsch. Gesundheitsw. **20**(34):1581-1583, 1965.

Kieser, C., and Rüttimann, A.: Arthroscopy of the knee joint, Schweiz. Med. Wochenschr. **106**(47):1631-1637, 1976.

Klimov, G. I.: Diagnosis of injuries of the knee joint menisci with the aid of arthrography with double contrasting, Ortop. Travmatol. Protez. **35**(3):40-43, 1974.

Klimov, G. E.: Diagnosis of injuries of the knee joint menisci with the aid of arthrography with double contrasting, Ortop. Travmatol. Protez. **34**(3):40-43, 1974.

Kobayashi, A.: Arthrography of the knee, J. Jpn. Orthop. Assoc. **42**(9):871-909, 1968.

Kolar, J., Drugov, A. B., and Babick, Y. A.: 133 XE arthrography for synovitis of the knee joint, R.O.E.F.O. **118**(1):77-81, 1973.

Komprda, J.: Importance of arthrography in the diagnosis of internal knee injuries, Acta Chir. Orthop. Traumatol. Cech. **34**(5):471-479, 1967.

Kormano, M., Schrank, W. W., and Swirsky, M.: Lymphatic filling during knee arthrography, Ann. Chir. Gynaecol. Fenn. **65**(6):382-384, 1976.

Kovesdi, J. M., Jr.: Arthroscopy of the knee: an 18-month review, J. Am. Osteopath. Assoc. **76**(3):186-188, 1976.

Kraus, M., and Charuzi, I.: Arthroscopy of the knee (editorial), Harefuah **91**(3):94-96, 1976.

Kreft, E.: Proceedings: arthroscopy: its place in the diagnosis of knee lesions, J. Bone Joint Surg. [Br.] **57**(2):258, 1975.

Kremer, H., Schierl, W., Schattenkirchner, M., Baumann, D., Metz, I., and Zollner, N.: Echography of knee joint cysts (author's transl.), Munch. Med. Wochenschr. **119**(37):1183-1186, 1977.

Kunitsch, G., Muhr, G., and Oestern, J. H.: Significance of arthrography in the diagnosis of meniscus, Arch. Orthop. Unfallchir. **79**(4):335-340, 1974.

Kus, W., and Salamon, Z.: Arthroscopy of the knee joint (preliminary report), Chir. Narzadow Ruchu Ortop. Pol. **41**(5):569-573, 1976.

Lapayowker, M. S., Cliff, M. M., and Tourtellotte, C. D.: Arthrography in the diagnosis of calf pain, Radiology **95**(2):319-323, 1970.

Larowe, P. C., Ormond, R. S., and Gutse, E.: Double contrast arthrography of the knee, Henry Ford Hosp. Med. J. **18**(2):107-114, 1970.

Leclerc, J., Aube, L., and Dionne, G.: Study of the meniscus in arthrography of the knee, Can. J. Surg. **11**(4):466-472, 1968.

Leven, H.: Evaluation of a modified method for arthrography of the knee, Acta Radiol. [Diagn.] (Stockh.) **18**(3):351-356, 1977.

Leven, H.: Arthrography of the knee with a modified technique, Acta Radiol. [Diagn.] (Stockh.) **15**(2):237-240, 1974.

Levinsohn, E. M.: A new simple restraining device for fluoroscopically monitored knee arthrography, Radiology **122**(suppl. 2): 827, 1977.

Levitin, P. M.: Dissecting popliteal cyst: an unusual complication of Reiter's syndrome, South Med. J. **69**(11):1522-1532, 1976.

Lewin, J. R., and Mulhern, L. M.: Lymphatic visualization during contrast arthrography of the knee, Radiology **103**(3):577-579, 1972.

Lindgren, P. G., and Willen, R.: Gastrocnemius-semimembranosus bursa and its relation to the knee joint. I. Anatomy and histology, Acta Radiol. [Diagn.] (Stockh.) **18**(5):497-512, 1977.

Magill, C. D.: Value of knee arthroscopy, Rocky Mt. Med. J. **74**(4):203-205, 1977.

Mason, W. T.: Study of the use of arthrography, U.S. Navy Med. **64**(3):34-39, 1974.

Massare, C., and Bard, M.: Gonalgia following meniscectomy. Arthrographic findings. Review of 200 case records and radio-clinical comparison, Rev. Chir. Orthop. **61**(4):295-310, 1975.

Massare, C., Bard, M., and Tristant, H.: Interest of arthrography of the knee in joint pain after meniscectomy. Review of 200 personal cases (author's transl.), J. Radiol. Electrol. Med. Nucl. **55**(5):401-405, 1974.

Mathias, K.: Clinical and arthrographic aspects of the popliteal cysts, Chirurg **48**(6):384-388, 1977.

Mayer, G.: Importance of double-contrast arthrography for the diagnosis of injuries of the meniscus, Beitr. Orthop. Traumatol. **22**(6):304-307, 1975.

McBeath, A. A., and Wirka, H. W.: Positive-contrast arthrography of the knee. Report of experience with 311 arthrograms, Clin. Orthop. **88**:70-75, 1972.

McDaniel, W. J.: Isolated partial tear of the anterior cruciate ligament, Clin. Orthop. (115):209-212, 1976.

McGinty, J. B., and Freedman, P. A.: Arthroscopy of the knee, Clin. Orthop. (121):173-180, 1976.

McIntyre, J. L.: Arthrography of the lateral meniscus, Radiology **105**(3):531-536, 1972.

McIntyre, D. T.: Arthrography of the knee, Can. J. Surg. **11**(3):324-328, 1968.

Meire, H., Lindsay, D. J., Swinson, D. R., and Hamilton, E. B.: Comparison of ultrasound and positive contrast arthrography in the diagnosis of popliteal and calf swellings, Ann. Rheum. Dis. **33**(4):408, 1974.

Meire, G. B., Lindsay, D. J., Swinson, D. R., and Hamilton, E. B.: Comparison of ultrasound and positive contrast arthrography in the diagnosis of popliteal and calf swellings, Ann. Rheum. Dis. **33**(3):221-224, 1974.

Menanteau, B., Camerlain, M., Lussier, A., and Etienne, J. C.: An unusual dissecting cyst of the knee in a patient with rheumatoid arthritis, J. Radiol. Electrol. Med. Nucl. **58**(3):215-218, 1977.

Mennet, P.: Potential and limits of knee arthroscopy, Schweiz. Med. Wochenschr. **101**(44):1591, 1971.

Merola, G., and Tuzi, T.: Opaque arthrography of the synovectomized rheumatoid knee, Reumatismo **20**(1):19-25, 1968.

Merola, G., and Tuzi, T.: Opaque arthrography in initial arthrosis of the knee, Reumatismo **27**(1):190-192, 1975.

Merola, G., and Tuzi, T.: Post-synovectomy arthrography, Reumatismo **20**(5):565-566, 1968.

Meurman, K.: Double-contrast arthrography of the knee, Duodecim **88**(10):712-716, 1972.

Miller, A. F.: Arthroscopy of the knee, Ariz. Med. **34**(8):553-556, 1977.

Minkoff, J.: Arthroscopy—its value and problems, Orthop. Clin. North Am. **8**(3):683-706, 1977.

Miotti, R.: Improvement of arthrography using Ronpacon 440. Control in a double-blind study, Radiologe **12**(3):86-87, 1972.

Mittler, S., Freiberger, R. H., and Harrison-Stubbs, M.: A method of improving cruciate ligament visualization in double-contrast arthrography, Radiology **102**(2):441-442, 1972.

Moes, C. A., and Munn, J. D.: The value of knee arthrography in children, J. Can. Assoc. Radiol. **16**(4):226-233, 1965.

Mollowitz, G., and Thiemann, K. J.: Arthrography of the knee joint following tibial-head fractures, Hefte Unfallheilkd. (126):230-231, 1975.

Mollowitz, G., Thiemann, K. J., and Fischer, J.: Contribution of double contrast arthrography for the indication of rearthrotomy of the knee joint, Chirurg **41**(8):365-370, 1970.

Montgomery, C. E.: Synovial recesses in knee arthrography, Am. J. Roentgenol. Radium Ther. Nucl. Med. **121**(1):86-88, 1974.

Moriya, H.: The use of arthroscopy and biopsy in the diagnosis of monarticular chronic arthritis of the knee joint, Ryumachi **16**(1):12-34, 1976.

Nahoda, J., Freyov, A. J., Rybka, V., and Vohralik, M.: The value of arthrography in the diagnosis of posttraumatic conditions of the knee (author's transl.), Acta Chir. Orthop. Traumatol. Cech. **41**(3):275-277, 1974.

Nicholas, J. A., Freiberger, R. H., and Killoran, P. J.: Double-contrast arthrography of the knee. Its value in the management of two hundred and twenty-five knee derangements, J. Bone Joint Sug. [Am.] **52**(2):203-220, 1970.

Nicks, A. J., and Mihalko, M.: A simple device to open the knee joint space during double contrast arthrography, Radiology **122**(suppl. 2):827-828, 1977.

Norwood, L. A., Jr., Shields, C. L., Jr., Russo, J., Kerlan, R. K., Jobe, F. W., Carter, V. S., Blazina, M. E., Lombardo, S. J., and Del Pizzo, W.: Arthroscopy of the lateral meniscus in knees with normal arthrograms, Am. J. Sports Med. **5**(6):271-274, 1977.

O'Connor, R. L.: Arthroscopy of the knee, Surg. Annu. **9**:265-289, 1977.

O'Connor, R. L.: Arthroscopy in the diagnosis and treatment of acute ligament injuries of the knee, J. Bone Joint Surg. [Am.] **56**(2):333-337, 1974.

Ohnsorge, J.: Arthroscopy of the knee joint by means of glass fibers, Z. Orthop. **106**(3):535-538, 1969.

Olson, R. W.: Knee arthrography, Am. J. Roentgenol. Radium Ther. Nucl. Med. **101**(4):897-914, 1967.

O'Malley, B. P.: Value of delayed films in knee arthrography, J. Can. Assoc. Radiol. **25**(2):144-146, 1974.

Otto, R., and Menninger, H.: The diagnosis of soft tissue alterations of the knee by means of xeroradiography (author's transl.), Roentgenblaetter **30**(2):79-83, 1977.

Otto, R., and Wellauer, J.: Possibilities and limits of xeroradiography. A statement (author's transl.), R.O.E.F.O. **127**(5):471-477, 1977.

Pallardy, G., Fabre, P., Ledoux-Lebard, G., and Delbarre, F.: Arthrography of the knee in the study of bursitis and synovial cysts, J. Radiol. Electrol. Med. Nucl. **50**(6):481-494, 1969.

Pallardy, G., Fabre, P., Ledoux-Lebard, G., Renoux, J. P., and Delbarre, F.: Diagnosis of popliteal bursitis and cysts by arthrography of the knee, Rev. Rhum. Mal. Osteoartic. **38**(5):345-360, 1971.

Parks, V. J.: Arthroscopy, Natnews **12**(9):8, 1975.

Parks, V. J.: Arthroscopy, Nurs. Times **71**(52):2058-2059, 1975.

Peck, S. M., and Butcher, C.: Apparatus for arthrography of the knee joint, Radiography **40**(470):46-47, 1974.

Pellegrini, V.: Arthrography of the knee, Rev. Sanid. Milit. Argent. **63**(3):234-236, 1964.

Poehling, G. G., Bassett, F. H., III, and Goldner, J. L.: Arthroscopy: its role in treating nontraumatic and traumatic lesions of the knee, South. Med. J. **70**(4):465-496, 1977.

Pokorn, Y. V., and Burysek, P.: Our experiences with arthroscopy in the diagnosis of injured menisci of the knee joint, Rozhl. Chir. **54**(2):108-115, 1975.

Rasmussen, F.: Arthroscopy of the knee joint, Ugeskr. Laeger **137**(9):501-502, 1975.

Resnick, D., Goergen, T. G., Kaye, J. J., Ghelman, B., and Woody, P. R.: Discoid medial meniscus, Radiology **121**(3 pt. 1):575-576, 1976.

Ringertz, H. G.: Arthrography of the knee. II. Isolated and combined lesions, Acta Radiol. [Diagn.] (Stockh.) **17**(2):235-248, 1976.

Ringertz, H. G.: Arthrography of the knee. I. Localization of lesions, Acta Radiol. [Diagn.] (Stockh.) 14(1):138-144, 1973.

Ringertz, H. G.: Statistical analysis of a knee arthrography material, Nord. Med. 85(43):1257, 1971.

Rizk, G. K., Mnaymneh, W. A., and Musallan, J. J.: Double contrast arthrography of the knee, J. Med. Liban. 24(5):497-503, 1971.

Roebuck, E. J.: Double contrast knee arthrography. Some new points of technique including the use of dimer X, Clin. Radiol. 28(3):247-257, 1977.

Roebuck, E. J.: Proceedings: contrast media in knee arthrography, Br. J. Radiol. 49(579):287, 1976.

Romaniuk, P. A., Luning, M., and Thomas, G.: The percutaneous insertion of a polyethylene catheter into the knee joint for combined arthrography, Radiol. Diagn. (Berl.) 10(2):223-228, 1969.

Romaniuk, P. A., and Thomas, G.: The diagnostic value of arthrography in diseases of the knee joint. III. Report on 135 double examinations (air and contrast positive arthrography of the same joint), Radiol. Diagn. (Berl.) 9(5):515-527, 1968.

Romaniuk, P. A., and Thomas, G.: The diagnostic value of arthrography in knee joint diseases. II. Positive contrast arthrography, Radiol. Diagn. (Berl.) 9(3):377-404, 1968.

Romaniuk, P. A., and Thomas, G.: The diagnostic value of arthrography in diseases of the knee joint. I. Pneumarthrography, Radiol. Diagn. (Berl.) 8(3):315-335, 1967.

Rüttimann, A., and Pruszynski, B.: Knee joint arthrography using double-contrast media. Technics and clinical significance, Pol. Przegl. Radiol. 38(4):401-412, 1974.

Savastano, A. A., Poirier, P. E., and Izzi, J. A.: Double contrast arthrography of the knee—a report of 135 consecutive studies at Rhode Island Hospital, R.I. Med. J. 56(10):423-426, 1973.

Schawelson, R. T.: Double contrast knee arthrography with horizontal beam, Radiol. Technol. 41(2):98-103, 1969.

Schmidt, H.: Arthrography of knee disorders with the double contrast method, Nord. Med. 85(9):291, 1971.

Schmidt, H.: Diagnostic possibilities of double-contrast arthrography in disorders of the knee, Acta Orthop. Scand. 42(5):461, 1971.

Scholz, O., and Tauchmann, R.: Results and experiences with double-contrast arthrography in the diagnosis of meniscus damages, Zentralbl. Chir. 96(31):1049-1053, 1971.

Schonholtz, G. J.: Arthroscopy of the knee joint, South. Med. J. 69(11):1493-1495, 1976.

Schulte, L. A.: Discoid knee menisci in children, Arch. Chir. Neerl. 28(2):115-122, 1976.

Simmons, M. J.: Proceedings: double contrast arthrography in knee injuries, Br. J. Radiol. 48(575):945-946, 1975.

Solares, R.: Radiodiagnosis of the rupture of the meniscus of the knee. Auxiliary maneuver without contrast medium. Preliminary report (author's transl.), Prensa Med. Mex. 40(11-12):331-335, 1975.

Sommer, J.: Arthrography in meniscal injuries of the knee joint, Acta Orthop. Scand. 39(2):217-222, 1968.

Sproance, S. L., Metcalf, R., Smith, C. B., Griffiths, M. M., and Ward, J. R.: Chronic arthropathy associated with rubella vaccination, Arthritis Rheum. 20(2):741-747, 1977.

Staple, T. W.: Extrameniscal lesions demonstrated by double-contrast arthrography of the knee, Radiology 102(2):311-319, 1972.

Stenstrom, R.: Diagnostic arthrography of traumatic lesions of the knee joint in children, Ann. Radiol. (Paris) 18(4):391-394, 1975.

Stenstrom, R.: Arthrography of the knee joint in children. Roentgenologic anatomy, diagnosis and the use of multiple discriminant analysis, Acta Radiol. [Diagn.] (Stockh.) suppl. 281:1, 1968.

Stoker, D. J.: Arthrography of the knee [letter], Br. Med. J. 1(6056):287-288, 1977.

Stuhler, T. H., Lattermann, D., Krisch, H., and Stringarts, K.: Ganglion recidives of the knee joint. Arthrography and clinic (author's transl.), Z. Orthop. **115**(3):334-341, 1977.

Swett, H. A., Jaffe, R. B., and McIff, E. B.: Popliteal cysts: presentation as thrombophlebitis, Radiology **115**(3):613-615, 1975.

Taylor, A. R.: Arthrography of the knee in rheumatoid arthritis, Br. J. Radiol. **42**(499):493-497, 1969.

Taylor, A. R., and Ansell, B. M.: Arthrography of the knee before and after synovectomy for rheumatoid arthritis, J. Bone Joint Surg. [Br.] **54**(1):110-115, 1972.

Taylor, A. R., and Ansell, B. M.: Arthrography of the knee following synovectomy, Ann. Rheum. Dis. **29**(2):198-199, 1970.

Thijn, C. J.: Double-contrast arthrography in meniscal lesions and patellar chondropathy, Radiol. Clin. (Basel) **45**(5):345-362, 1976.

Thijn, C. J.: Arthrography in lesions of both menisci in one knee joint, Arch. Chir. Neerl. **26**(2):147-155, 1974.

Thijn, C. J.: Double contrast arthrography in degenerative lesions of the meniscus, Ned. Tijdschr. Geneeskd. **115**(14):604-606, 1971.

Thomas, M. L., and Andress, M. R.: Angioma of the knee demonstrated by angiography and arthrography, Acta Radiol. [Diagn.] (Stockh.) **12**(2):219-220, 1972.

Thomas, R. H., Resnick, D., Alazraki, N. P., Daniel, D., and Greenfield, R.: Compartmental evaluation of osteoarthritis of the knee. A comparative study of available diagnostic modalities, Radiology **116**(3):585-594, 1975.

Tubielewicz, J., and Gietka, J.: Importance of arthrography in gonarthrosis for the detection of non-traumatic lesions of the knee joint meniscus, Reumatologia **7**(1):39-43, 1969.

Tubielewicz, J., Gietka, J., and Mastalerski, J.: Technic of arthrography of the knee joint by means of double contrast media, Wiad. Lek. **22**(4):357-361, 1969.

Turner, A. F., and Budin, E.: Arthrography of the knee. A simplified technique, Radiology **97**(3):505-508, 1970.

Vajarapongse, K., Vongsathaporn, A., Chienpradit, K., and Limpaphayom, M.: Double contrast arthrography in the diagnosis of internal derangement of the knee, J. Med. Assoc. Thai. **60**(9):413-417, 1977.

Vanrens, J. G.: Knee arthroscopy, Ned. Tijdschr. Geneeskd. **119**(49):1943-1944, 1975.

Villiger, K. J.: Chondropathy of the patella. Experiences with 100 medializations, Chirurg **47**(10):547-554, 1976.

Wang, J. B., and Marshall, J. L.: Acute ligamentous injuries of the knee. Single contrast arthrography—a diagnostic aid, J. Trauma **15**(5):431-440, 1975.

Wershra, M., Dalinka, M. K., Coren, G. S., and Cotler, J.: Double contrast knee arthrography in the evaluation of osteochondritis dissecans, Clin. Orthop. (107):81-86, 1975.

Westall, D. R.: Arthrography: a critical study of the technique and possible improvement of knee arthrograms, Radiol. Technol. **45**(5):311-321, 1974.

Wiener, S. N.: Contrast arthrography of the knee joint: a comparison of positive and negative methods, Radiology **89**(6):1083-1086, 1967.

Wieser, C., Steiger, U., and Zinn, W.: Cystic pseudotumors of the popliteal fossa in knee arthrography, Radiol. Clin. (Basel) **36**(4):232-236, 1967.

Wolfe, R. D., and Gioliano, V. J.: Double-contrast arthrography in the diagnosis of pigmented villonodular synovitis of the knee, Am. J. Roentgenol. Radium Ther. Nucl. Med. **110**(4):793-799, 1970.

Wolfers, H.: Arthrography of the knee joint using a fluid contrast medium and nitrous oxide, Radiologe **9**(7):229-233, 1969.

Wruhs, O.: Arthroscopy of tibial-head fractures, Hefte Unfallheilkd. (126):234-236, 1975.

Wruhs, O.: Arthroscopy of the knee joint, Z. Orthop. **111**(4):664-665, 1973.

Wruhs, O.: Arthroscopy and endophotography for diagnosis and documentation of knee joint injuries, Wien. Med. Wochenschr. **120**(8):126-133, 1970.

Yates, D. B.: Arthroscopy of the knee after the injection of 90Y, Ann. Rheum. Dis. **32**(suppl.):48-50, 1973.

Zullig, R., Kieser, C., Raschle, R., and Rüttimann, A.: Reliability of arthrography in the diagnosis of postmeniscectomy complaints—comparison of 50 rearthrotomy findings, Z. Unfallmed. Berufskr. **70**(3):118-137, 1977.

Index

340